ANNALS OF
THE NEW YORK ACADEMY
OF SCIENCES

Volume 946

EDITORIAL STAFF

Executive Editor
BARBARA M. GOLDMAN

Managing Editor
JUSTINE CULLINAN

Associate Editor
JOYCE HITCHCOCK

The New York Academy of Sciences
2 East 63rd Street
New York, New York 10021

HIV-ASSOCIATED CARDIOVASCULAR DISEASE

Clinical and Biological Insights

ANNALS OF THE NEW YORK ACADEMY OF SCIENCES
Volume 946

HIV-ASSOCIATED

CARDIOVASCULAR DISEASE

Clinical and Biological Insights

Edited by
Giuseppe Ippolito, Nicola Petrosillo,
Giuseppe Barbaro, and Steven E. Lipshultz

The New York Academy of Sciences
New York, New York
2001

Library of Congress Cataloging-in-Publication Data

HIV-associated cardiovascular disease : clinical and biological insights / edited by Giuseppe Ippolito ... [et al.].
    p. ; cm. — (Annals of the New York Academy of Sciences, ISSN 0077-8923 ; v. 946)
    Includes bibliographical references and index.
    ISBN 1-57331-354-8 (cloth : alk. paper) — ISBN 1-57331-355-6 (paper)
    1. Cardiological manifestations of general diseases—Congresses. 2. AIDS (Disease)—Complications—Congresses. I. Ippolito, Giuseppe. II. New York Academy of Sciences. III. Series.
    [DNLM: 1. Acquired Immunodeficiency Syndrome—complications—Congresses. 2. Cardiovascular Diseases—complications—Congresses. 3. Cardiovascular Diseases—etiology—Congresses. WC 503.5 H67637 2001]
    Q11 .N5 vol. 946
    [RC682]
    616.1'071—dc21
    [617.9'5]

    2001044075
    CIP

K-M Research/PCP
Printed in the United States of America
ISBN 1-57331-354-8 (cloth)
ISBN 1-57331-355-6 (paper)
ISSN 0077-8923

ANNALS OF THE NEW YORK ACADEMY OF SCIENCES

Volume 946
November 2001

HIV-ASSOCIATED CARDIOVASCULAR DISEASE
Clinical and Biological Insights

Editors
GIUSEPPE IPPOLITO, NICOLA PETROSILLO,
GIUSEPPE BARBARO, AND STEVEN E. LIPSHULTZ

This volume is the result of a colloquium entitled **Clinical and Biological Insights in HIV-Associated Cardiovascular Disease**, sponsored by the Lazzaro Spallanzani Institute—IRCCS and held December 5, 2000, in Rome, Italy.

CONTENTS

Part III. Clinical Insight

Financial support was received from:

• THE ITALIAN MINISTRY OF PUBLIC HEALTH

HIV-Associated Cardiovascular Disease: Clinical and Biological Insights

Preface

This volume of the *Annals of the New York Academy of Sciences* is the result of the international colloquium **HIV-Associated Cardiovascular Disease: Clinical and Biological Insights** held in Rome on December 5, 2000, which addressed the most recent clinical and biological knowledge concerning HIV-associated cardiovascular disease.

Although cardiac involvement during the course of HIV infection was recognized early in the AIDS epidemic, the incidence of this manifestation has not been fully assessed, owing mostly to underreporting, underclassification, and several confounding factors, including the characteristics of patients and the standard of care found in clinical centers. Cardiac abnormalities were detected through non-invasive techniques more often than would have been expected from clinical symptoms and/or after physical examination. Nevertheless, cardiac involvement continues to present diagnostic and therapeutic challenges not only for clinicians specializing in infectious diseases and cardiologists, but also for virologists and basic scientists.

Clinical manifestations of cardiac involvement are multifarious: pericarditis with or without tamponade, pulmonary hypertension with right ventricular failure, focal or diffuse myocarditis, dilated cardiomyopathy, Kaposi's sarcoma and non-Hodgkin's lymphoma involving the heart and pericardium, nonbacterial thrombotic endocarditis, and infective endocarditis. The use of potentially cardiotropic drugs, including ones used in the treatment of HIV infections, may also cause cardiac abnormalities.

Although highly active antiretroviral therapy (HAART) has dramatically modified the survival rate and quality of life for HIV$^+$ patients in the past decade, there are suggestions that the likelihood of cardiac involvement, particularly cardiomyopathy, may increase as patients live longer lives with HIV disease.

Moreover, the etiology of cardiac abnormalities is still unclear, and although it can be related to infection with HIV, many other possible causes have been proposed such as: alcohol, cocaine, and injection drug use, as well infections/superinfections by bacterial, fungal, parasitic, and viral organisms. In particular, host–parasite interaction plays a crucial role.

With this in mind, the (Italian) National Institute for Infectious Diseases "Lazzaro Spallanzani" designed a multidisciplinary forum to encourage scientific exchange among scientists and physicians working in infectious diseases, epidemiology, cardiology, virology, molecular biology, and public health.

Papers in this issue of the *Annals* should achieve the following:

- disseminate knowledge on epidemiology, pathogenesis, and clinical manifestations of cardiac involvement in HIV$^+$ patients;

- evaluate risk factors for cardiovascular disease in the HAART era, including metabolic disorders in patients treated with HAART since their primary HIV infection;

- analyze the role of host-parasite interaction and of drugs in cardiac manifestations;

- aid clinicians in recognizing and managing the problem;

- analyze nosocomial and occupational risks for employees and patients during health care procedures and provide strategies for minimizing the risks; and finally,

- furnish a framework to define guidelines for the management of cardiac involvement.

This volume provides evidence for the rapidly growing knowledge in this field and confirms that a variety of problems need to be addressed when discussing this complex disease.

—GIUSEPPE IPPOLITO, M.D.

The Changing Picture of the HIV/AIDS Epidemic

GIUSEPPE IPPOLITO, VINCENZO GALATI,
DIEGO SERRAINO, AND ENRICO GIRARDI

*Dipartimento di Epidemiologia, Istituto Nazionale per le Malattie Infettive
"Lazzaro Spallanzani"– IRCCS, 00149 Rome, Italy*

ABSTRACT: Twenty years after it was first recognized, the HIV/AIDS epidemic
continues to expand, but its impact varies greatly in different parts of the
World. The worst of the epidemic is now centered in developing countries,
especially sub-Saharan Africa, and areas such as Eastern Europe, which was
only marginally involved a few years ago but has recently experienced the largest growth in the epidemic. In industrialized countries Highly Active Antiretroviral Therapy (HAART) has changed the natural history of HIV/AIDS,
causing a reduction in mortality and morbidity due to HIV/AIDS and related
diseases. Many interlocking factors determine the impact of HAART at the
population level, including reduction of morbidity and mortality, changes in
the natural history of HIV/AIDS and associated illnesses, and the effects of
HAART on HIV transmission. To fully appreciate the potential benefits of
HAART, the epidemic should continue to be monitored in the future, and the
effects of HAART on reducing HIV transmission should also be evaluated.
Interventions addressed to encourage the adoption of safer sex practices are
badly needed, since a "rebound" in risky sexual behaviors was recently reported among high risk groups, which is, at least in part, attributable to the optimism about new treatments.

KEYWORDS: HIV infection; acquired immunodeficiency syndrome (AIDS);
epidemiology; highly active antiretroviral therapy (HAART)

INTRODUCTION

Twenty years ago, the first cases of a newly recognized disease, then also called
Gay Related Immunodeficiency Syndrome (GRID), were reported in the United
States among a population of homosexual males. At that time, nobody anticipated
that the world would be facing a new pandemic, the like of which present generations
had never experienced. In fact, Acquired Immunodeficiency Syndrome (AIDS), as
the disease was renamed, was revealed earlier as a widespread epidemic, silently dis-
seminating through other risk populations, including injection drug users (IDUs)
hemophiliacs, blood transfusion recipients and high-risk heterosexuals. By the end
of 2000, there was no part of the world that was not been affected by the HIV/AIDS
epidemic. The extent of the infection throughout the world varies: the worst of the

Address for correspondence: Dr. Giuseppe Ippolito, Dipartimento di Epidemiologia, Istituto Nazionale per le Malattie Infettive "Lazzaro Spallanzani"– IRCCS, Via Portuense 292,
00149 Rome, Italy. Voice: +39 065594223; fax +39 065594224.
    ippolito@inmi.it

epidemic is now centered in developing countries, especially sub-Saharan Africa, which accounts for around three-quarters of all HIV-related deaths, and two-thirds of all people living with HIV/AIDS.[1]

In developed countries, where highly active antiretroviral therapy (HAART) has been available since 1996, the implementation of HAART deeply modified the features of infection and the epidemic of HIV/AIDS. Several clinical trials showed the efficacy of HAART in reducing viral replication and reconstituting immunity, leading to a prolonged time of symptom-free disease, prolonged survival after AIDS diagnosis, and changes in the natural history of HIV-associated illnesses.[2–4] Observational studies confirmed these results at the population level, reporting decreased HIV-related deaths and AIDS-defining opportunistic infection over time.[5,6] Owing to the decrease of HIV/AIDS mortality and AIDS morbidity, if levels of new HIV infections remain stable, the total impact of HAART in developed countries in the years to come is expected to result in an overall increase of the prevalence of HIV infection.

HAART's impact on the incidence of HIV infection is less clear, but some possible effects have been suggested. In fact, HAART may decrease HIV transmission by diminishing HIV RNA shedding in biological fluids, such as semen and cervicovaginal secretions of treated subjects.[7,8] On the other hand, prolonged survival of HIV$^+$ subjects can increase the incidence of HIV infection in the susceptible population and a rebound in unsafe sexual behaviors has been reported among high risk groups [especially men who have sex with men (MSM)], possibly related to less concern about HIV transmission from HAART-treated persons.[9] These factors could counterbalance an effective role of HAART in diminishing HIV transmission.

Therefore, the effect of HAART on HIV/AIDS at the population level results from a number of related factors, including reduced morbidity and mortality as well as changes in the natural history of HIV-associated illnesses and its effects on HIV transmission. The aim of this paper is to briefly review the evolving global picture of the HIV/AIDS epidemic and to describe some of the factors affecting the impact of HAART at the population level.

A GLOBAL VIEW OF HIV/AIDS EPIDEMIC

An estimated 36 million people are living with HIV/AIDS world-wide and 22 million people have already died due to HIV/AIDS; therefore to date nearly 60 million people have been infected. During 2000, 5 million new HIV infections were estimated to occur, and 3 million deaths due to HIV/AIDS.[1] Predictions by the World Health Organization proved optimistic, as they predicted in 1991 that the total number of HIV infections would be 40 million by the year 2000.[10] It is now clear that life expectancy and economic growth in most developing countries, mainly in sub-Saharan Africa, are closely dependent on the future of HIV/AIDS epidemic.[11]

In Western Europe and North America, an estimated 30,000 adults and 45,000 children became infected with HIV during the year 2000. The total number of persons living with HIV in these regions was estimated to be 1.46 million.[1] In these countries, the epidemic has changed in recent years. A persistent relatively low level of incidence, combined with longer survival, produced a modest increase of the prevalence of HIV infection. Notably, the marked falls in mortality in 1996 and 1997, which were attributed to the favorable effects of HAART on disease progression and deaths, have leveled off in the past two years.

Eastern Europe, only marginally involved a few years ago, has recently experienced the largest growth in the epidemic. In 2000, more new infections occurred than in all of the previous years combined. The estimate of the actual number of persons living with HIV by the end of 2000 is 300,000, which is more than twice as many as there were in 1999. So far, the epidemic has been predominantly confined to IDUs, but conditions still exist for a broader spread of infection.[11]

Sub-Saharan Africa is suffering the worst devastation compared to the rest of the world, with an increasing impact due to the epidemic. In 2000, the total number of people (adults and children) living with HIV/AIDS was 25.3 million, and of these estimated new infections accounted for 3.8 million. The average prevalence of HIV infection in the adult population of sub-Saharan Africa is 8.8%, with peaks of 20% in some countries in the southern cone, whose infection rates have overtaken East Africa. Heterosexual sex is the major transmission route, together with a persistent level of mother-to-child transmission.

East Asia and the Pacific include some of the world's most populous countries. The HIV epidemic is still confined to injection drug users, whose numbers are increasing in many regions.[12] There is increasing concern about the possible spread of infection in countries like China, where a recent steep rise in sexually transmitted diseases (STDs) has been reported.[13]

In South and Southeast Asia 700,000 new HIV infections were estimated to have occurred in 2000, mostly among men. The major routes of infection are injectable drug use and sexual transmission, both through commercial sex and sex between men.

Latin America had an estimated 150,000 new infections in 2000. Some 1.4 million adults and children were estimated to be living with HIV/AIDS by the end of 2000. The total incidence rate does not seem to have increased, but several Central American countries are facing a rise in epidemic levels. Infection rates are generally high in the Caribbean, where HIV/AIDS prevalence rates in the adult population exceeded 5%.[1]

Different patterns of transmission exist in different parts of the world.[14,15] A "concentrated" pattern of HIV transmission is found in Western European countries, North America, Australia, and some parts of Latin America and Asia, where the infection is endemic, but mostly occurs in so-called "high-risk" population groups, such as MSM and IDUs, with a low prevalence of infection in the general population (generally less than 1%) and a high prevalence (5 to 50%) in affected minorities. A "generalized" transmission pattern, characterized by a wide spread of the epidemic among the adult population and a predominance of heterosexually transmitted infections, is a typical pattern of east and central African countries, where prevalence was much greater than 1%. Moreover, some countries show a mixed transmission pattern, with an initial spread of infection among at-risk groups and a subsequent involvement of a broader part of the population. Such a situation can be observed in countries such as Brazil or India, where the infection first hit male homosexuals and female sex workers, and a broader spread in the general population followed.

4 　　　　　　　ANNALS NEW YORK ACADEMY OF SCIENCES

IMPACT OF HAART AT A POPULATION LEVEL

Reduced Morbidity and Mortality

Since the introduction of zidovudine treatment in HIV/AIDS patients, improved morbidity and mortality were reported in persons with advanced disease.[16] However, later studies on zidovudine monotherapy did not show clear long-term benefits in terms of reducing mortality.[17] The standard of care shifted from monotherapy to sequential therapy with nucleoside reverse transcriptase inhibitors (NRTI), followed by combined NRTI therapy, after large trials had shown a marked decrease in morbidity and mortality rates in comparison to zidovudine monotherapy.[18,19] The highest increase in survival rates for HIV+ individuals was obtained by using triple combination therapy, including protease inhibitors.[2,3,6]

Observational studies provided confirmation of the results of clinical trials at the population level, showing a decreased risk of AIDS-defining opportunistic infections and death, over time.[2,3,6,19,20] This resulted in changes in the natural history of HIV infection, with several implications for epidemiological studies of the disease.

Before the HAART era, cohort studies on individuals with known seroconversion dates reported that the median time from primary infection to AIDS diagnosis was about 10 years. The average survival after AIDS diagnosis was considered to be nearly 1.5 years. A median survival of 12.5 years was reported among patients aged 12–24 years at seroconversion, and of 7.9 years among those aged 45–54 years. The major determinants of progression to AIDS and death in industrialized countries, were age at seroconversion and time from seroconversion.[21]

After a generalized diffusion of HAART in developed countries, the face of HIV/AIDS has changed; there is now a prolonged asymptomatic period after infection, as well as prolonged survival time after an AIDS-defining disease is diagnosed. Reduction of morbidity and mortality without a reduction in the rates of new infections, should result in an increased prevalence of HIV infection. In fact, an increase in the number of persons estimated to be living with HIV/AIDS was reported in the United States at the end of 1997.[22]

Whether the total impact of HAART will continue to be increasingly advantageous at the population level in coming years is difficult to predict. This depends on several factors, such as sustained viral suppression, patient adherence to prescribed treatments, emergence of further resistant viral strains and their transmission to uninfected subjects, HAART toxicity, and the effects of antiretroviral therapy on HIV transmission.

Longitudinal studies are needed to evaluate both the incubation period and the survival time in HIV+ persons, in order to better understand changes due to the widespread use of HAART, together with the therapies for HIV-associated disorders. Surveillance of changes in the epidemic still requires focused attention on all HIV+ persons, not only on those developing AIDS, since treatment will delay the development of AIDS in most persons. Therefore, improvements in the surveillance of new cases of HIV infection are urgently needed.

Impact of HAART on HIV-associated Illnesses

Since 1996, data from cohort studies and surveillance systems clearly show a decreasing trend in the incidence of nearly all opportunistic infections among HIV$^+$ persons in industrialized countries. For example, among persons enrolled in the Adult and Adolescent Spectrum of Disease (ASD) Project in the United States, the incidence of *Pneumocystis carinii* pneumonia declined by 21.5% per year in 1996–1998; in the same period the incidence of *Mycobacterim avium* complex disease decreased by 39.9% per year and that of candida esophagitis by 16.7% per year.[23]

Furthermore, the natural history of opportunistic infections occurring since the widespread availability of HAART, may have changed significantly. In Italy, survival at 24 months after diagnosis of an AIDS-defining disease more than doubled for patients diagnosed after 1995, in comparison to those diagnosed before the end of 1995. In addition, a reduction of the risk of death ranging from 55% to 80% was observed for all AIDS-defining illnesses, except lymphomas.[24]

The impact of HAART at the population level on the incidence of HIV-associated opportunistic infections can be exemplified by the case of tuberculosis. Tuberculosis is the only HIV-associated respiratory infection that can readily be transmitted to HIV$^-$ persons. Moreover, HIV infection is one of the factors contributing to the resurgence of tuberculosis in several parts of the world. This is due to both the high risk of developing active tuberculosis in HIV$^+$ persons and the increased risk of tuberculosis infection from them to non-HIV-infected persons. In the United States, the number of tuberculosis cases increased in 1985–1990, and 28,000 cases of tuberculosis were reported in excess to what was expected from the historical trends.[25] It was estimated that at least 30% of the excess cases could be directly attributed to the HIV epidemic.[26] Since 1992, however, the number of reported cases has started to decrease and, compared to 1992, a 34% decrease in the incidence of tuberculosis was observed in 1999. In this context the decrease of HIV-associated tuberculosis was even more pronounced. In fact, the proportion of tuberculosis cases with HIV infection between 1993–1994 and 1998 decreased from 15% to 10% among persons of all ages and from 29% to 20% among those aged 15–44 years.[27] This downward trend appears to reflect in part the intensification of control measures, including those specifically targeted to HIV$^+$ persons.[28–30] However, the widespread use of HAART appears to have significantly contributed to the decline of HIV-associated tuberculosis. In San Francisco, since 1991, several tuberculosis interventions were intensified.[31] The overall tuberculosis incidence rate dropped from 46.0 to 29.8 per 100,000 population between 1991 and 1997 and an even larger reduction was observed among HIV$^+$ persons (from 491.8 to 65.6). Interestingly, tuberculosis incidence decreased by 5–15% each year between 1991 and 1996 while an 80% decrease (from 295.1 to 65.6 per 100,000 HIV$^+$ persons) was recorded between 1996 and 1997, when HAART became available. This observation is confirmed in studies in which data on antiretroviral use in individual patients were analyzed. In the United States, among HIV$^+$ persons enrolled in the ASD project, a more than twofold decrease in the overall incidence of tuberculosis was observed from 1992 to 1997,[23] and the risk of tuberculosis was reduced by 80% in persons on HAART and by 40% in persons on other antiretroviral therapies, compared to those who received no antiretrovirals.[32] Similar results are reported in a cohort study from Italy in which patients who took dual combination therapy had an 80% reduction in the risk of tuberculosis, while in those on triple combination therapy the risk of tuberculosis was reduced by 91% compared to patients who did not receive combination therapy.[33] Another study from Italy analyzed changes in the clinical presentation and outcome of HIV-associated tuberculosis, before and after the widespread implementation of HAART. Compared to patients diagnosed in 1995–96, those diagnosed in 1997–98 were more likely to have tuberculosis as the first AIDS-defining illness (78% vs. 58%), to have HIV diagnosed less than two months before tuberculosis (33% vs. 7%), to have "typical" chest X-ray pattern (45% vs. 25%), and they had a higher CD4+ count. Moreover, survival was significantly prolonged for those diagnosed in 1997–98, and a decreased risk of death was observed in patients starting HAART after tuberculosis diagnosis.[34] Finally, a temporary exacerbation of tuberculosis symptoms and lesions after initiation of therapy for tuberculosis, often referred to as paradoxical reaction and considered a rare occurrence, has been reported with increasing frequency among patients starting HAART while on antituberculosis therapy.[35]

A more complex interaction seems to exists between HAART and HIV-associated malignancies. The available epidemiological evidence linking HAART and cancer among HIV+ individuals in Western countries derives from a few single investigations and from a large meta-analysis of longitudinal studies on time trends of HIV-related neoplasms, comparing cancer incidence rates in the pre- and in the post-HAART periods.

A reduction in Kaposi's sarcoma (KS) incidence has been reported by the Multicenter AIDS Cohort Study (MACS), where a nested case control study assessed a positive effect of HAART showing that none of the 14 KS cases diagnosed since July 1995 was in a person treated with HAART.[36] Patients involved in the AIDS Clinical Trial Group (ACTG) had a statistically significant 88% reduction in KS incidence in the post-HAART period.[37] Similarly, the ASD study[38] clearly indicated that the incidence of KS was lower in persons for whom any antiretroviral therapy was prescribed (11/1,000 person-years), than among persons not taking antiretroviral therapy (82/1,000 person-years).

In the above-mentioned studies, the effect of HAART on the incidence of non-Hodgkin's lymphoma (NHL) appeared to be less consistent than that registered for KS. Two studies suggested an increase in the incidence of NHL in the post-HAART period. Between 1985 and 1997, incidence rates of NHL reported by the MACS had risen by nearly 20% per year,[36] even though only one out of eight NHL cases had actually received HAART. Findings from the ASD study[38] showed that the incidence of NHL was more than twofold higher in HIV-positive individuals treated with HAART, but a statistically significant decrease over time restricted to primary brain lymphoma (PBL) was registered.

On the contrary, NHL incidence declined from 1992–95 to 1996–97 by 26% among a total of 6,587 ACTG participants,[37] while in the San Francisco City Clinic Cohort[39] NHL incidence remained relatively constant from 1993 to 1996 (about 1.5/100 person-years). No significant trends were observed in the incidence of other lymphomas, including Hodgkin's disease (HD), apart from a lower incidence of HD in persons treated with HAART, documented by Jones and colleagues.[38]

At least part of the difficulty in highlighting the effect of HAART on NHLs is related to the role of the immune reconstitution attributable to HAART, which in contrast to the case of KS may not be sufficient to prevent the occurrence of most types of NHL.[4]

The effect of HAART on cancer occurrence among HIV[+] patients has been extensively studied by pooling cancer incidence data from 23 prospective investigations. These 23 studies included 47,936 HIV-seropositive individuals residing in the USA, Europe, or Australia and they represented over 80% of the available epidemiological evidence from developed countries regarding cancer incidence in HIV[+] people since the introduction of HAART.[40] Incidence rates for KS, NHL, HD, cervical cancer and other cancer types or sites were calculated and rate ratios were estimated, comparing the incidence rates in 1997 through 1999 with rates in 1992 through 1996, adjusting for study, age, sex and HIV transmission group.

For the period 1992 through 1999, 2704 incident cancers were reported in 138,000 person-years of observation. The adjusted incidence rate for KS fell from 15.2 per 1000 person-years in 1992 through 1996 to 4.9 per 1000 person-years in 1997 through 1999 (rate ratio = 0.32) and the corresponding incidence rates for NHL also fell, from 6.2 to 3.6 per 1000 person-years, respectively (rate ratio = 0.58). Interestingly, this picture was not consistent for all types of NHL, since the rate ratios for incidence rates in 1997 through 1999 compared to 1992 through 1996 were 0.42 for PBL, 0.57 for immunoblastic lymphoma, and 1.18 for Burkitt's lymphoma.

There were no significant changes between the two time periods in the incidence of HD or of cervical cancer, and the adjusted incidence rates for all other cancers combined was 1.7 per 1000 person-years in each time period.[40]

In conclusion, the epidemiological evidence is consistent in showing substantial reductions in the incidence of KS since the widespread use of HAART, whereas for NHL, only the decline of PBL has been clearly ascertained. Since HAART has been in widespread use in developed countries for only a short period, cancer incidence rates in HIV[+] people should continue to be monitored in the future to fully appreciate its potential benefits.

HAART and Infectiousness

A clear correlation has been shown between high viral levels of HIV-1 found in the source and the probability of HIV transmission, regardless of the transmission route.[41–44] A low CD4[+] count and an advanced stage of the disease also correlate with the HIV transmission rate.[42,45] Other sexually transmitted diseases can also enhance viral shedding in the genital tract, both in men and in women.[46,47]

Antiretroviral therapies, leading to reduced plasma HIV RNA levels and increased CD4[+] cell counts, might play an important role in reducing infectiousness.

Evidence of a decreased transmission of HIV-1 related to antiretroviral use originally derived from the results obtained in a two-thirds decrease in the rate of mother-to-child transmission by means of a complex regimen of zidovudine, given both to HIV[+] women during pregnancy and delivery, and to the newborn for a few weeks.[42] Since these results were reported, an increasing number of pregnant women in developed countries have received antiretroviral treatment. More recently these treatments have been based mainly on antiretroviral combinations,[48] together with the adoption of other prophylactic interventions with a proven efficacy in reducing vertical transmission, such as avoiding breast feeding and vaginal delivery. This resulted in a dramatic reduction in vertical transmission rates at the population level.

For example, a recently published European study reported a decline of HIV vertical transmission rate from 15.5% prior to 1994 to 2.6% after 1998. At the same time, the use of antiretroviral treatment during pregnancy increased, including both the 076 full regimen of zidovudine (from 28% in 1995 to 89% by 1999) and the use of triple therapy started in pregnancy (from less than 1% in 1997 to 44% in 1999).[49] Similarly, in the United States, data from the Women and Infants Transmission Study showed a decrease in the vertical transmission rate from 19.5% prior to 1994 to 7% among women receiving zidovudine since 1994. Moreover, no cases of transmission were recorded among the 70 women who received a combination regimen that included protease inhibitors.[50]

Prophylaxis regimens used in industrialized countries are too costly and complex to be used routinely in resource-poor settings. Trials of simplified regimens were conducted using shorter zidovudine regimens, more suitable for developing countries, which showed maintained efficacy.[51] Similar results were obtained in a trial of single-dose nevirapine given to mothers and newborns in Uganda.[52] A multicenter trial evaluating prophylaxis regimens combining zidovudine and lamivudine was conducted in Uganda, Tanzania, and South Africa. Three regimens of combined zidovudine and lamivudine were adopted: prepartum, intrapartum, and postpartum; intrapartum and postpartum; intrapartum only. A preliminary analysis showed a 52% efficacy in the reduction of transmission rates for the full regimen.[53]

Studies on the effects of antiretroviral therapy on the sexual transmission of HIV-1 are more difficult to accomplish, mostly owing to the difficulty of conducting population studies, which require the identification of all of one person's potential sources of exposure to HIV.[54] Although evidence exists of viral compartmentalization, with different HIV-1 variants detected in plasma and in the genital secretions,[55] a positive correlation between the plasma virus load and virus shedding in genital secretions was shown. Indeed, several studies have suggested that a decrease in virus levels in genital secretions paralleled that recorded in the peripheral blood after HAART treatment.[7,8,56] Plasma viral load was identified as the major predictor of the risk of heterosexual transmission in a community-based randomized trial, which also observed rare transmission to the partners of HIV+ persons with levels of less than 1500 copies of HIV RNA per milliliter.[57] On the other hand, replication-competent virus was detected in seminal cells of subjects with undetectable levels of HIV RNA in the blood plasma, and HIV-1 DNA remained commonly detectable in the anorectal mucosa of homosexual men receiving HAART and with HIV plasma viremia less than 50 copies/ml.[58,59] Perhaps to a lesser extent, persistent infectiousness may therefore remain, despite a good virological response to HAART. Taken together, these observations suggest that a decreased level of infectiousness is probably achieved by the use of potent antiretroviral therapy. Together with the adoption of safer sexual practices and the aggressive STD diagnosis and treatment, HAART may represent a primary tool in decreasing the further spread of sexually acquired HIV.

However, after years of prevention efforts addressed to reduce sexual high-risk behaviors, concerns have been raised regarding a "rebound" of unsafe sexual behaviors, especially among high risk groups like MSM. In particular, this was reported after HAART became a generalized standard of care for HIV/AIDS. Studies showing an increased pattern of "safe sex fatigue" were conducted among MSM in different contexts,[60,61] and there was an association between optimism about new treatments and risk practices in MSM.[9] Moreover, findings from a study on sexual risk behaviors among heterosexual discordant couples conducted from 1996 in California showed a decreased concern about HIV transmission especially among seronegative partners, even if patients taking protease inhibitor therapy were less likely to report unprotected sex compared with those not taking protease inhibitors.[62] Recently, findings by a computerized match of people in the San Francisco STD and AIDS registries, showed that among a population of mainly homosexual men in San Francisco, people on HAART were more likely to develop an STD, an epidemiological marker of unsafe sex.[63] In a simulation model designed to evaluate the possible future scenario of HIV/AIDS epidemic in the gay community in San Francisco, it has been estimated that a wide use of HAART could effect a significant decrease in the incidence of new infections, even in the presence of higher levels of drug resistance and incomplete adherence to treatments. However, a mere increase of 10% in the prevalence of risky behaviors would completely abrogate the beneficial effects of HAART.[64]

Therefore, there is no place for complacency, and it will be of paramount importance to keep encouraging the adoption of safer sex practices, both among HIV+ subjects and their partners, as well as among other people, more or less aware of the actual risk related to their own sexual behavior.

Advances in HIV/AIDS treatments, aimed at maximizing improvements in the quality of life of HIV+ individuals, might also play an important role in decreasing the possibility of HIV transmission to uninfected people and produce the need for further studies to monitor the impact of new treatments in the general population. Moreover, they should be accompanied by preventive interventions targeted to populations at higher risk of acquiring infection, so as to avoid a paradoxical effect of increased risky behavior, which is at least partly attributable to the general awareness of a better quality of care, resulting in a decreased concern for acquiring HIV.

REFERENCES

1. JOINT UNITED NATIONS PROGRAMME ON HIV/AIDS AND WORLD HEALTH ORGANIZA-TION. 2000. AIDS Epidemic Update: December 2000–UNAIDS, Geneva.
2. CAMERON, D.W., M. HEATH-CHIOZZI, S. KRAVCIC, *et al.* 1996. Prolongation of life and prevention of AIDS complications in advanced HIV immunodeficiency with ritonavir: update. Collected abstracts of the XI International Conference on AIDS. Vancouver, July 1996 vol. 1: 24 [abstract MoB411].
3. HAMMER, S.M., K.E. SQUIRES, M.D. HUGHES, *et al.* 1997. A controlled trial of two nucleoside analogues plus indinavir in persons with human immunodeficiency virus infection and CD4 cell counts of 200 per cubic millimeter or less. N. Engl. J. Med. **337:** 725–733.
4. PALELLA, F.J. JR., K.M. DELANEY, A.C. MOORMAN, *et al.* 1998. Declining morbidity and mortality among patients with advanced human immunodeficiency virus infection. HIV Outpatient Study Investigators [see comments]. N. Engl. J. Med. **338:** 853–860.
5. MOUTON, Y., S. ALFANDARI & M. VALETTE. 1997. Impact of protease inhibitors on AIDS-defining events and hospitalizations in 10 French AIDS reference centres. AIDS **11:** F101–F106.
6. PEZZOTTI, P., P.A. NAPOLI, S. ACCIAI, *et al.* 1999. Increasing survival time after AIDS in Italy: the role of new combination antiretroviral therapies. AIDS **13:** 249–255.
7. VERNAZZA, P.L., J.J. ERON, S.A. FISCUS, *et al.* 1999. Sexual transmission of HIV: infectiousness and prevention. AIDS **13:** 155–166.

8. CU-UVIN, S., A.M. CALIENDO, S. REINERT, *et al.* 2000. Effect of highly active antiretroviral therapy on cervicovaginal HIV-1 RNA. AIDS **14:** 415–421.
9. BOLDING, G. *et al.* 2000. International differences among gay men in HIV optimism and sexual risk behaviour—a report from London, Melbourne, Sydney and Vancouver. Abstract LbPp 105, XIIIth International AIDS Conference, Durban, South Africa.
10. GLOBAL PROGRAMME ON AIDS. 1991. Current and Future Dimensions of the HIV/AIDS Pandemic—World Health Organization, Geneva.
11. PIOT, P., M. BARTOS, P.D. GHYS, *et al.* 2001. The global impact of HIV/AIDS. Nature **410:** 968–973.
12. BEYRER, C, M.H. RAZAK, K. LISAM, *et al.* 2000. Overland heroin trafficking routes and HIV-1 spread in south and south-east Asia. AIDS **14:** 75–83.
13. CHEN, X.S., X.D. GONG, G.J. LIANG, *et al.* 2000. Epidemiologic trends of sexually transmitted diseases in China. Sex. Transm. Dis. **27:** 138–142.
14. MONITORING THE AIDS PANDEMIC (MAP). 1998. The status and trends of the HIV/AIDS epidemics in the world. Geneva MAP, pp. 1–27.
15. NICOLL, A. & O.N. GILL. The global impact of HIV infection and disease. 1999. Commun. Dis. Public Health. **2:** 85–89.
16. FISCHL, M.A., D.D. RICHMAN, M.H. GRIECO, *et al.* 1987. The efficacy of azydothymidine (AZT) in the treatment of patients with AIDS and AIDS-related complex: a double blind, placebo controlled trial. N. Engl. J. Med. **317:** 185–191.
17. CONCORDE COORDINATING COMMITTEE. 1994. Concorde: MRC/ANRS randomised double blind controlled trial of immediate and deferred zidovudine in symptom-free HIV infection. Lancet. **343:** 871–881.
18. HAMMER, S.M., D.A. KATZENSTEIN, M.D. HUGHES, *et al.* 1996. A trial comparing nucleoside monotherapy with combination therapy in HIV-infected adults with CD4+ cell counts from 200 to 500 per cubic millimeter. N. Engl. J. Med. **335:** 1081–1090.
19. DELTA COORDINATING COMMITTEE. 1996. Delta: a randomised double-blind controlled trial comparing combinations of zidovudine plus didanosine or zalcitabine with zidovudine alone in HIV-infected individuals. Lancet **348:** 283–291.
20. BRODT, H.R., B.S. KAMPS, P. GUTE, *et al.* 1997. Changing incidence of AIDS-defining illnesses in the era of antiretroviral combination therapy. AIDS **11:** 1731–1738.
21. COLLABORATIVE GROUP ON AIDS INCUBATION AND HIV SURVIVAL INCLUDING THE CASCADE EU CONCERTED ACTION. 2000. Time from HIV-1 seroconversion to AIDS and death before widespread use of highly-active antiretroviral therapy: a collaborative re-analysis. Lancet **355:** 1131–1137.
22. CENTERS FOR DISEASE CONTROL AND PREVENTION. 1998. HIV/AIDS Surveillance Report. **10:** 1–43.
23. JONES, J.L., D.L. HANSON, M.S. DWORKIN, *et al.* 1999. Surveillance for AIDS-defining opportunistic illnesses, 1992-1997. MMWR **48** (No. SS-2): 1–22.
24. CONTI, S., M. MASOCCO, P. PEZZOTTI, *et al.* 2000. Differential impact of combined antiretroviral therapy on the survival of Italian patients with specific AIDS-defining illnesses. J. Acquir. Immune Defic. Syndr. **25:** 451–458.
25. JEREB, J.A., G.D. KELLY, S.W. DOOLEY, *et al.* 1991. Tuberculosis morbidity in the United States: final data 1990. MMWR **40**(SS-3): 23–27.
26. BLOOM, B.R. & C.L. MURRAY. 1992. Tuberculosis. Commentary on a reemergent killer. Science **257:** 1055–1064.
27. CENTERS FOR DISEASE CONTROL AND PREVENTION. 2000 August. Reported Tuberculosis in the United States, 1999.
28. FRIEDEN, T.R., P.I. FUJIWARA, R.M. WASHKO, *et al.* 1995. Tuberculosis in New York City—turning the tide. N. Engl. J. Med. **333:** 229–233.
29. BUCHER, H.C., L.E. GRIFFITH, G.H. GUYATT, *et al.* 1999. Isoniazid prophylaxis in HIV infection: a meta-analysis of randomized controlled trials. AIDS **13:** 501–507.
30. GRAHAM, N.M.H., N. GALAI, K.E. NELSON, *et al.* 1996. Effect of isoniazid chemoprophylaxis on HIV-related mycobacterial disease. Arch. Intern. Med. **156:** 889–894.

31. JASMER, R.M., J.A. HAHN, P.M. SMALL, *et al.* 1999. A molecular epidemiologic analysis of tuberculosis trends in San Francisco, 1991–1997. Ann. Intern. Med. **130:** 971–978.
32. JONES, J.L., D.L. HANSON, M.S. DWORKIN, *et al.* 2000. HIV-associated tuberculosis in the era of highly active antiretroviral therapy. Int. J. Tuberc. Lung Dis. **4:** 1026–1031.
33. GIRARDI, E., G. ANTONUCCI, P. VANACORE, *et al.* [GRUPPO ITALIANO DI STUDIO TUBERCOLOSI E AIDS (GISTA)]. 2000. Impact of combination antiretroviral therapy on the risk of tuberculosis among persons with HIV infection. AIDS **14:** 1985–1991.
34. GIRARDI, E., F. PALMIERI, A. CINGOLANI, *et al.* 2001. Changing clinical presentation and survival in HIV-associated tuberculosis after highly active antiretroviral therapy. J. Acquir. Immune Defic. Syndr. **26:** 326–331.
35. NARITA, M., D. ASHKIN, E.S. HOLLENDER, *et al.* 1998. Paradoxical worsening of tuberculosis following antiretroviral therapy in patients with AIDS. Am. J. Respir. Crit. Care Med. **158:** 157–161.
36. JACOBSON, L.P., T.E. YAMASHITA, R. DETELS, *et al.* 1999. Impact of potent antiretroviral therapy on the incidence of Kaposi's sarcoma and non-Hodgkin's lymphomas among HIV-1-infected individuals. J. Acquir. Immune. Defic. Syndr. **21**(Suppl.1): S34–S41.
37. RABKIN, C.S., M.A. TESTA, J. HUANG, *et al.* 1999. Kaposi's sarcoma and non-Hodgkin's lymphoma incidence trends in AIDS Clinical Trial Group study participants. J. Acquir. Immune Defic. Syndr. **21**(suppl.1): S31–S33.
38. JONES, J.L., D.L. HANSON, M.S. DWORKIN, *et al.* 1999. Effect of antiretroviral therapy on recent trends in selected cancers among HIV-infected persons. J. Acquir. Immune Defic. Syndr. **21**(Suppl.1): S11–S17.
39. BUCHBINDER, S.P., S.D. HOLMBERG, S. SCHEER, *et al.* 1999. Combination antiretroviral therapy and incidence of AIDS-related malignancies. J. Acquir. Immune Defic. Syndr. **21**(suppl.1): S23–S26.
40. INTERNATIONAL COLLABORATION ON HIV AND CANCER. 2000. The impact of highly active anti-retroviral therapy on the incidence of cancer in people infected with the human immunodeficiency virus. Collaborative reanalysis of individual data on 47,936 HIV-infected people from 23 cohort studies in 12 developed countries. J Natl. Cancer Inst. **92:** 1823–1830.
41. BUSCH, M.P., E.A. OPERSKALSKI, J.W. MOSLEY, *et al.* 1996. Factors influencing human immunodeficiency virus type 1 transmission by blood transfusion. J. Infect. Dis. **174:** 26–33.
42. CONNOR, E. M., R.S. SPERLING, R. GELBER, *et al.* 1994. Reduction of maternal-infant transmission of human immunodeficiency virus type 1 with zidovudine treatment. N. Engl. J. Med. **331:** 1173–1180.
43. LEE, T.H., N. SAKAHARA, E. FIEBIG, *et al.* 1996. Correlation of HIV-1 RNA levels in plasma and heterosexual transmission of HIV-1 from infected transfusion recipients (letter). J. Acquir. Immune Defic. Syndr. **12:** 427–428.
44. RAGNI, M.V., H. FARUKI & L.A. KINGSLEY. 1998. Heterosexual HIV-1 transmission and viral load in haemophilic patients. J. Acquir. Immune Defic. Syndr. **17:** 42–45.
45. SEAGE, G.R., K.H. MAYER & C.R. MORSBURGH. 1993. Risk of human immunodeficiency virus infection from unprotected receptive anal intercourse increases with decline in immunologic status of infected partners. Am. J. Epidem. **137:** 899–908.
46. DYER, J.R., J.J. ERON, I.F. HOFFMAN, *et al.* 1998. Association of CD4 cell depletion and elevated blood and seminal plasma human immunodeficiency virus type 1 (HIV-1) RNA concentrations with genital ulcer disease in HIV-infected men in Malawi. J. Infect. Dis. **177:** 224–227.
47. MOSTAD, S.B., J.OVERBAUGH, D.M. DE VANGE, *et al.* 1997. Hormonal contraception, Vitamin A deficiency, and other risk factors for shedding of HIV-1 infected cells from the cervix and vagina. Lancet **350:** 922–927.
48. PECKHAM, C. & M.L. NEWELL. 2000. Preventing sexual transmission of HIV Infection. N. Engl. J. Med. **343:** 1036–1037.
49. EUROPEAN COLLABORATIVE STUDY. 2001. HIV-infected pregnant women and vertical transmission in Europe since 1986. AIDS **15:** 761–770.

50. COOPER, E.R., M. CHARURAT, D.N. BURNS, *et al.* 2000. Trends in antiretroviral therapy and mother-infant transmission of HIV. J. Acquir. Immune Defic. Syndr. **24:** 45–47.
51. DABIS, F, P. MSELLATI, N. MEDA, *et al.* 1999. 6-Month efficacy, tolerance, and acceptability of a short regimen of oral zidovudine to reduce vertical transmission of HIV in breastfed children in Côte d'Ivoire and Burkina Faso: a double-blind placebo-controlled multicentre trial. Lancet **353:** 781–785.
52. GUAY, L.A., P. MUSOKE, T. FLEMING, *et al.* 1999. Intrapartum and neonatal single-dose nevirapine compared with zidovudine for prevention of mother-to-child transmission of HIV-1 in Kampala, Uganda: HIVNET 012 randomised trial. Lancet **354:** 795–802.
53. SABA, J. 1999. Current Status of PETRA Study. *In* 2nd Conference of Global Strategies for the Prevention of HIV Transmission From Mother to Infant: Montreal, Quebec.
54. WEIDLE, P.J., S.D. HOLMBERG & K.M. DE COCK. 1999. Changes in HIV and AIDS epidemiology from new generation antiretroviral therapy. AIDS **13**(Suppl.A): S61–S68.
55. ZHU, T, N. WANG, A. CARR, *et al.* 1996. Genetic characterization of human immunodeficiency virus type 1 in blood and genital secretions: evidence for viral compartmentalization and selection during sexual transmission. J. Virol. **70:** 3098–3107.
56. GUPTA, P., J. MELLORS, L. KINGSLEY, *et al.* 1997. High viral load in semen of human immunodeficiency virus type 1–infected men at all stages of disease and its reduction by therapy with protease and nonnucleoside reverse transcriptase inhibitors. J. Virol. **71:** 6271–6275.
57. QUINN, T.C., M.J. WAWER, N. SEWAKAMBO, *et al.* 2000. Viral load and heterosexual transmission of human immunodeficiency virus type 1. N. Engl. J. Med. **342:** 921–929.
58. ZHANG, H., G. DORNADULA, M. BEAUMONT, *et al.* 1998. Human immunodeficiency virus type 1 in the semen of men receiving highly active antiretroviral therapy. N. Engl. J. Med. **339:** 1803–1809.
59. LAMPINEN, M.T., C.W. CRITCHLOW, J.M. KUYPERS, *et al.* 2000. Association of antiretroviral therapy with detection of HIV-1 RNA and DNA in the anorectal mucosa of homosexual men. AIDS **14:** F69–F75.
60. VALLEROY, L.A., D.A. MACKELLAR, J.M. KARON, *et al.* 2000. HIV prevalence and associated risks in young men who have sex with men. JAMA **284:** 198–204.
61. DODDS, J.P., A. NARDONE, D.E. MERCEY, *et al.* 2000. Increase in high risk sexual behaviour among homosexual men, London 1996–8: cross sectional, questionnaire study. [see comments]. Br. Med. J. **320:** 1510–1511.
62. VAN DER STRATEN, A., C.A. GOMEZ, J. SAUL, *et al.* 2000. Sexual risk behaviors among heterosexual HIV serodiscordant couples in the era of post-exposure prevention and viral suppressive therapy. AIDS **14:** F47–F54.
63. SCHEER, S., P. LEE CHU, J.D. KLAUSNER, *et al.* 2001. Effect of highly active antiretroviral therapy on diagnoses of sexually transmitted diseases in people with AIDS. Lancet **357:** 432–435.
64. BLOWER, S.M., H.B. GERSHENGORN & R.M. GRANT. 2000. A tale of two futures: HIV and antiretroviral therapy in San Francisco. Science **287:** 650–654.

Epidemiology of Cardiovascular Involvement in HIV Disease and AIDS

STACY D. FISHER[a] AND STEVEN E. LIPSHULTZ[b]

[a]*Department of Medicine, Cardiology Unit,*
University of Rochester Medical Center and the Department of Medicine,
University of Rochester School of Medicine and Dentistry,
Rochester, New York 14642, USA

[b]*Division of Pediatric Cardiology, University of Rochester Medical Center and*
Strong Children's Hospital, and the Department of Pediatrics,
University of Rochester School of Medicine and Dentistry,
Rochester, New York 14642, USA

ABSTRACT: The epidemiology of cardiac complications related to HIV including cardiomyopathy, increased left ventricular mass, myocarditis, pericardial effusion, endocarditis, and malignancy are discussed. A large number of HIV-infected individuals will present with cardiac complications in the next decade as chronic viral infection, co-infections, drug therapy, and immunosuppression affect the heart. Understanding the nature and course of cardiac illness related to HIV infection will allow appropriate monitoring, early intervention and therapy, and will provide a baseline to evaluate the effects of new therapeutic regimens such as highly active antiretroviral therapy on the cardiovascular system.

KEYWORDS: cardiomyopathy; HIV infection; pericardial effusion

BACKGROUND

Cardiac illness related to HIV infection tends to occur late in the disease course and is therefore becoming more prevalent as therapy of the viral infection and longevity improve. Autopsy series and retrospective analyses suggest that cardiac lesions are present in 25–75% of patients with AIDS. As 36.1 million adults and children are estimated to be living with HIV/AIDS and 5.3 million adults and children are estimated to have been newly infected with HIV during the year 2000,[1] HIV-associated symptomatic heart failure is becoming one of the leading causes of heart failure worldwide. Regional HIV/AIDS statistics and features (see TABLE 1) reflect the high prevalence of disease among selected populations, specifically in sub-Saharan Africa and the Caribbean.[1] The predominance of infection is currently in men in most populations, whereas new infections are occurring disproportionately in women.[1]

Address for correspondence: Steven E. Lipshultz, M.D., 601 Elmwood Avenue, Box 631, Cardiology Unit, University of Rochester Medical Center, Rochester, NY 14642. Voice: 716-275-6096; Fax: 716-275-7436.
steve_lipshultz@urmc.rochester.edu

TABLE 1. Selected UNAIDS/WHO estimated regional HIV/AIDS statistics, end of year 2000

Region	Living with AIDS	New Infections	Adult Prevalence	Percent Female
Africa				
Sub-Saharan	25.3 m	3.8 m	8.8%	55
North and Middle East	400,000	80,000	0.2%	40
Asia				
South/SE	5.8 m	780,000	0.56%	35
East/Pacific	640,000	130,000	0.07%	13
America				
North	920,000	45,000	0.6%	20
South	1.4 m	150,000	0.5%	25
Europe				
Eastern/Central Asia	700,000	250,000	0.35%	25
Western	540,000	30,000	0.24%	25
Caribbean	390,000	60,000	2.3%	35
Australia/New Zealand	15,000	500	0.13%	10

NOTE: m denotes million.

The spectrum of HIV-associated cardiovascular illness in the era before highly active antiretroviral therapy (HAART) is described in TABLE 2.

PROSPECTIVE STUDIES OF CARDIOVASCULAR INVOLVEMENT IN HIV-INFECTED ADULTS

The first prospective study suggested high levels of cardiac involvement, with 6/12 patients having abnormal cardiac function or pericardial effusion. Electrocardiographic abnormalities were found in 9/12 (75%) patients and included low voltage QRS complexes. Radionuclide ventriculography revealed 2 patients with a left ventricular ejection fraction less than 1 standard deviation below the normal population and 1 patient with a right ventricular ejection fraction less than 1 standard deviation below normal.

Subsequent larger prospective trials include a trial of 429 HIV[+] patients. Of 256 patients with a normal baseline echocardiogram and sequential studies performed, new abnormalities developed in 53 (21%) over a period of 24 ± 17 months.[3] Abnormalities included LV dilation in 22 patients, both LV dilation and hypokinesis in 8 patients, isolated pericardial effusion in 8 patients, diastolic dysfunction in 9 patients, right heart dilation in 1 patient, left ventricular hypertrophy in 3 patients, and intracardiac mass in 2 patients.

AUTOPSY STUDY OF CARDIOVASCULAR
ABNORMALITIES IN HIV-INFECTED ADULTS

A recent autopsy study of adults who died of AIDS by the Gruppo Italiano per lo Studio Cardiologico dei pazienti affetti da AIDS (GISCA) found that 82/440 (19%) had cardiac abnormalities related to HIV infection. Abnormalities included dilated cardiomyopathy in 12 patients, lymphocytic interstitial myocarditis in 30 (10/12 with dilated cardiomyopathy), infective endocarditis in 28, pericardial effusion in 53, myocardial Kaposi's sarcoma in 2, and myocardial B-cell immunoblastic lymphoma in 1 patient. HIV nucleic acid sequences were detected in the myocytes of 29 patients, 25 who had an active myocarditis.[4]

LEFT VENTRICULAR DYSFUNCTION IN HIV-INFECTED ADULTS

In a prospective study of asymptomatic HIV+ adults, 76 of 952 (8%) patients had significant left ventricular dysfunction over 60 months follow-up.[5] Cardiomyopathy was diagnosed 28 ± 10 months after enrollment. All patients with dilated cardiomyopathy had symptoms and signs of heart failure; 84% were New York Heart Association (NYHA) class III and 16% were class IV. Of the 12 patients who were in NYHA functional class IV, 5 died of congestive heart failure a mean of 9 ± 2.1 months after the diagnosis of cardiomyopathy.

Patients with asymptomatic left ventricular dysfunction (fractional shortening less than 28%, with global left ventricular hypokinesis) may have transient disease by echocardiographic criteria. In one serial echocardiographic study, 3/6 patients with initial abnormal fractional shortening had normal readings after a mean of 9 months. All 3 with persistently depressed left ventricular function died within 1 year of baseline.[6]

Dilated cardiomyopathy was strongly associated with a depressed CD4 T-cell count.[5,7] Also associated with accelerated left ventricular dysfunction was the onset of encephalopathy, which heralds cardiac demise.[7,8]

Mortality in HIV+ patients with cardiomyopathy is increased independent of CD4 count, age, sex, and risk group. The median survival to AIDS-related death was 101 days in patients with left ventricular dysfunction and 472 days in patients with a normal heart, and at similar infection stage.[9] Isolated right ventricular dysfunction or borderline left ventricular dysfunction did not place patients at risk in this cohort.[9]

Compared to ischemic or idiopathic cardiomyopathy, HIV-related cardiomyopathy has an extremely poor prognosis.[10] HIV+ patients who have asymptomatic left ventricular dysfunction may have a transient course of disease.[6]

LEFT VENTRICULAR DYSFUNCTION IN HIV-INFECTED CHILDREN

Left ventricular dysfunction is a common consequence of HIV infection in children. In a study of 205 vertically HIV+ children (median age 22 months, echocardiographic follow-up every 4–6 months, electrocardiography, Holter monitoring, and chest radiography yearly), decreased left ventricular function had a prevalence of

TABLE 2. **Spectrum of HIV-related cardiovascular abnormalities**

Type	Possible Etiologies and Associations	Incidence
Dilated cardiomyopathy	Infectious: HIV, toxoplasma, coxsackievirus group B, Epstein-Barr virus, cytomegalovirus, adenovirus Autoimmune response to infection Drug-related: cocaine, possibly AZT, IL-2, doxorubicin, interferon Metabolic/Endocrine: nutritional deficiency/wasting (selenium, B12, carnitine), thyroid hormone, growth hormone, adrenal insufficiency, hyperinsulinemia Cytokines: TNF-α, nitric oxide, TGF-β, endothelin-1 Immunodeficiency	Estimated 15.9 patients/1000 asymptomatic HIV-infected persons.[5]
Pericardial effusion	Bacteria: Staphylococcus, Streptococcus, Proteus, Nocardia, Pseudomonas, Klebsiella, Enterococcus, Listeria Mycobacteria Viral Pathogens: HIV, herpes simplex virus (HSV), cytomegalovirus Other Pathogens: cryptococcus, toxoplasma, histoplasma Malignancy Capillary leak/Wasting/Malnutrition Hypothyroidism Prolonged Acquired Immunodeficiency	11%/year[13] Spontaneous resolution in up to 42% of affected patients.[6,13]
Infective Endocarditis	Autoimmune response to infection Bacterial: *Staphylococcus aureus* or *epidermidis*, *Salmonella* species, *Streptococcus* species (Enterococcus), *Hemophilous parainfluenza*, *Pseudalleschira boydii* Fungal/Yeast: *Aspergillus fumigatus*, *Candida* species, *Cryptococcus neoformans*	Up to 6% incidence[9]
Non-Bacterial Thrombotic Endocarditis (generally tricuspid valve)	Underlying valvular endothelial damage, Vitamin C deficiency, disseminated intravascular coagulation, hypercoagulable state, malnutrition, wasting, prolonged acquired immunodeficiency	Rare incidence[9,30]

TABLE 2/continued.

Type	Possible Etiologies and Associations	Incidence
Malignancy (Kaposi's sarcoma, Non-Hodgkin's lymphoma, Leiomyosarcoma)	Prolonged immunodeficiency, low CD4 count Viral associations: human herpesvirus-8, Epstein-Barr virus	1% incidence (3/440)[18]
Right Ventricular and Pulmonary Disease	Recurrent bronchopulmonary infections, pulmonary arteritis, microvascular pulmonary emboli due to thrombus or drug injection.	0.5% incidence[16]
Primary Pulmonary Hypertension	Plexogenic pulmonary arteriopathy Mediator release from endothelium	0.5% incidence[16]
Vasculitis (all types)	Drug therapy (antibiotic and antiretroviral)	Case reports
Accelerated atherosclerosis	Protease inhibitor therapy, atherogenesis by virus-infected macrophages, chronic inflammation	Up to 8% prevalence by autopsy and case reports[22,24]
Autonomic Dysfunction	Associated nervous system disease Drug therapy side effects Prolonged immunodeficiency Malnutrition	Common in late-stage disease[28]
Arrhythmias	Drug therapy Pentamidine Autonomic dysfunction	Unknown

5.7%.[11] The 2-year cumulative incidence was 15.3%. The cumulative incidence of symptomatic congestive heart failure and/or the use of cardiac medications was 10% over 2 years.

Rapid onset congestive heart failure bears a grim prognosis in HIV+ adults and children, with over half of patients dying of cardiac failure within 6–12 months of diagnosis.[12] Chronic onset heart failure may respond better to medical therapy in this patient population.[9,12]

PERICARDIAL EFFUSION IN HIV-INFECTED ADULTS

A 5-year prospective evaluation of cardiac involvement in AIDS found 16/231 patients had or developed pericardial effusions.[13] Patients had asymptomatic HIV ($n = 59$), AIDS-related complex ($n = 62$), and AIDS ($n = 74$). Three subjects had an effusion on enrollment, and 13 developed effusions during follow-up (12/13 with AIDS at enrollment). Pericardial effusions were generally small (80%) and asymptomatic (87%). The calculated incidence of pericardial effusion among those with

AIDS was 11%/year. The prevalence of effusion in AIDS patients rises over time, reaching an estimated mean in asymptomatic patients of 22% after 25 months of follow-up.

Another prospective study found 71/256 HIV[+] patients developed pericardial effusions that were classified as large in 13, moderate in 10, and small in 48.[14] There was no association found between age, race, or interval after seroconversion and the development of pericardial effusion. Advanced HIV disease state (AIDS) was associated with the development of pericardial effusion. In this study, 78% with AIDS versus 26% with earlier stages of HIV infection had effusion on at least 1 echocardiogram. Those with effusion had smaller body surface area and lower CD4 counts (mean 119 cells/ml) than those without effusion (333 cells/ml). Follow-up echocardiography revealed resolution of the effusion in 9, increased effusion size in 3, and an unchanged effusion in 15 patients studied.

Among subjects with AIDS and a pericardial effusion, 36% were alive after 6 months of follow-up, whereas 93% of those without effusion were alive at 6 months.[13] Two patients developed pericardial tamponade by clinical and echocardiographic criteria.[13] Several studies have suggested spontaneous resolution of pericardial effusion over time in 13–42% of affected patients.[6,13] However, mortality remains markedly increased in patients who had developed an effusion whether or not the effusion resolved.[6,13]

In a retrospective series of cardiac tamponade cases in a U.S. city hospital, 13 of 37 patients (35%) had HIV infection. HIV infection should be suspected whenever young patients present with pericardial effusion or tamponade.[15]

RIGHT VENTRICULAR DYSFUNCTION AND PULMONARY HYPERTENSION IN HIV-INFECTED ADULTS

Isolated right ventricular hypertrophy with or without right ventricular dilation is generally related to pulmonary diseases that increase pulmonary vascular resistance such as recurrent bronchopulmonary infections in HIV[+] patients. Primary pulmonary hypertension has been described in a disproportionate number of HIV[+] individuals and is estimated to occur in 0.5% of hospitalized AIDS patients.[16] Primary pulmonary hypertension has been reported in HIV[+] patients without a history of thromboembolic disease, intravenous drug use, or pulmonary infections.

INFECTIVE ENDOCARDITIS

Intravenous drug users are at greater risk than the general population for infective endocarditis, chiefly of right-sided heart valves. Surprisingly, HIV[+] patients may not have a higher incidence of endocarditis than people with similar risk behaviors.[17]

NONBACTERIAL THROMBOTIC ENDOCARDITIS

Friable clumps of platelets and red blood cells adhere to the cardiac valves in nonbacterial thrombotic endocarditis (NBTE). NBTE was reported in approximately

TABLE 3. **Nonbacterial thrombotic endocarditis**

Author	Year	Cases/Autopsy	Valve(s)	Symptom
Garcia	1983	Case report	Mitral/aortic	Emboli
Snider	1983	2/50	—	Emboli
Fink	1984	1/4	Tricuspid/pulmonic	None
Guarda	1984	2/13	1) Tricuspid/ mitral	DIC
			2) Aortic, tricuspid, mitral	Emboli
Cammarosano/ Lewis	1985	3/41	1)Tricuspid	Emboli
			2) Mitral	Emboli
			3) All	—
Roldan	1987	4/54	Tricuspid/mitral (3)	
Klatt	1988	7/187		
Currie	1995	0/110		

10% of U.S. autopsies in AIDS patients before 1989. A large autopsy series in the United Kingdom found only 1/110 cases of mitral valve NBTE.[17] There have been no case reports since 1989 (see TABLE 3). NBTE should be suspected in the case of emboli from an unknown source and in disseminated intravascular coagulation.

CARDIOVASCULAR MALIGNANCY

Malignancy affects many AIDS patients, generally in the later stages of disease. Cardiac malignancy is usually related to metastatic disease. Kaposi's sarcoma affects up to 35% of AIDS patients, particularly homosexuals, with an incidence inversely related to the CD4 count.[18,19]

Primary cardiac malignancy associated with HIV infection is generally due to cardiac lymphoma. Non-Hodgkin's lymphomas are 25 to 60 times more common in HIV⁺ individuals. HIV⁺ patients with widespread Kaposi's sarcoma had frequent cardiac involvement. Lymphomas are the first manifestation of AIDS in up to 4% of new cases.[20,21]

ATHEROSCLEROSIS

Accelerated atherosclerosis has been observed in young HIV⁺ individuals without traditional coronary risk factors.[22–24] Intimal thickening due to smooth muscle cell proliferation and characteristic atherosclerotic plaque in the setting of increased tumor necrosis factor and IL-1 production has been described as mamillated vegetations with endoluminal protrusions on histologic examination.[22] Significant coronary lesions were discovered at autopsy in 8 HIV⁺ subjects ages 23–32 who died unexpectedly.[23] Cytomegalovirus was present in 2 and hepatitis B virus was found in 2. None of the 8 patients had evidence of cocaine use.

Premature cerebrovascular disease is common in AIDS patients. An 8% stroke prevalence in AIDS patients was estimated in an autopsy study in the 1980s.[25] Of the patients with stroke, 4/13 had evidence of cerebral emboli and 3 of those 4 had a clear cardiac source of embolus.

Protease inhibitor therapy significantly alters lipid metabolism and may be associated with premature atherosclerotic disease.[26] Angiographically proven advanced symptomatic coronary artery disease has been reported in men under age 40 treated with protease inhibitors.[26] Chronic inflammatory states have also been associated with premature atherosclerotic vascular disease.

CONGENITAL CARDIOVASCULAR MALFORMATIONS IN HIV-INFECTED CHILDREN

Most pediatric patients with HIV are infected in the perinatal period. Rates of congenital cardiovascular malformations in cohorts of HIV-uninfected and HIV$^+$ children born to HIV$^+$ mothers range from 5.6% to 8.9%. These rates are 5 to 10 times higher than reported in population-based epidemiological studies, but not higher than in normal populations similarly screened.[27]

AUTONOMIC DYSFUNCTION/ HEMODYNAMIC ABNORMALITIES

Early clinical signs of autonomic dysfunction in HIV$^+$ patients include syncope and presyncope, diminished sweating, diarrhea, bladder dysfunction, and impotence. In one study comparing 26 patients with AIDS or AIDS-related complex to age- and gender-matched controls, heart rate variability, Valsalva ratio, cold pressor testing, isometric exercise (increase in diastolic blood pressure), hemodynamic response to tilt table testing, and hemodynamic response to standing showed that autonomic dysfunction was present in AIDS-related complex, but was pronounced in AIDS patients.[28] Patients with HIV-associated nervous system disease had the greatest abnormalities in autonomic function.[28]

Non-cardiac predictors of serious cardiac events (congestive heart failure, cardiac arrest, dysrhythmias, and tamponade) include advanced stage of HIV-infection, encephalopathy, CMV serology, EBV serology, wasting, and lymphocytic interstitial pneumonitis.[29]

SUMMARY

Global estimates of the number of people living with HIV infection range from 33.4 to 120 million worldwide between the years 1998 and 2000. If there is a 10% incidence of symptomatic congestive heart failure over 2 years, then there are 3.34 to 12 million cases of congestive heart failure expected during a 2-year interval.

As people live longer with HIV infection, long-term manifestations of infection and immunosuppression such as heart disease are emerging as important health concerns and important etiologies of late morbidity and mortality. The effects of

HAART therapy on the incidence and course of HIV-related cardiovascular diseases are yet to be determined.

REFERENCES

1. CENTERS FOR DISEASE CONTROL AND PREVENTION. 2000. HIV/AIDS Surveillance Rep. **12**(No. 1).
2. RAFFANTI, S.P., A.J. CHIARAMIDA, P. SEN, *et al.* 1988. Assessment of cardiac function in patients with the acquired immunodeficiency syndrome. Chest **93**: 592–594.
3. HSIA J. & L.B. MCQUINN. 1993. AIDS cardiomyopathy. Resident Staff Physician **39**: 21–24.
4. BARBARO, G., G. DI LORENZO, B. GRISORIO, *et al.* 1998. Cardiac involvement in the acquired immunodeficiency syndrome: a multicenter clinical-pathological study. AIDS Res. **14**: 1071–1077.
5. BARBARO, G., G. DILORENZO, B. GRISORIO, *et al.* 1998. Incidence of dilated cardiomyopathy and detection of HIV in myocardial cells of HIV-positive patients. N. Engl. J. Med. **339**: 1093–1099.
6. BLANCHARD, D.G., C. HAGENHOFF, L.C. CHOW, *et al.* 1991. Reversibility of cardiac abnormalities in human immunodeficiency virus (HIV)-infected individuals: a serial echocardiographic study. J. Am. Coll. Cardiol. **17**: 1270–1276.
7. LIPSHULTZ, S.E., K.A. EASLEY, E.J. ORAV, *et al.* 1998. Left ventricular structure and function in children infected with human immunodeficiency virus. The Prospective P^2C^2 HIV Multicenter Study. Circulation **97**: 1246–1256.
8. BARBARO, G., G. DI LORENZO, M. SOLDINI, *et al.* 2000. Clinical course of cardiomyopathy in HIV-infected patients with or without encephalopathy related to the myocardial expression of tumour necrosis factor-alpha and nitric oxide synthase. GISCA. AIDS **14**: 827–838.
9. CURRIE, P.F., A.J. JACOB, A.R. FOREMAN, *et al.* 1994. Heart muscle disease related to HIV infection: prognostic implications. Br. Med. J. **309**: 1605–1607.
10. FELKER, G.M., R.E. THOMPSON, J.M. HARE, *et al.* 2000. Underlying causes and long-term survival in patients with initially unexplained cardiomyopathy. N. Engl. J. Med. **342**: 1077–1084.
11. STARC, T.J., S.E. LIPSHULTZ, S. KAPLAN, *et al.* 1999. Cardiac complications in children with human immunodeficiency virus infection. Pediatric pulmonary and cardiac complications of vertically transmitted HIV infection (P^2C^2 HIV) study group, National Heart, Lung, and Blood Institute. Pediatrics **104**: 2,e14. URL: http://www.pediatrics.org/cgi/content/full/104/2/e14
12. SHEARER, W.T., S.E. LIPSHULTZ, K.A. EASLEY, *et al.* 2000. Alterations in cardiac and pulmonary function in pediatric rapid human immunodeficiency virus type 1 disease progressors. Pediatric pulmonary and cardiac complications of vertically transmitted HIV infection study group. Pediatrics **105**: 1,e9. URL: http://www.pediatrics.org/cgi/content/full/105/1/e9
13. HEIDENREICH, P.A., M.J. EISENBERG, L.L. KEE, *et al.* 1995. Pericardial effusion in AIDS. Incidence and survival. Circulation **92**: 3229–3234.
14. HSIA, J. & A.M. ROSS. 1994. Pericardial effusion and pericardiocentesis in human immunodeficiency virus infection. Am. J. Cardiol. **74**: 94–96.
15. KWAN, T., M.M. KARVE & O. EMEROLE. 1993. Cardiac tamponade in patients infected with HIV. A report from an inner-city hospital. Chest **104**: 1059–1062.
16. HIMELMAN, R.B., M. DOHRMANN, P. GOODMAN, *et al.* 1989. Severe pulmonary hypertension and cor pulmonale in the acquired immunodeficiency syndrome. Am. J. Cardiol. **64**: 1396–1399.
17. CURRIE, P.F., G.R. SUTHERLAND, A.J. JACOB, *et al.* 1995. A review of endocarditis in acquired immunodeficiency syndrome and human immunodeficiency virus infection. Eur. Heart J. **16**: 15–18.
18. JENSON, H.B. & B.H. POLLOCK. 1998. Cardiac cancers in HIV-infected patients. *In* Cardiology in AIDS. S.E. Lipshultz, Ed.: 255–263. Chapman & Hall. New York.

19. SILVER, M.A., A.M. MACHER, C.M. REICHERT, *et al.* 1984. Cardiac involvement by Kaposi's sarcoma in acquired immune deficiency syndrome (AIDS). Am. J. Cardiol. **53:** 983–985.
20. BERAL, V., T. PETERMAN, R. BERKELMAN, *et al.* 1991. AIDS-associated non-Hodgkin lymphoma. Lancet **337:** 805–809.
21. DUONG, M., C. DUBOIS, M. BUISSON, *et al.* 1997. Non-Hodgkin's lymphoma of the heart in patients infected with human immunodeficiency virus. Clin. Cardiol. **20:** 497–502.
22. TABIB, A., C. LEROUX, J.F. MORNEX & R. LOIRE. 2000. Accelerated coronary atherosclerosis and arteriosclerosis in young human-immunodeficiency-virus-positive patients. Coronary Artery Dis **11:** 41–46.
23. CAPRON, L., Y.U. KIM, C. LAURIN, *et al.* 1992. Atheroembolism in HIV-positive individuals. Lancet **340:** 1039–1040.
24. CONSTANS, J., J.M. MARCHAND, C. CONRI, *et al.* 1995. Asymptomatic atherosclerosis in HIV-positive patients: a case-control ultrasound study. Ann. Intern. Med. **27:** 683–685.
25. BERGER, J.R., J.O. HARRIS, J. GREGORIOS, *et al.* 1990. Cerebrovascular disease in AIDS: a case-control study. AIDS **4:** 239–244.
26. HENRY, K., H. MELROE, J. HUEBSCH, *et al.* 1998. Severe premature coronary artery disease with protease inhibitors. Lancet **351:** 1328.
27. LAI, W.W., S.E. LIPSHULTZ, K.A. EASLEY, *et al.* 1998. Prevalence of congenital cardiovascular malformations in children of human immunodeficiency virus-infected women: the prospective P^2C^2 HIV Multicenter Study. J. Am. Coll. Cardiol. **32:** 1749–1755.
28. FREEMAN, R., M.S. ROBERTS, L.S. FRIEDMAN, *et al.* 1990. Autonomic function and human immunodeficiency virus infection. Neurology **40:** 575–580.
29. BJOLLER, A.M., I AL-ATTAR, E.J. ORAV, *et al.* 1998. Cardiovascular morbidity and mortality in pediatric HIV infection. *In* Cardiology in AIDS. S.E. Lipshultz, Ed.:77–94. Chapman & Hall. New York.
30. LOPEZ, J.A., R.S. ROSS, M.C. FISHBEIN & R.J. SIEGEL. 1987. Nonbacterial thrombotic endocarditis: a review. Am. Heart J. **113:** 773–784.

Pathological Findings of HIV-Associated Cardiovascular Disease

GIULIA D'AMATI, CIRA R.T. DI GIOIA, AND PIETRO GALLO

Department of Experimental Medicine and Pathology,
"La Sapienza" University, Rome, Italy

ABSTRACT: More effective therapies have improved survival times of HIV$^+$ patients, resulting in a higher prevalence of long-term complications of the disease. This review focuses on HIV-associated cardiovascular pathology, correlating the morphologic findings to clinical syndromes of HIV disease/AIDS.

KEYWORDS: AIDS; HIV; cardiac pathology; cardiomyopathy; endocarditis; myocardium

With the increasing survival of patients, a growing number of clinical and pathological reports have described cardiac involvement in the course of human immunodeficiency virus (HIV) infection. The prevalence of cardiac abnormalities has not been exactly defined. Autopsy studies show cardiovascular involvement in up to 40% of AIDS patients. However, clinical and echocardiographic data indicate a higher prevalence of cardiac disease in the course of HIV infection.[1–4]

MYOCARDIAL PATHOLOGY

According to published clinical and autopsy reports, the prevalence of myocardial abnormalities in HIV$^+$ patients ranges from 25% to 75%. This wide range probably reflects differences in methodology, patient's risk factors, disease stage and environmental factors, such as drug addiction or therapeutic agents. Myocardial involvement in HIV$^+$ patients includes dilated cardiomyopathy, myocarditis, ischemic heart disease, and neoplastic invasion from lymphoma or Kaposi's sarcoma. In addition, the right ventricle can be involved as a consequence of AIDS-related pulmonary disease.

Dilated Cardiomyopathy

Since the first report by Cohen *et al.* in 1986,[5] an increasing number of clinical and echocardiographic studies have documented dilated cardiomyopathy in HIV$^+$ patients. The reported prevalence of this heart condition ranges between 5% and 23%.[2,6–11]

Address for correspondence: Giulia d'Amati, M.D., Department of Experimental Medicine and Pathology, University "La Sapienza," Viale Regina Elena 324, 00161, Rome, Italy. Voice/fax: 39-06-4461484.

giulia.damati@uniroma1.it

Pathologic Features

Pathologic features of AIDS-related cardiomyopathy are similar to those observed in seronegative patients. At autopsy, the heart shape is modified, because of ventricular dilation and apical rounding (see FIGURE 1 A). Heart weight is generally increased, owing to fibrosis and myocyte hypertrophy. On average, long-term survivors have significantly heavier hearts than those dying after a brief disease course. The epicardium is usually normal and coronary arteries do not show significant atherosclerosis. The myocardium is rather flabby and the ventricular wall usually collapses on section.

On cut surface, the ventricles show an *eccentric hypertrophy*, that is, a mass increase with chamber volume enlargement (FIG. 1B). Although hypertrophy is demonstrated by the increase in cardiac weight, this is not always grossly evident owing to ventricular dilation; the free wall width may be normal, or even thinner than normal, as happens in short-term survivors.

Endocardial fibrosis is a common finding, as well as mural thrombi, mainly located at the apex. On histology (see FIGURE 2), myocytes show variable degrees of hypertrophy and degenerative changes, such as myofibril loss, causing hydropic changes within the myocell. An increase in interstitial and endocardial fibrillar collagen is a constant feature in this cardiomyopathy.

Inflammatory cells may infiltrate the myocardium. In fact, some authors report the presence of active lymphocytic myocarditis in up to 83% of patients with a clinical diagnosis of dilated cardiomyopathy.[11] Several studies show evidence of HIV nucleic acid sequences in endomyocardial biopsies from HIV patients with dilated cardiomyopathy.[11–13] This finding is frequently associated either with interstitial lymphocytic infiltration or with foci of active myocarditis.

Dilated cardiomyopathy can be associated with pericardial effusion or infective endocarditis, especially in intravenous drug abusers.[11,14]

Myocarditis

Myocarditis is documented at autopsy in up to 50% of AIDS patients dead from non-cardiac causes[15–17] and in 31%–83% [11,18] of patients with clinical signs of congestive heart failure. It can be part of a disseminated infection, resulting from opportunistic microorganisms, such as *Candida albicans, Cryptococcus neoformans*, and *Toxoplasma gondii*. It most often shows histological features of a lymphocytic myocarditis, suggestive of a viral etiology. In fact, the presence of coxsackievirus B3, cytomegalovirus and Epstein-Barr virus has been reported in endomyocardial biopsies from seropositive patients.[11] In addition, HIV-1 nucleic acid sequences have been detected by *in situ* hybridization in endomyocardial biopsies of patients with left ventricular dysfunction.[11,13] Most of them had active myocarditis on histology.

Pathologic Findings

On gross examination a marked dilation of the cardiac chambers is almost always present. In most cases, owing to the focal distribution of inflammation and myocyte necrosis, the myocardium is not flabby as in hearts with a diffuse inflammatory response. Heart weight is within normal limits. According to the Dallas criteria,[19]

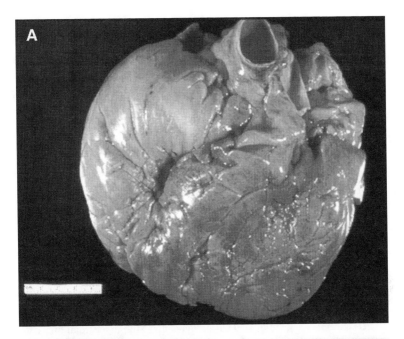

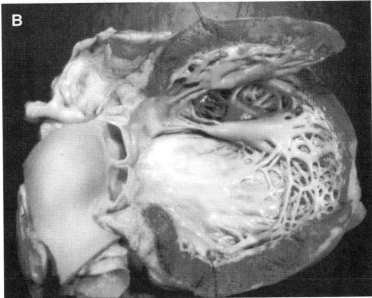

FIGURE 1. Dilated cardiomyopathy in HIV-negative (**A**) and in HIV-positive (**B**) patients. In both cases the heart has a globular shape with rounded apex, due to ventricular dilation. On the cut surface the left ventricular cavity is enlarged with mild myocardial hypertrophy and diffuse endocardial fibrosis. (FIGURE 1A is reprinted from The Internet Pathology Laboratory for Medical Education <http://medstat.med.utah.edu> with the kind permission of Dr. Edward C. Klatt, Florida State University College of Medicine.)

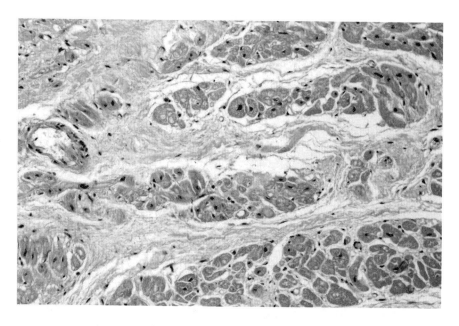

FIGURE 2. AIDS-related dilated cardiomyopathy. Mild myocardial hypertrophy and vacuolization. Interstitial collagen is increased (hematoxylin-eosin, 20×).

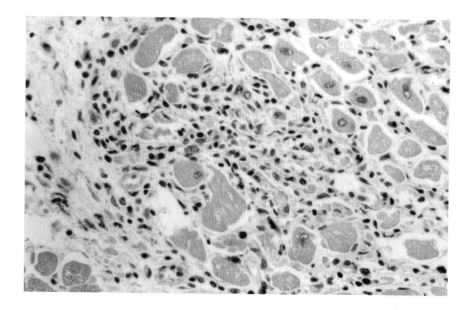

FIGURE 3. AIDS-related active lymphocytic myocarditis. There is a marked interstitial lymphocytic infiltrate with myocyte necrosis (hematoxylin-eosin, 20×).

active myocarditis is characterized by multifocal or diffuse interstitial inflammatory infiltrates associated with degenerative changes or frank myocyte necrosis (see FIGURE 3). Histological findings in HIV-affected patients with myocarditis do not substantially differ from those observed in seronegative patients. However, the degree of inflammatory infiltrate is generally milder. This is believed to result from the impaired efficiency of cell-mediated immunity. In addition, the inflammatory infiltrate is mainly made by CD8+ lymphocytes, and aberrant expression of HLA class II antigens by cardiac myocytes is much rarer than in HIV-negative myocarditis. The severity of clinical symptoms is not always related to the degree of myocardial inflammation and damage. Autopsy studies of AIDS patients dead of acute left ventricular dysfunction almost invariably show a marked inflammatory infiltrate.[10] However, mild and focal mononuclear infiltrates are frequently observed in hearts of AIDS patients, irrespective of the presence of cardiac symptoms.

Histology and immunohistochemistry rarely detect the presence of viruses in the myocardium. However, *in situ* hybridization studies reveal a high frequency of either cytomegalovirus or HIV-1 (see FIGURE 4) or both, in AIDS patients with lymphocytic myocarditis and severe left ventricular dysfunction.[2,11] These data support the hypothesis that, at least in a subset of patients, HIV-1 has a pathogenic action and possibly influence the clinical evolution towards dilated cardiomyopathy.

Opportunistic myocardial infection is generally part of systemic infections. Fungal lesions are visible on gross examination as multiple, small, rounded plaques of whitish color, often hemorrhagic (see FIGURE 5A). On histology, pathogens most frequently observed are protozoa, such as *Toxoplasma gondii*, or fungi, such as

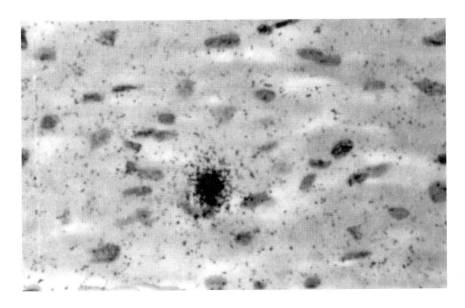

FIGURE 4. Endomyocardial biopsy from a HIV-1-positive patient with dilated cardiomyopathy. *In situ* hybridization with a HIV-1-specific probe, labeled with S35 reveals a positive myocyte. Note the absence of inflammation (hematoxylin-eosin, 40×).

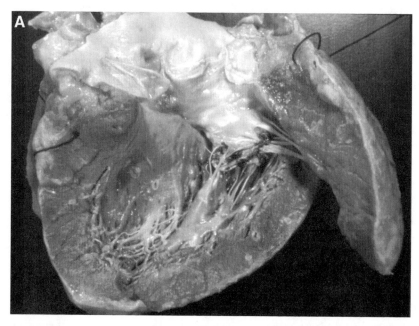

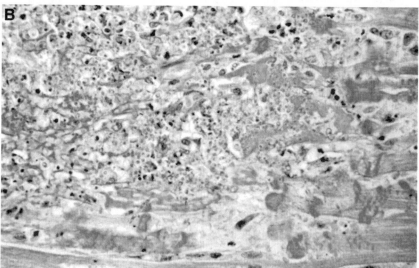

FIGURE 5. Embolic myocarditis complicating *Candida* spp. myocarditis. The ventricular myocardium shows multiple rounded small lesions of whitish color (**A**). On histology, the presence of fungal spores is associated to diffuse myocyte necrosis (**B**) (hematoxylin-eosin, 20×).

Candida albicans (FIG. 5 B), *Cryptococcus neoformans* (see FIGURE 6), and *Aspergillus* spp. (see FIGURE 7).[9] Myocardial and cerebral toxoplasmosis are often associated; histological examination shows "pseudocysts" packed with the protozoa within cardiac myocytes (see FIGURE 8).

Bacterial myocarditis is not infrequent in HIV-positive drug addicts with infective endocarditis. It is a consequence of coronary embolization from valve vegetations.

Ischemic Heart Disease

The prevalence of ischemic heart disease is apparently increasing among HIV+ patients. This can be related to their longer survival, to the higher incidence of herpes virus infection among these patients or, as recently described, to administration of highly active antiretroviral therapy (HAART), including protease inhibitors. Lipodystrophy, hyperlipidemia and hyperglycemia have been described during treatment with protease inhibitors.[20] These side effects may partly account for the increase of cardiovascular accidents in HIV patients treated with HAART.

Pathologic examination of coronary arteries generally reveals eccentric fibro-atheromasic plaques, with variable degrees of chronic inflammatory infiltrates. Lesions with morphologic features similar to accelerated arteriosclerosis were recently described at autopsy of young HIV+ patients.[21] However, clinical and pathological reports dealing with acute coronary syndromes in HIV+ patients treated with HAART are quite scarce.

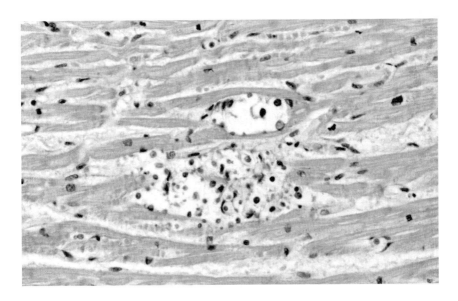

FIGURE 6. Myocardial cryptococcosis. The microorganisms are visible within the myocytes. Note the absence of inflammatory infiltrates (hematoxylin-eosin, 40 ×).

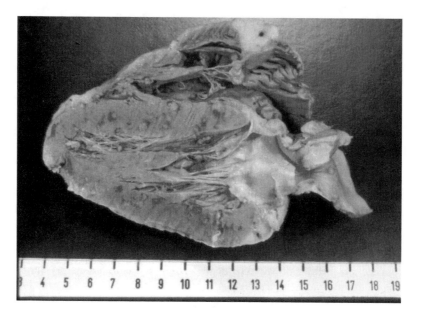

FIGURE 7. Myocardial invasive aspergillosis. Myocardial lesions appear as multiple whitish nodules of variable size, with a hemorrhagic halo.

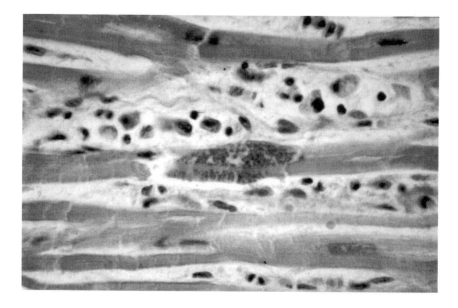

FIGURE 8. Myocardial toxoplasmosis. Bradyzoites are visible within a myocyte surrounded by a bland inflammatory infiltrate (hematoxylin-eosin, 40×).

Conduction System Involvement

Conduction tissue damage can be due to lymphocytic myocarditis, opportunistic infections, and drug cardiotoxicity or to the localization of HIV within the conduction system myocytes. Histological examination may reveal a lymphomonocytic infiltration, myocyte degenerative changes and fibrosis. These changes can be associated with electrocardiographic abnormalities, most frequently first degree atrioventricular block, left anterior hemiblock and left bundle block.[2]

Malignancies

Lymphomas

AIDS-related lymphomas are high-grade B-cell tumors, consisting of large-cell immunoblastic or small noncleaved-cell (Burkitt's or Burkitt-like) lymphomas in approximately 80–90% of cases.[22] Typically the AIDS lymphomas present in extra nodal sites, such as the central nervous system, gastrointestinal tract and bone marrow. Malignant lymphoma presenting as a primary cardiac tumor is rare; however, its incidence is apparently increasing in HIV+ patients.[23–28]

Clinical presentation of cardiac lymphomas, either primitive or secondary, is varied. Symptoms range from dyspnea to chest pain. Many patients have intractable congestive heart failure, arrhythmias or pericardial effusions, but others do not show clinical evidence of cardiac involvement, at least in the initial phase of the disease.

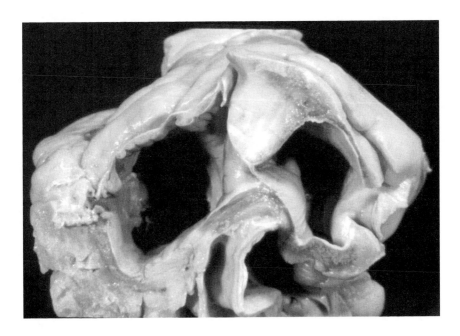

FIGURE 9. AIDS-related large cell B immunoblastic lymphoma involving the atrial septum.

Clinical suspicion of heart involvement by malignant lymphoma should be confirmed by endomyocardial biopsy.

Pathologic Findings. On gross examination (see FIGURE 9), multiple firm nodules of white tissue within the myocardium characterize primary cardiac lymphomas. The right atrium is most frequently affected, followed by the right ventricle, left ventricle, left atrium, atrial septum and ventricular septum. Pericardial involvement is typical, while extension onto valves is rare. Heart weight is often increased. On histology, the nodular masses are composed of large cells of B phenotype, with peripheral myocardial infiltration (see FIGURE 10).

Secondary cardiac involvement by extra-nodal lymphomas may present as direct extension from a mediastinal mass through the pericardium, or as lymphatic or hematogenous spread.

Kaposi's Sarcoma

Kaposi's sarcoma is a low-grade malignancy derived from mesenchymal or endothelial cells. It is the most common AIDS-related neoplasm, occurring in approximately 30% of patients, mostly male homosexuals.

At autopsy, heart involvement is observed in 5–8% of patients with cutaneous and visceral forms of Kaposi's sarcoma.[1,2] Rarely, the heart is the sole site of involvement.[29] Clinical signs of the disease are scarce and non-specific. However, pericardial hemorrhage with fatal cardiac tamponade has been described as a complication of Kaposi's sarcoma.[30]

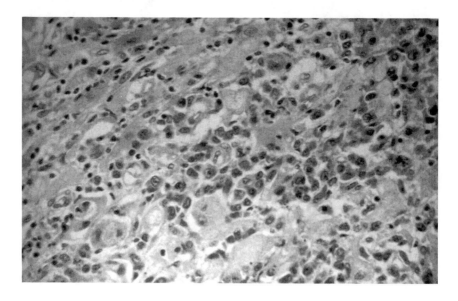

FIGURE 10. Myocardial infiltration by large cell lymphoma, associated with diffuse myocardial damage (hematoxylin-eosin, 40×).

Pathologic Features. At autopsy, the epicardium and pericardium are most frequently involved. Coronary wall infiltration and myocardial involvement are rare. Nodular coalescent dark-red plaques and nodules are the characteristic features of Kaposi's sarcoma (see FIGURE 11).

As seen by histology, early lesions are formed by irregularly shaped capillary vessels surrounded by a mixed inflammatory infiltrate. As the lesions evolve, there is a decrease in the inflammatory infiltrate and interstitial spindle-shaped cells become more evident. In the late stage, the lesions are nodular, formed by spindle cells surrounding slit-like capillary vessels (see FIGURE 12). The histological features of cardiac Kaposi's sarcoma are usually those of a late-stage lesion, because they are rarely diagnosed during life.

Isolated Right Ventricular Hypertrophy and Dilation

Right ventricular hypertrophy and/or dilation, often associated with pericardial effusion, can be observed in the clinical course of HIV infection. This finding is related to the presence of pulmonary hypertension, which can be due to pulmonary infections, to diffuse alveolar damage, or to recurrent pulmonary emboli from intravenous debris acquired through drug abuse. The clinical outcome of right ventricular dysfunction is related to the degree of pulmonary hypertension, varying from a mild asymptomatic condition to severe cardiac impairment with cor pulmonale and death.[31] In addition, the occurrence of right-sided infective endocarditis related to the high frequency of intravenous drug use among HIV-positive patients may explain right ventricular overload or recurrent pulmonary embolic events.

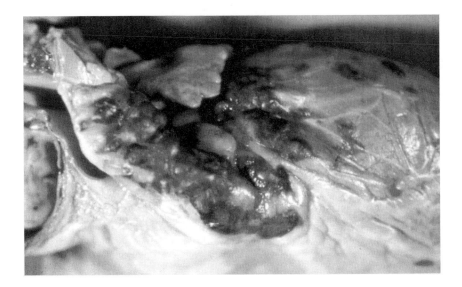

FIGURE 11. Cardiac Kaposi's sarcoma. The epicardial lesions appear as red purple coalescent plaques.

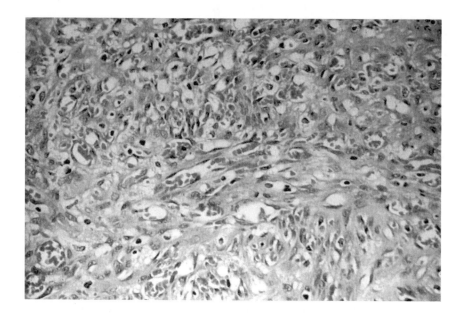

FIGURE 12. Myocardial involvement by Kaposi's sarcoma. Histology shows spindle cells surrounding slit-like capillary vessels (hematoxylin-eosin, 40×).

ENDOCARDIAL DISEASE

Nonbacterial Thrombotic Endocarditis

Nonbacterial thrombotic endocarditis has been reported with increasing frequency in HIV[+] patients in the terminal stage of the disease.[32] This process, commonly associated with chronic severe wasting diseases, particularly malignancies, and severe inanition, is observed in 10–15% of AIDS patients at autopsy.[17,18] Small valvular vegetations can be detected on echocardiography in asymptomatic patients.

Pathologic Findings

Nonbacterial thrombotic endocarditis can involve all four cardiac valves.[17,33] On gross examination one sees thrombi adherent to the endocardial surface of the valve cusps, consisting microscopically of platelets within a fibrin mesh with few inflammatory cells. Thrombotic vegetations may be either single or multiple polypoidal masses, along the cusp apposition lines. The valve often shows changes due to previous inflammatory or dystrophic lesions.

Thrombotic vegetations of nonbacterial thrombotic endocarditis are similar to those found in infective endocarditis; the differential diagnosis is based on the absence of the other typical features of infective endocarditis, such as destruction and erosion of the cusp edges with tears and perforations through the body of the cusp itself, and valvular leaflet aneurismal sacs. In addiction, no infective pathogens are detected on histological examination. Systemic or pulmonary embolization of vegetations is usually detected at autopsy (more than 40% of patients with nonbacterial thrombotic endocarditis) and is underestimated clinically. Often, clinical symptoms of systemic thromboembolization (cerebral, pulmonary, renal, and splenic infarcts) make the valvular lesions clinically obvious. However, systemic thromboembolic disease due to nonbacterial thrombotic endocarditis is a rare cause of death (7%) in AIDS patients.[17]

The vegetations in nonbacterial thrombotic endocarditis may be infected by pyogenic or fungal pathogens during a transient bacteremia, bringing about a typical infective endocarditis.

Infective Endocarditis

Infective endocarditis may be due to either pyogenic or opportunistic pathogens. In the latter case, they are often part of a systemic opportunistic infection with multiple organ localizations. Fungal endocarditis has been reported with increasing frequency as the AIDS epidemic has gained momentum, helped by the compromise of cell-mediated immunity in patients with HIV infection.

Infective endocarditis occurs more frequently in intravenous drug abusers with AIDS, who comprise the second largest risk group for HIV infection after male homosexuals. These patients have frequent bacteremias, owing to the introduction of skin pathogens and talcum powder by unsterile intravenous injection, causing a higher risk of endocardial infection of right-sided cardiac valves (see FIGURE 13). Infective endocarditis is higher in intravenous drug addicts who abuse multiple drugs (cocaine used intravenously in combination with heroin) in addition to alcohol.

The spectrum of pathogens responsible of endocardial infection in intravenous drug abusers with AIDS is not significantly different from that in non-infected drug

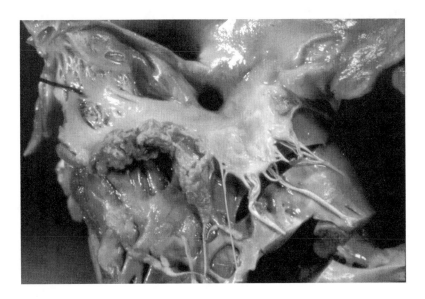

FIGURE 13. Infective endocarditis of the tricuspid valve in a HIV-positive drug abuser. A large polypoid thrombotic lesion is observed on the posterior leaflet.

abusers. However, owing to the deficit in cellular immunity, the pathogens are more virulent, leading to more significant cardiac structural damage and functional deterioration. Pyogenic bacteria more commonly causing infective endocarditis in AIDS are *Staphylococcus aureus, S. epidermidis, Streptococcus pneumoniae* and *Haemophilus influenzae.* Infective endocarditis by Gram-negative bacteria, especially *Pseudomonas* species, has become more common in patients with AIDS, perhaps owing to their repeated hospitalizations that promote the acquisition of resistant organisms.[34] Austrian's syndrome, which is characterized by acute *S. pneumoniae* endocarditis, pneumococcal pneumonia and meningitis, has been noted more commonly in HIV-positive intravenous drug abusers, although this syndrome was originally described in alcoholics. Avirulent bacteria, as the HACEK group (*Haemophilus* species, *Actinobacillus actinomycetemcomitans, Cardiobacterium hominis, Eikenella corrodens* and *Kingella kingae*), which are often part of the endogenous flora of the mouth, can cause endocarditis in seropositive patients. These bacteria are also difficult to culture from endocardial vegetations.[35] Failure to obtain positive blood cultures in the patients with AIDS with strong clinical evidence for infective endocarditis should suggest prior antibiotic therapy or endocarditis by unusual bacteria (as well as HACEK organisms) or fungi. *Candida* species are cultured in less than 50% of patients and *Aspergillus* can rarely be cultured from blood.

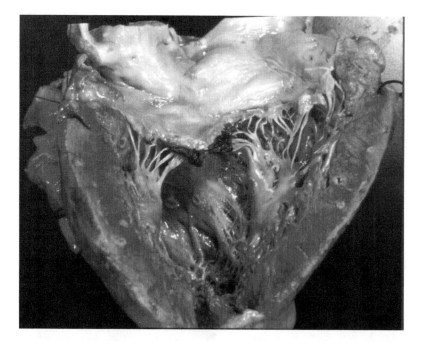

FIGURE 14. *Candida* spp. endocarditis in an AIDS patient. Two polypoid thrombotic lesions are observed on the anterior mitral leaflet; little abscesses are also evident in the myocardial wall.

Fungal endocarditis, especially from C*ryptococcus neoformans* or *Candida albicans*, is common in AIDS, particularly in intravenous drug abusers (see FIGURE 14). It is generally related to systemic spread of fungal infection from extracardiac foci. Candidiasis of the oropharynx and esophagus is most often the primary focus, often progressing to systemic infection (see FIGURE 15).[36] Systemic cryptococcosis is one of the most common infections in AIDS patients. Although meningitis and encephalitis are the most frequent manifestations of cryptococcosis, cardiac involvement, particularly with pericardial effusion, is common. Fungal myocarditis or myocardial abscesses may also occur in association with valve destruction. As cryptococcal meningitis is often the focus of clinical attention, cardiac involvement may be overlooked. Conversely, neurologic complications secondary to cerebral embolization from primary cardiac infection may be the initial presenting complain. *Aspergillum fumigatus* endocarditis associated with disseminated aspergillosis may also occur in AIDS.[37] With aspergillosis, as well as other fungi, signs of systemic or cerebral embolism may indicate the presence of endocarditis because of the absence of positive blood cultures and unobtrusive clinical evidence of heart disease.

Pathologic Features

Infective endocarditis is an ulcerative-polypous lesion due to a destructive valve process with thrombotic stratifications. Thrombotic vegetations are usually gray, but their color is very variable depending on the pathogen involved. They are generally located on the endocardial surface of valve cusps but can be found also on mural endocardium. Their consistence is variable: they are friable at first and later become compact and adherent to the endocardium, owing to their organization. The friability

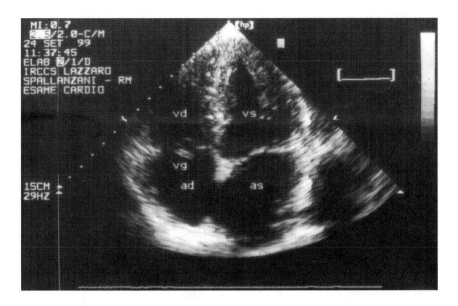

FIGURE 15. Apical four-chamber echocardiographic view showing tricuspid endocardial vegetation in an AIDS patient with esophageal candidiasis.

is increased by lithic effects of bacteria and polymorphonuclear leukocytes. Valvular tissue destruction may involve the tensive appparatus with chordae tendinous rupture. Endocardial ulcerations at the cusp apposition lines are frequent, resulting in leaflets with a moth-eaten look. On histology, thrombotic vegetations consist of fibrin and agglutinated platelets with inflammatory infiltration. In the acute stage of endocardial infection there is an infiltration with polymorphonuclear leukocytes with valve tissue necrosis; later there is a chronic inflammatory infiltration, made up of macrophages, lymphocytes and plasma cells, neoformed capillary vessels, and a fibroblastic proliferation that replaces the necrotic tissue and spreads at the base of thrombotic vegetation. In fungal endocarditis, however, the vegetations are made up essentially of fungal colonies without much fibrin (see FIGURE 16), and they may be so bulky that they obstruct the valve ostium (see FIGURE 17). The presence of colonies of microrganisms is very important for differential diagnosis with marantic endocarditis. Histological identification of pathogens responsible for valve lesions is not always possible, especially in cases with prior antibiotic therapy.

When the left-side cardiac valves are involved, endocarditis can have a galloping course, with rapid onset of heart failure due to acute valvular insufficiency secondary to perforation of valve leaflets or a rupture of tendineous chordae or papillary muscles. Other complications are due to myocardial involvement with possible perforation of the ventricular septum or myocardial abscesses. The infection can extend to the pericardium with purulent pericarditis. The higher frequency of right-sided infectious endocarditis in HIV[+] intravenous drug abusers can explain the pulmonary embolic events with possible pulmonary cavitations and abscesses.[38]

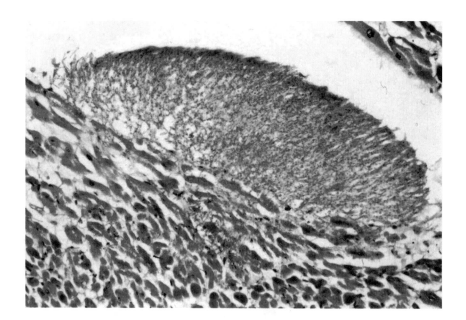

FIGURE 16. Mural thrombus in fungal endocarditis. The thrombus is essentially made by mycetes with scarce fibrin (hematoxylin-eosin, 20×).

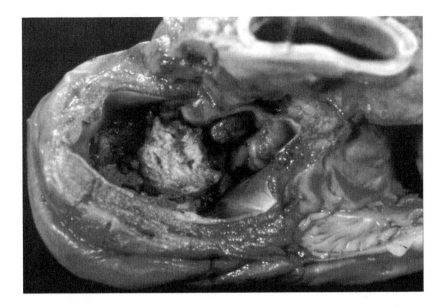

FIGURE 17. Infective endocarditis of the mitral valve. A bulky thrombotic mass obstructs the valve ostium.

If antibiotic therapy is efficacious and the patient does not have rapidly fatal complications, endocarditis can heal. The outcome is thrombous organization and fibrous repair. Residual bulky thrombotic polypi are often seen as calcific masses leaning out of both endocardic surfaces of valvular leaflets.

PERICARDIAL PATHOLOGY

The pericardium is commonly involved in a variety of pathologic cardiac states associated with AIDS. In fact pericardial involvement is described either by echocardiography or at autopsy in up to one-third of AIDS patients.[14] In contrast to isolated myocardial involvement,[9] pericardial disease is the most common cause of clinical cardiovascular symptoms and signs in AIDS patients.

The clinical spectrum of pericardial disease in AIDS includes effusions with or without cardiac tamponade, constrictive pericarditis, and neoplastic infiltration by lymphoma and Kaposi's sarcoma. There is no apparent correlation between clinical stage of HIV infection and severity of pericardial involvement.[7,39]

Pericardial Effusions

Pericardial effusions are rather common, occurring in from 38% to 46% of AIDS patients with cardiac involvement.[14,32,33,36,39,40–44]

Most pericardial effusions are idiopathic.[17] Infections, neoplasias, myocarditis, endocarditis or myocardial infarct have been described as possible etiologies. Little is known about the pathogenesis of pericardial effusions in AIDS patients. However, in the absence of cardiac infection or malignancy, the pathogenesis is likely to be multifactorial. The causes can be metabolic or hemodynamic alterations,[1] dysproteinemias, or pulmonary hypertension due to chronic lung disease (i.e., cytomegalovirus pneumonia).[6] The presence of HIV-1 in macrophages inside the pericardium suggests that the virus may play a rule in pathogenesis of pericardial effusions in AIDS patients.[45]

Pericarditis

Pericarditis is found at autopsy in 30% of AIDS patients.[33] It can be serous, fibrinous, serofibrinous, purulent, or hemorrhagic. Pericardial symptoms and clinical signs can be the first clinical finding of cardiac disease in the course of HIV infection. Common symptoms are pericardial murmurs that disappear with increasing effusion. Other symptoms are chest pain, fever, and dyspnea. Cardiac tamponade may occur. Echocardiography is the most appropriate way of detecting pericarditis (see FIGURE 18).

Pericardial flogosis may be caused by a wide array of pathogens, always in conjunction with disseminated infection. *Mycobacterium tuberculosis hominis* and *M. avium-intracellulare*,[46] herpes simplex (by culture only),[47] *Actinomycetales* (*Nocardia asteroides*)[48] and bacteria such as *Staphylococcus aureus* and *Salmonella typhimurium.* may be identified in pericardial fluid even though in a few cases no pathogens can be isolated.[32] Fungal infections by *Candida albicans, Cryptococcus neoformans* and *Aspergillus fumigatus,* do not often involve the pericardium.[49,50–52]

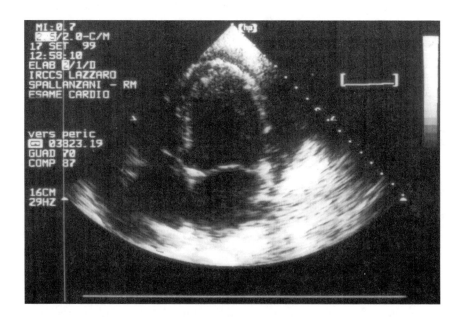

FIGURE 18. Apical four-chamber echocardiographic view showing a mild pericardial effusion in an AIDS patient with *M. avium* intracellulare infection.

Mycobacterium tuberculosis and *M. avium-intracellulare* have become major opportunistic infections in AIDS, especially in populations with high rates of endemic mycobacterial infection, such as intravenous drug abusers and low-income, minority populations. Since *Mycobacterium* has a strong tropism for pericardium, pericarditis has long been recognized as a classic manifestation of *M. tuberculosis* infection in patients with AIDS. Tuberculosis in AIDS is often atypical, with a high prevalence of extra-pulmonary manifestations, atypical chest radiograph features, and high rates of disseminated disease. Recurring pericardial effusion, pericardial abscess, and pericarditis are frequently encountered.[34]

An acute pericardial effusion is usually found on echocardiography; at autopsy multiple necrotizing granulomas are found both on the epicardium and pericardium.[53] The pericardium may also be involved by nonmycobacterial infections such as *Actinomycetales* (*Nocardia asteroides* or *Streptomyces species*).[48] In contrast to tuberculosis, infection with nontuberculous mycobacteria occurs more commonly in homosexuals and in younger patients.[54]

Whereas pericardial disease in the immunocompetent host may be associated with a variety of viruses, most commonly coxsackievirus, pericardial involvement in AIDS is more frequently related to infection with other common viral pathogens, especially herpes simplex virus type 1 and 2.[47,55] Pericardial effusions found in immunocompromised patients may be caused by reactivation of viral infections that are usually self-limited in immunocompetent individuals. Disseminated cytomegalovirus infection is common in AIDS and may involve the heart. Pericardial disease may occur, although it is not a prominent clinical or pathologic finding in cytomegalovirus infection.

Pathologic Features

The most common type of pericarditis is fibrinous or serofibrinous. There is a variable amount of fibrin on the epicardium (see FIGURE 19), while pericardial effusion may be absent or present in variable degree. Many cases of fibrinous pericarditis resolve without residual effects. In other instances, the fibrin deposits organize and form fibrous pericardial adhesions.

Bacterial pericarditis is characterized by a fibrinopurulent exudate. On histology an infiltrate of polymorphonuclear leukocytes is seen in the epicardial connective tissue. Cardiac tamponade often occurs. Fibrous adhesions may result, leading to pericardial constriction.

Hemorrhagic pericarditis shows a serofibrinous or suppurative exudate associated with the presence of serosanguinous fluid in the pericardium. It is typical of tuberculosis, severe bacterial infections, or pericardial malignancy.

Malignancies

Lymphomas

The association of non-Hodgkin's lymphoma and AIDS has been well documented (see above). Malignant lymphomas are usually clinically silent. They may show clinical symptoms such as heart failure, pericardical effusion, and arrhythmias.[6,56]

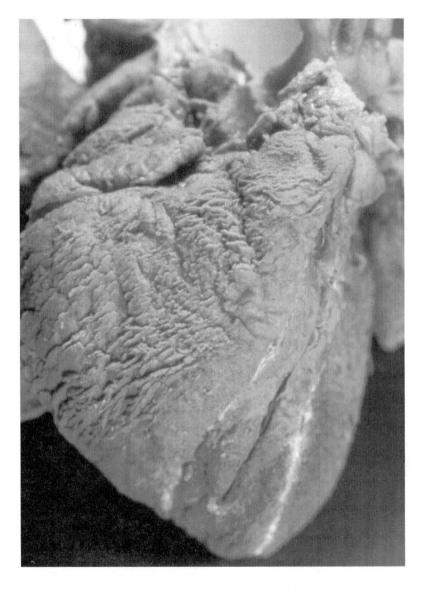

FIGURE 19. Fibrinous pericarditis. The epicardial surface shows a focal fibrous thickening.

In contrast to lymphomas in seronegative patients, which are epicardial or pericardial in location, in AIDS patients the tumor is most often located within the myocardium or in the subendocardial layer. There may be pericardial effusion with a mass lesion of the heart sometimes prolapsing across the tricuspid valve or involving the inferior portions of both ventricles.[57]

Kaposi's Sarcoma

When Kaposi's sarcoma involves the heart (see above), the epicardial surface is a common site of involvement. Echocardiography shows a significant pericardial effusion with clinical signs of cardiac tamponade. At autopsy the pericardium and the epicardial fat show the typical nodular coalescent dark-red lesions or violaceous plaques.[58,59] Occasionally the myocardium may also be involved. Typically, the neoplastic infiltration then extends along the great vessels and the coronary vessels with spread of tumor through the lymph channels along the vasa vasorum.

REFERENCES

1. LEWIS, W. 1989. Cardiac findings from 115 autopsies. Prog. Cardiovasc. Dis. **32:** 207–215.
2. BARBARO, G., G. DI LORENZO, *et al.* 1998. Cardiac involvement in the acquired immunodeficiency syndrome. A multicenter clinical-pathological study. AIDS Res. Hum. Retroviruses **14:** 1071–1077.
3. YUNIS, N.A. & V.E. STONE. 1998. Cardiac manifestations of HIV/AIDS: a review of disease spectrum and clinical management. J. AIDS Human Retrovirol. **18:** 145–154.
4. RERKPATTANAPIPAT, P., N. WONGPRAPARUT, *et al.* 2000. Cardiac manifestations of acquired immunodeficiency syndrome. Arch. Intern. Med. **160:** 602–608.
5. COHEN, I.S., D.W. ANDERSON, *et al.* 1986. Congestive cardiomyopathy in association with the acquired immunodeficiency syndrome. N. Engl. J. Med. **315:** 628–630.
6. MILEI, J., D. GRANA, *et al.* 1998. Cardiac involvement in acquired immunodeficiency syndrome. A review to push action. Clin. Cardiol. **21:** 465–472.
7. LEVY, W.S., G.L. SIMON, *et al.* 1989. Prevalence of cardiac abnormalities in human immunodeficiency virus infection. Am. J. Cardiol. **63:** 86–89.
8. HIMELMAN, R.B., W.S. CHUNG, *et al.* 1989. Cardiac manifestations of human immunodeficiency virus infection: a two-dimensional echocardiographic study. J. Am. Coll. Cardiol. **13:** 1030–1036.
9. HERSKOWITZ A., D. VLAHOV, *et al.* 1993. Prevalence and incidence of left ventricular dysfunction in patients with human immunodeficiency virus infection. Am. J. Cardiol. **71:** 955–958.
10. DE CASTRO, S., G. D'AMATI, *et al.* 1994. Frequency of development of acute global left ventricular dysfunction in human immunodeficiency virus (HIV) infection. J. Am. Coll. Cardiol. **24:** 1018–1024.
11. BARBARO, G., G. DI LORENZO, *et al.* 1998. Incidence of dilated cardiomyopathy and detection of HIV in myocardial cells of HIV-positive patients. N. Engl. J. Med. **339:** 1093–1099.
12. GRODY, W.W., L. CHENG & W. LEWIS. 1990. Infection of the heart by the human immunodeficiency virus. Am. J. Cardiol. **66:** 203–206.
13. HERSKOWITZ, A., T.C. WU, *et al.* 1994. Myocarditis and cardiotropic viral infection associated with severe left ventricular dysfunction in late-stage infection with human immunodeficiency virus. J. Am. Coll. Cardiol. **24:** 1025–1032.
14. FERGUSON, D.W. & B. VOLPP. 1994. Cardiovascular complications of AIDS. Heart Dis. Stroke **3:** 388–394.
15. BAROLDI, G., S. CORALLO & M. MORONI. 1988. Focal lymphocitic myocarditis in acquired immunodeficiency syndrome (AIDS): a correlative morphologic and clinical study in 26 consecutive fatal cases. J. Am. Coll. Cardiol. **12:** 463–469.
16. BARBARO, G., G. DI LORENZO, *et al.* 1996. Clinical meaning of ventricular ectopic beats in the diagnosis of HIV-related myocarditis: a retrospective analysis of Holter electrocardiographic recordings, echocardiographic parameters, histopathological and virologic findings. Cardiologia **41:** 1199–1207.
17. ANDERSON, D.W. & R. VIRMANI. 1990. Emerging patterns of heart disease in human immunodeficiency virus infection. Hum. Pathol. **21:** 253–259.

18. ROLDAN, E.O., L. MOSKOWITZ & G.T. HENSLEY. 1987. Pathology of the heart in acquired immunodeficiency syndrome. Arch. Pathol. Lab. Med. **111:** 943–946.
19. ARETZ, H.T., M.E. BILLINGHAM, *et al.* 1987. Myocarditis: a histopathologic definition and classification. Am. J. Cardiovasc. Pathol. **1:** 3–14.
20. PERIARD, D., A. TELENTI, *et al.* 1999. Atherogenic dyslipidemia in HIV-infected individuals treated with protease inhibitors. Circulation **100:** 700–705.
21. TABIB, A., C. LEROUX, *et al.* 2000. Accelerated coronary atherosclerosis and arteriosclerosis in young human-immunodeficiency-virus-positive patients. Coronary Artery Dis. **11:** 41–46.
22. LEVINE, A.M. 1994. Malignant lymphoma complicating immunodeficiency disorders. Ann. Oncol. **5:** S29–S35.
23. BALASUBRAMANYAM, A., M. WAXMAN, *et al.* 1986. Malignant lymphoma of the heart in acquired immune deficiency syndrome. Chest **90:** 243–246.
24. GUARNER, J., R.K. BRYNES, *et al.* 1987. Primary non-Hodgkin's lymphoma of the heart in two patients with the acquired immunodeficiency syndrome. Arch. Pathol. Lab. Med. **111:** 254–256.
25. COSTANTINO, A., T.E. WEST, *et al.* 1987. Primary cardiac lymphoma in a patient with acquired immunodeficiency syndrome. Cancer **60:** 2801–2807.
26. HOLLADAY, A.O., R.J. SIEGEL & D.A. SCHWARTZ. 1992. Cardiac malignant lymphoma in acquired immune deficiency syndrome. Cancer **70:** 2203–2207.
27. DUONG, M., C. DUBOIS & M. BUISSON. 1997. Non-Hodgkin lymphoma of the heart in patients infected with human immunodeficiency virus. Clin. Cardiol. **20:** 497–502.
28. MCDONNEL, P.J., R.B. MANN & B.H. BULKLEY. 1982. Involvement of the heart by malignant lymphoma: a clinicopathologic study. Cancer **49:** 944–951.
29. AUTRAN, B.R., I. GORIN, *et al.* 1983. AIDS in a Haitian woman with cardiac Kaposi's sarcoma and Whipple disease. Lancet **1:** 767–768.
30. BURKE, A. & R. VIRMANI. 1995. Tumors of the heart and great vessels, 3rd edit. Armed Forces Institute of Pathology, Washington, DC.
31. HIMELMAN, R.B., M. DOHRMANN, *et al.* 1989. Severe pulmonary hypertension and cor pulmonale in acquired immunodeficiency syndrome. Am. J. Cardiol. **64:** 1396–1399.
32. KAUL, S., M.C. FISHBEIN & R.J. SIEGEL. 1991. Cardiac manifestations of acquired immune deficiency syndrome. A 1991 update. Am. Heart J. **122** (2): 535–544.
33. CAMMAROSANO, C. & W. LEWIS. 1985. Cardiac lesions in acquired immune deficiency virus (AIDS). J. Am. Coll. Cardiol. **5:** 703–706.
34. FRANCIS, C.K. Cardiac involvement in AIDS. 1990. Current problems in Cardiology. Mosby-Year Book, Inc. St. Louis.
35. ELLNER, J.J., M.S. ROSENTHAL, *et al.* 1979. Infective endocarditis caused by slow growing fastidious, Gram-negative bacteria. Medicine **58:** 145–158
36. GUARDA, L.A., M.A. LUNA, *et al.* 1984. Acquired immune deficiency syndrome: postmortem findings. Am. J. Clin. Pathol. **81:** 549–557.
37. HENOCHOWICZ, S., M. MUSTAFA, *et al.* 1985. Cardiac aspergillosis in acquired immune deficiency syndrome. Am. J. Cardiol. **55:** 1239–1240.
38. DE CASTRO, S., G. D'AMATI, *et al.*1997. Myocardial aspects of HIV infection. Cardiologia **42:** 337–341.
39. MONSUEZ, J.J., E.L. KINNEY, *et al.* 1988. Comparison among acquired immune deficiency syndrome patients with and without clinical evidence of cardiac disease. Am. J. Cardiol. **62:** 1311–1313.
40. KINNEY, E.L., D. BRAFMAN & R.J. WRIGHT. 1989. Echocardiographic findings in patients with acquired immunodeficiency (AIDS) and AIDS-related complex (ARC). Cath. Cardiovasc. Diagn. **16:** 182-185.
41. BESTETTI, R.B. 1989. Cardiac involvement in the acquired immune deficiency syndrome. Int. J. Cardiol. **22:** 143–146.
42. FINK, L., N. REICHEK & M.G. SUTTON. 1984. Cardiac abnormalities in acquired immune deficiency syndrome. Am. J. Cardiol. **54:** 1161–1163.
43. MINARDI, G., M. DI SEGNI, *et al.* 1991. Valutazione ecocardiografica in soggetti HIV positivi. G. Ital. Cardiol. **21:** 273–280.
44. CORALLO, S., M.R. MUTINELLI, *et al.* 1988. Echocardiography detects myocardial damage in AIDS: prospective study in 102 patients. Eur. Heart J. **9:** 887–892.

45. KOVACS, A., D.R. HINTON, *et al.* 1996. Human immunodeficiency virus type 1 infection of the heart in three infants with acquired immunodeficiency syndrome and sudden death. Pediatr. Infect. Dis. J. **15:** 819–824.
46. WOODS, G. & J. GOLDSMITH. 1989. Fatal pericarditis due to mycobacterium avium-intracellulare in acquired immune deficiency syndrome. Chest **95:** 1355–1357.
47. FREEDBERG, R.S., A.J. GINDEA, *et al.* 1987. Herpes simplex pericarditis in AIDS. N.Y. State J. Med.:304–306.
48. HOLTZ, M.A., D.P. LAVERY & R. KAPILA. 1985. Actinomycetales infection in the acquired immunodeficiency syndrome. Ann. Intern. Med. **102:** 203–205.
49. BRIVET, F., J. LIVARTOWSKI, *et al.* 1987. Pericardial cryptococcal disease in acquired immune deficiency syndrome [Letter]. Am. J. Med. **82:** 1273.
50. ZUGER, A., E. LOUIE, *et al.* 1986. Cryptococcal disease in patients with the acquired immunodeficiency syndrome. Ann. Intern. Med. **104:** 234–240.
51. SCHUSTER, M., F. VALENTINE & R. HOLTZMAN. 1985. Cryptococcal pericarditis in an IVDA. J. Infect. Dis. **152:** 842.
52. SCHWARTZ, D.A. 1989. Aspergillus pancarditis following bone marrow transplantation for chronic myelogenous leukemia. Chest **95:** 1338–1339.
53. D'CRUZ, I.A., E.E. SENGUPTA, *et al.* 1986. Cardiac involvement, including tubercolosis pericardial effusion, complicanting acquired immune deficiency syndrome. Am. Heart J. **112:** 1100–1102.
54. FOURNIER, A.M., G.M. DICKINSON, *et al.* 1988. Tuberculosis and nontuberculous mycobacteriosis in patients with AIDS. Chest **93:** 772–777.
55. TOMA, E., M. POISSON, *et al.* 1989. Herpes simplex type 2 pericarditis and bilateral facial palsy in a patient with AIDS. J. Infect. Dis. **160:** 553.
56. STEFFEN, H.M., R. MULLER, *et al.* 1990. The heart in HIV-1 infection: preliminary results of a prospective echocardiographic investigation. Acta Cardiologica **XLV:** 529–535.
57. GILL, P.S., A.N. CHANDRARATNA, et al. 1987. Malignant lymphoma: cardiac involvement at initial presentation. J. Clin. Oncol. **5:** 216–224.
58. STEIGMAN, C.K., D.W. ANDERSON, *et al.* 1986. Fatal cardiac tamponade in acquired immune deficiency syndrome with epicardial Kaposi's sarcoma. Am. Heart J. **116:** 1105–1107.
59. STOTKA, J.L., C.B. GOOD, *et al.* 1989. Pericardial effusion and tamponade due to Kaposi's sarcoma in acquired immunodeficiency syndrome. Chest **95:** 1359–1361.

AIDS Cardiomyopathy

Physiological, Molecular, and Biochemical Studies in the Transgenic Mouse

WILLIAM LEWIS

Department of Pathology and Laboratory Medicine,
Emory University School of Medicine, Atlanta, Georgia 30322, USA

ABSTRACT: Cardiomyopathy in AIDS (AIDS CM) is an important and prevalent clinical problem. Mechanisms of AIDS CM are not completely understood. Among the potential etiologies of AIDS CM are HIV-1, various opportunistic infections, inflammatory reactions, cytokine effects, and cardiotoxicity of prescribed or illicit drugs. The transgenic mouse (TG) offers a unique *in vivo* way to elucidate mechanisms of AIDS CM. Structural and functional effects of HIV-1 and specific HIV-1 gene products on heart tissue can be addressed by TGs. Selective effects of HIV-1 and antiretroviral therapy may be defined in controlled studies. We utilized AIDS TGs with generalized expression of HIV-1 gene products in CM models. We treated those TGs with individual and combined antiretroviral therapeutics (HAART) to compare cardiovascular effects of AIDS per se and its therapy. We next developed cardiac-specific TGs in which selected HIV-1 genes are driven by α-myosin heavy chain promoter to target the selected HIV-1 gene to the cardiac myocyte to define effects of specific HIV-1 gene products on the cardiac myocyte. Each transgenic approach is a model system that affords a distinct opportunity to explore the pathogenesis and pathophysiology of AIDS CM.

KEYWORDS: cardiomyopathy; AIDS; HAART; transgenic mice

INTRODUCTION

It is clear that an important way to investigate the complex clinical problems of cardiomyopathy (CM) in the acquired immunodeficiency syndrome (AIDS CM) is to generate authentic models of AIDS, its therapy, and environmental factors that may have an impact on cardiac performance. Physiological events, pathological features, and consequences of AIDS CM are then dissected and monitored in a relevant way.

Unfortunately, few authentic murine models recapitulate HIV-1 infection, particularly of the heart, or of CM in AIDS. Conversely, although HIV-1 infection of the heart has been reported, it may not be very prevalent. Over the past two decades, my laboratory has focused (and continues to focus) on models of AIDS CM. Reviews of mechanisms of human AIDS CM have been published.[1] They may help in relating

Address for correspondence: William Lewis, M.D., Department of Pathology and Laboratory Medicine, Emory University School of Medicine, 7117 Woodruff Memorial Research Building, 1639 Pierce Drive, Atlanta, GA 30322. Voice: 404-712-9005; fax: 404-727-8540.
wlewis@emory.edu

the significant primary publications that have arisen since the inception of the epidemic nearly 20 years ago.

All clinical evidence suggests that combined anti-HIV-1 chemotherapy (HAART), usually including AZT and other nucleoside reverse transcriptase inhibitors (NRTIs), is a formidable way of combatting HIV-1 infection and treating AIDS.[2,3] Because of the relatively recent advent of HAART, its cardiovascular side effects may not yet be fully appreciated.

Cardiac effects of HAART and HAART's role in AIDS CM are addressed experimentally in my laboratories. The contribution of other cardiotoxins, such as alcohol and cocaine, may have an effect on AIDS CM and therefore must also be evaluated in the complex analysis of AIDS CM.

TGs AND VIRAL PATHOGENESIS OF HIV

Transgenic mice are useful in the study of viral gene function and pathogenesis in AIDS and other viral illnesses.[4-9] An advantage to their use is the cellular incorporation of viral sequences into selected (or non-selected) cells. Problems associated with viral administration are obviated because the viral sequences are contained within every target cell, although they may be variably expressed in tissues. The practicality of the mouse in the laboratory, its extensive use in cardiovascular research, and the power of transgenesis provide a unique experimental system to dissect complex aspects of AIDS CM.

TGs may show pathologic changes that are relatively rare in infected humans. By its very nature, the TG approach offers the advantage (and the disadvantage) of permanent incorporation of the transgene into murine genetic material. This biological fact enables the investigator to evaluate direct effects (from the TG) and allows monitoring of disease progression from preclinical development throughout its natural history to death. It obviates any immunological or other systemic input that could potentially affect cardiac performance.

TGs may manifest phenotypic changes relatively early in the natural history; in contrast, human disease frequently reveals itself in later stages. With HIV-1 infection, manifestations of immunodeficiency frequently are marked by opportunistic infections that occur after variable durations of immune dysfunction. As mentioned, immunological dysfunction may or may not be manifested in such TGs.

Although the power and appeal of the transgenic mouse system is evident, drawbacks also exist. *In vitro* studies with transfected cells lines showed that mouse cells supported HIV-1 gene expression driven by the HIV-1 long terminal repeat (LTR).[10,11] However, the transfected HIV-1 clones produced low levels of progeny virions compared to human cells. This observation may reflect a weak or nonexistent transactivation capability of Tat on its own LTR in rodent cells.[12,13] Low virus production could be the result of basal LTR activity in the absence of strong Tat function in rodent cells. Weaker activity of Tat may be due to less efficient, or lack of, interaction of Tat with rodent cellular protein(s). In human cells their counterpart(s) cooperate more effectively with Tat through the *trans*-acting response element (TAR) to increase the steady state levels of HIV-1 mRNA.

One potential concern in a TG model is that a relatively low level of expression of HIV-1 genes *in vitro* is seen in rodent-derived cells compared to human-derived cells. The level of expression of any particular viral protein in TGs may not approach the threshold required to induce acute pathological changes and may not closely or accurately mimic human disease.

Chronically or persistently low levels of expression may permit the development of phenotypes similar to those in humans, but may require extended development time. The extended time window provides opportunities for development of effects. Slowly developing disorders, like CM, may be allowed to appear.

TRANSGENIC STRATEGIES TO DEFINE AIDS CM

As alluded to above, various transgenic strategies are available to dissect the role of HIV-1 infection in the pathogenesis and pathophysiology of AIDS CM. Each has its strengths and weaknesses. In general, two overall approaches are utilized in my laboratories. The first employs non-specific transgenic models of HIV-1 with phenotypic similarities to AIDS. In the second more recent approach, organ-specific, targeted transgenesis is employed.

NON-TARGETED TGS

Related TGs are relevant for use in models of AIDS CM. Iwakura and colleagues[14] developed TGs harboring a defective provirus with a deletion within the pol gene. RNase protection assays demonstrated the highest level of transgene expression in eye, slightly less in spleen, and barely detectable levels in the brain and thymus. No signal was detected in the heart, kidney, liver, or bone marrow.

The alternative approach to targeted transgenes is employed in the author's laboratory uses established TG models of AIDS in which cardiac-specific targeting was not used, but generalized expression of the transgene allows for "systemic" effects.

The heterozygous NL4-3Δ gag/pol TG mouse became available from collaborator Paul Klotman (Mount Sinai Medical Center, New York, NY). He developed a heterozygous TG containing a construct with an internal deletion that eliminated much of the gag/pol coding sequence.[15] None of the founder mice that carried this transgene developed disease during their lifespan. Three founders (Tg22, Tg25, and Tg26) produced progeny that developed renal disease, and one (Tg26) developed skin lesions[16] as well as myopathy/myositis.[17] Tissue distribution and level of expression of the viral transgene varied between the three lines.

In each case, three distinct mRNA species could be detected corresponding to full-length, singly spliced, and doubly spliced messages. Highest mRNA expression was in skin and muscle. Expression could be detected in thymus, gastrointestinal tract, kidney, eye, brain, and spleen. Cardiac expression was low. Aside from widespread but varied tissue distribution, NL4-3Δ gag/pol TGs demonstrate nephropathy, wasting, and skin diseases that phenotypically resemble clinical counterparts in AIDS.

Klotman showed different patterns of protein expression in different TG tissues (by immunoblotting). Analysis of protein extracts from TG skin demonstrated specific staining of HIV-1 proteins, including the gp41, gp120, and gp160 env proteins, while kidney extracts were shown only to contain gp41. In contrast, skeletal muscle only showed the presence of the Nef protein. The disparate patterns of protein expression could be explained by differences in Rev function between tissues. It is possible that some tissue, for example, skin, contains essential Rev cofactors while others do not. Histopathological examination of the kidneys from the Tg22 and Tg25 lines revealed diffuse global glomerulosclerosis, microcystic tubular dilation, and sparse monocytic infiltrates within the interstitium.

Tg26 animals showed a spectrum of pathological changes including segmental and global glomerulosclerosis, tubular dilation, atrophy of the tubular epithelium, proteinaceous casts, and a monocytic interstitial infiltrate.[18] Use of antibodies specific for Rev, Tat, Nef, gp41, or gp 120 demonstrated the accumulation of Rev protein only within sclerotic glomeruli[18] in contrast to the immunoblotting results, which demonstrated only the presence of gp41 in kidney lysates.[15] This apparent contradiction may be explained if the Rev protein were found in the circulation and deposited in the sclerotic glomeruli. Nevertheless, expression of HIV-1 mRNA was documented only in the three independent lines that developed the characteristic renal nephropathology of AIDS nephropathy, and this implicated HIV-1 as the causative agent.[18]

PHARMACOLOGICAL CM USING TGS

Pharmacologically induced CM occurs with AZT treatment of rats and mice.[19–21] AZT CM enables the investigators to define the role of anti-HIV-1 chemotherapy in the pathogenesis and pathophysiology of AIDS CM[20–27] (see FIGURE 1).

Altered mtDNA replication is linked to mitochondrial toxicity of nucleoside agents used in treatment of viral illnesses.[28] AZT and fialuridine (FIAU, 1-2-deoxy-2-fluoro-β-D-arabinofuranosyl-5-iodouracil) serve as tools in AIDS CM models since they inhibit DNA pol-γ. We proposed the DNA pol-γ hypothesis to address mechanisms of pharmacological AIDS CM.[27] In pharmacological AIDS CM, changes in mtDNA replication reflect combined effects. These include subcellular availability and abundance of the nucleoside analog in the target, the ability of the nucleoside analog to become phosphorylated intracellularly, the ability of the nucleoside analog triphosphate to inhibit DNA pol-γ (possibly reflected in its K_i *in vitro*), and tissue requirement for oxidative phosphorylation.

Using FIAU as a model compound, members of this class possess 3′-hydroxyl groups and compete with the native nucleotide (e.g., FIAUTP competes with dTTP). The nucleoside analog monophosphate incorporates into mtDNA and extends the nascent mtDNA chain. The second type is represented by some dideoxynucleosides including AZT used in AIDS treatment. With agents that resemble AZT structurally, the 5′-triphosphates are used as substrates for DNA pol-γ and compete with the natural dNTP. However, they also terminate nascent mtDNA chains because they lack 3′-hydroxyl groups for mtDNA extension.

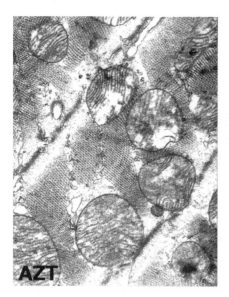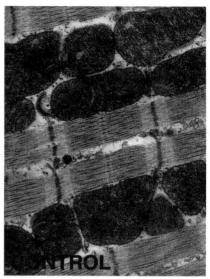

FIGURE 1. Transmission electron microscopy of samples of hearts from Sprague Dawley rats treated with AZT for 35d. (**A**) In control, the sarcomeres are registered and mitochondria are essentially unremarkable. (**B**) in AZT-treated, mitochondrial structural damage was found. Changes included cristae dissolution (*arrow*) and disruption (magnification 14,000×).

TG studies performed in our laboratory addressed the relative impact of HIV-1 and AZT on CM in AIDS. TGs and inbred FVB/n mice received water *ad libitum* with and without AZT (0.7 mg/ml) for 21 or 35d. After 21d, echocardiographic studies were performed and abundance of mRNAs for cardiac sarcoplasmic reticulum calcium ATPase (SERCA2), sodium calcium exchanger (NCX1), and atrial natriuretic factor (ANF) were determined individually using Northern analysis of extracts of left ventricles (LVs). After 35d, contractile function and relaxation were analyzed in isolated work performing hearts. Histopathological and ultrastructural (TEM) changes were identified. After 21d, molecular indicators of cardiac dysfunction were identified. Depressed SERCA2 and increased ANF mRNA abundance were found in LVs from AZT-treated TGs. NCX1 abundance was unchanged. Eccentric LV hypertrophy was determined echocardiographically. After 35d, cardiac dysfunction was worst in AZT-treated and -untreated TGs. Decreases in the first derivative of the maximal change in LV systolic pressure with respect to time (+dP/dt) occurred at baseline in TGs with and without AZT treatment. Increased half-time of relaxation and ventricular relaxation (−dP/dt) occurred in AZT-treated and -untreated TGs. Increased time to peak pressure was found only in AZT-treated TGs. In AZT-treated FVB/n, −dP/dt was decreased. Ultrastructurally, mitochondrial destruction was most pronounced in AZT-treated TGs, but also was found in AZT-treated FVB/n (see FIGURE 2). Transgenic mice that express HIV-1 demonstrate cardiac dysfunction. AZT treatment of

FVB/n causes mitochondrial ultrastructural alterations and alterations in −dp/dt. In TGs, AZT treatment worsens CM.

Treatment with certain NRTIs (stavudine/lamivudine) results in anion gap acidosis.[29] HAART combinations have been implicated in and may be involved in the development of the cardiovascular and metabolic changes that include elevated plasma lactate (LA). To determine the effects of HAART on the development of LA and organ dysfunction, a "2 by 2" protocol was created using 8-week-old TGs (NL4-3Δ gag/pol) and age-matched wild type FVB/n with HAART treatment or with vehicle. The HAART regimen included 35-day treatment of combined zidovudine (~150 mg/kg/d) + lamivudine (0.8mg/kg/d) + indinavir (32 mg/kg/d) or vehicle controls. At termination, mice underwent echocardiographic monitoring as we have done in the past and retro-orbital blood sampling for plasma lactate determinations using commercial assays. TG + HAART developed elevated LA compared to any other cohorts. LV mass normalized to body weight in TG + HAART was greatest compared to all other cohorts. This HAART regimen administered to transgenic AIDS mice results in elevation in LA and cardiac dysfunction.

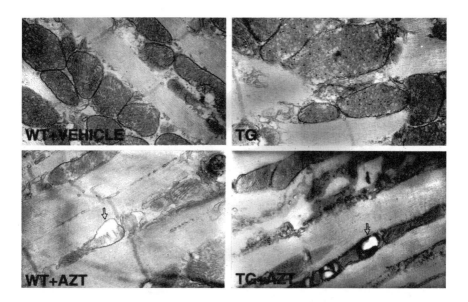

FIGURE 2. TEM changes in cardiac myocytes from FVB/n and AIDS TG mice (NL4-3D gag/pol) with and without AZT treatment. LV myocardial samples were processed from of WT + vehicle (*upper left*), WT + AZT (*upper right*), TG + vehicle (*lower left*), TG + AZT (*lower right*) after 35d. In TG + AZT, significant mitochondrial structural damage was found. Mitochondrial damage also was observed in WT + AZT, but to a lesser extent. Other cohorts revealed minimal mitochondrial damage. Changes included cristae dissolution (*arrow*); magnification 14,000× for each.

TARGETING TGs TO THE HEART IN AIDS

For the past few years, members of my laboratory have selected a less complex, potentially easier, alternative approach to determine the pathological consequences from expression of an individual viral gene product.

With the targeted transgenic approach, we have successfully targeted selected HIV-1 transgenes to mice cardiac ventricular myocytes. This cardiac-targeted TG approach was established principally by Jeff Robbins through the development of and use of the cardiac-specific α myosin-heavy-chain promoter (α-MyHC).[30,31] By creating single-gene TGs with cardiac-specific expression of individual HIV-1 genes driven by the α-MyHC promoter, members of my laboratory are defining structural and functional effects of HIV-1 gene products on cardiac performance and myocyte structure.

TGs expressing HIV-1 Tat have been created where HIV-1 tat is driven by LTR.[32] This contrasts with TGs generated recently in my laboratory in which cardiac-specific expression of HIV-1 Tat was accomplished.[33] In the former case, TGs with non-specific expression of Tat develop a high incidence of hepatocellular carcinomas,[34] endothelial proliferation, and skin lesions that resemble Kaposi's Sarcoma.[35,36] Many other tumors were present in 29% of TGs37 along with non-neoplastic diseases. One tat TG line driven by the chicken β-actin promoter demonstrated B cell lymphoma.[38]

In some TGs, HIV-1 Tat potentiates AZT-induced cellular toxicity[39] and a mechanism of oxidative damage was suggested. This may relate to decreased GSH found in Tat TG livers[40] and to observations of increased apoptosis *in vitro*, possibly mediated by oxidative stress.[41,42]

We created lines of AIDS TGs that express HIV-1 tat in ventricular cardiac myocytes with different levels of tat expression. Progeny of founders demonstrate expression of HIV-1 tat polyadenylated mRNA in cardiac myocytes (Northern) but not in other selected tissues. Hemizygotes demonstrate left ventricle hypertrophy pathologically and defects in the structure of mitochondrial cristae with enlarged, bizarre mitochondria. We found that the hemizygous, high expressor α-MyHC-tat TG demonstrates abnormal mitochondrial structure.

At present, we also have developed two lines of TGs expressing Nef in the cardiac myocytes. The TGs each express approximately 1–2 copies of the TG. Phenotypic analysis is under way. Other TG constructs being generated include HIV-1 vpr and vpu. Together, these TGs may be effective tools to deduce the mechanisms of AIDS CM and the role of HIV-1 gene products in its development.

As may be deduced, a disadvantage of the single gene targeted transgenesis approach may be the fact that several viral proteins may be required to interact with each other to induce pathological or physiological (phenotypic) changes. Additionally, as a gene is removed from its genomic context, *cis*-acting control elements may be altered or omitted, a situation that could potentially affect gene expression.

ALTERNATIVE APPROACHES TO TARGETED TGs—
ADVANTAGES AND DISADVANTAGES

A potential, related TG approach localizes complete, infectious HIV-1 to murine cardiac myocytes. Such a transgene contains all viral transcriptional and post-transcriptional control elements such as the LTR, TAR, and RRE. In addition, the whole genomic transgene has the potential to express all encoded viral proteins and should allow for protein:protein interactions. However, a system employing an intact human provirus in rodents is worrisome. Mice expressing intact HIV-1,[43] may be animal reservoirs for virus.[44] The system could be potentially infectious to humans.

Recombination with endogenous retroviruses also is a concern with an intact HIV-1 TG. This may include physical recombination, such as phenotypic mixing and pseudotyping, and genetic recombination. Phenotypic mixing would occur if the envelope proteins of one virus intermingled among the envelope proteins of another virus. This would give the recombinant virus a dual tropism. Pseudotyping results when one virus provides all of the envelope proteins for a second virus. The recombinant may infect a cell type normally refractory to the core virus. However, in order to propagate the virus in the new cell type, pseudotyping must occur with every subsequent infection. Both physical recombinants may occur in the mouse and could be potential health threats to humans.[45,46]

A third possibility, genetic recombination between HIV-1 and a mouse virus, may create a hybrid virus with unknown species specificity.[47] Potential for infection with this class of TG requires proper containment (BSL3). Given the above concerns and drawbacks, and with the clinical and pathological data available about AIDS CM, one approach chosen for my laboratory uses a TG with a replication defective HIV-1 (with deletion of one or more of the structural genes). This is particularly suitable for one experimental line of TGs. In AIDS CM experiments undertaken in my laboratories, the defective retrovirus (NL4-3Δ gag/pol) or selected HIV-1 genes (e.g., tat) would be incapable of unilaterally producing viral particles in the TG. However, since most of the genome is complete, a murine retrovirus may still be capable of pseudotyping the subgenomic HIV-1 RNA molecule.

As mentioned previously, pseudotypes may allow infection of other cells but must be maintained by a subsequent pseudotyping event. In this case, the defective virus could not reproduce to yield virions, even if the pseudotyped virus infected human cells, and thus would not be a practical safety concern. Mature viral particles could, theoretically, only be produced as a result of genetic recombination. Although the subgenomic TGs may not *a priori* warrant high level containment, the possibility of recombination makes additional measures a precaution. The subgenomic TG may have additional advantages over whole genomic TG in that it is less complex and codes fewer viral genes. Fewer genes may eliminate a potential phenotype that may be seen in whole genomic TG. This may be beneficial if late-onset phenotypes were unmasked by eliminating earlier or more severe ones.

SUMMARY

TGs are useful to model some aspects of AIDS CM and other cardiovascular diseases in AIDS. The utility of such approaches is particularly important as combinations of HAART change so that toxic mechanisms and retroviral contributions can be addressed in a scientifically meaningful and clinically relevant way.

ACKNOWLEDGMENTS

Research reported here was supported by NIH NHLBI Grants R01 HL59798 and R01 HL65167.

REFERENCES

1. LEWIS, W. 2000. Cardiomyopathy in AIDS: a pathophysiological perspective. Prog. Cardiovasc. Dis. **43:** 151–170.
2. SPOONER, K.M., H.C.LANE & H. MASUR. 1996. Guide to major clinical trials of antiretroviral therapy administered to patients infected with human immunodeficiency virus. Clin. Infect. Dis. **23:** 15–27.
3. CARPENTER, C.C., M.A. FISCHL, S.M. HAMMER, et al. 1996. Antiretroviral therapy for HIV infection in 1996. Recommendations of an international panel. International AIDS Society-USA. JAMA **276:** 146–154.
4. SMALL, J.A., G.A. SCANGOS, L. CORK, et al. 1986. The early region of human papovavirus JC induces dysmyelination in transgenic mice. Cell **46:** 13–18.
5. HINRICHS, S.H., M. NERENBERG, R.K. REYNOLDS, et al. 1987. A transgenic mouse model for human neurofibromatosis. Science **237:** 1340–1343.
6. GREEN, K.Y. & P.H. DORSETT. 1986. Virus antigens: localization of epitopes involved in hemagglutination and neutralization by using monoclonal antibodies. J. Virol. **57:** 893–898.
7. KIM, C.M., K. KOIKE, I. SAITO, et al. 1991. HBx gene of hepatitis B virus induces liver cancer in transgenic mice. Nature **351:** 317–320.
8. KLOTMAN, P.E. & A.L. NOTKINS. 1996. Transgenic models of human immunodeficiency virus type-1. Curr. Top. Microbiol. Immunol. **206:** 197–222.
9. TINKLE, B.T., H. UEDA & G. JAY. 1995. The pathogenic role of human immunodeficiency virus accessory genes in transgenic mice. Curr. Top. Microbiol. Immunol. **193:** 133–156.
10. ADACHI, A., H.E. GENDELMAN, S. KOENIG, et al. 1986. Production of acquired immunodeficiency syndrome-associated retrovirus in human and nonhuman cells transfected with an infectious molecular clone. J. Virol. **59:** 284–291.
11. LEVY, J.A., C. CHENG-MAYER, D. DINA & P.A. LUCIW. 1986. AIDS retrovirus (ARV-2) clone replicates in transfected human and animal fibroblasts. Science **232:** 998–1001.
12. KHILLAN, J.S., K.C. DEEN, S.H. YU, et al. 1988. Gene transactivation mediated by the TAT gene of human immunodeficiency virus in transgenic mice. Nucleic Acids Res. **16:** 1423–1430.
13. ALONSO, A., D. DERSE & B.M. PETERLIN. 1992. Human chromosome 12 is required for optimal interactions between Tat and TAR of human immunodeficiency virus type 1 in rodent cells. J. Virol. **66:** 4617–4621.
14. IWAKURA, Y., T. SHIODA, M. TOSU, et al. 1992. The induction of cataracts by HIV-1 in transgenic mice. AIDS **6:** 1069–1075.
15. DICKIE, P., J. FELSER, M. ECKHAUS, et al. 1991. HIV-associated nephropathy in transgenic mice expressing HIV-1 genes. Virology **185:** 109–119.

16. KOPP, J.B., J.F. ROONEY, C. WOHLENBERG, *et al.* 1993. Cutaneous disorders and viral gene expression in HIV-1 transgenic mice. AIDS Res. Hum. Retroviruses **9**: 267–275.

17. ADLER, S.H., L.A. BRUGGEMAN, J.B. KOPP, *et al.* 1992. Transcription of HIV-1 genes in transgenic mice is associated with myopathy and myositis. International Conference on AIDS, A48.

18. KOPP, J.B., M.E. KLOTMAN, S.H. ADLER, *et al.* 1992. Progressive glomerulosclerosis and enhanced renal accumulation of basement membrane components in mice transgenic for human immunodeficiency virus type 1 genes. Proc. Natl. Acad. Sci. USA **89**: 1577–1581.

19. LAHDEVIRTA, J., C.P. MAURY, A.M. TEPPO & H. REPO. 1988. Elevated levels of circulating cachectin/tumor necrosis factor in patients with acquired immunodeficiency syndrome. Am. J. Med. **85**: 289–291.

20. LEWIS, W., T. PAPOIAN, B. GONZALEZ, *et al.* 1991. Mitochondrial ultrastructural and molecular changes induced by zidovudine in rat hearts. Lab. Invest. **65**: 228–236.

21. LEWIS, W., B. GONZALEZ, A. CHOMYN & T. PAPOIAN. 1992. Zidovudine induces molecular, biochemical, and ultrastructural changes in rat skeletal muscle mitochondria. J. Clin. Invest. **89**: 1354–1360.

22. LEWIS, W., J.F. SIMPSON & R.R. MEYER. 1994. Cardiac mitochondrial DNA polymerase-gamma is inhibited competitively and noncompetitively by phosphorylated zidovudine. Circ. Res. **74**: 344–348.

23. LEWIS, W., R.R. MEYER, J.F. SIMPSON, *et al.* 1994. Mammalian DNA polymerases alpha, beta, gamma, delta, and epsilon incorporate fialuridine (FIAU) monophosphate into DNA and are inhibited competitively by FIAU Triphosphate. Biochemistry **33**: 14620–14624.

24. LEWIS, W., E.S. LEVINE, B. GRINIUVIENE, *et al.* 1996. Fialuridine and its metabolites inhibit DNA polymerase gamma at sites of multiple adjacent analog incorporation, decrease mtDNA abundance, and cause mitochondrial structural defects in cultured hepatoblasts. Proc. Natl. Acad. Sci. USA **93**: 3592–3597.

25. LEWIS, W., B. GRINIUVIENE, K.O. TANKERSLEY, *et al.* 1997. Depletion of mitochondrial DNA, destruction of mitochondria, and accumulation of lipid droplets result from fialuridine treatment in woodchucks (*Marmota monax*). Lab. Invest. **76**: 77–87.

26. D'AMATI, G. & W. LEWIS. 1994. Zidovudine causes early increases in mitochondrial ribonucleic acid abundance and induces ultrastructural changes in cultured mouse muscle cells. Lab. Invest. **71**: 879–884.

27. LEWIS, W. & M.C. DALAKAS. 1995. Mitochondrial toxicity of antiviral drugs. Nature Med. **1**: 417–422.

28. SWARTZ, M.N. 1995. Mitochondrial toxicity—new adverse drug effects [editorial; comment]. N. Engl. J. Med. **333**: 1099–1105.

29. MOORE, R., J. KERULY & R. CHAISSON. 2000. Differences in Anion Gap with Different Nucleoside RTI Combinations. 7th Conference on Retroviruses and Opportunistic Infections. San Francisco, CA.

30. NG, W.A., I.L. GRUPP, A. SUBRAMANIAM & J. ROBBINS. 1991. Cardiac myosin heavy chain mRNA expression and myocardial function in the mouse heart. Circ. Res. **68**: 1742–1750.

31. PALERMO, J., J. GULICK, M. COLBERT, *et al.* 1996. Transgenic remodeling of the contractile apparatus in the mammalian heart. Circ. Res. **78**: 504–509.

32. VOGEL, J., S.H. HINRICHS, R.K. REYNOLDS, *et al.* 1988. The HIV tat gene induces dermal lesions resembling Kaposi's sarcoma in transgenic mice. Nature **335**: 606–611.

33. RAIDEL, S. & W. LEWIS. 2000, Abstract. HIV-1 Tat Construct targeted to adult cardiac ventricular myocytes alters heart structure and function. 2000 Keystone Symposia. Keystone, CO.

34. VOGEL, J., S.H. HINRICHS, L.A. NAPOLITANO, *et al.* 1991. Liver cancer in transgenic mice carrying the human immunodeficiency virus tat gene. Cancer Res. **51**: 6686–6690.

35. CORALLINI, A., G. ALTAVILLA, L. POZZI, *et al.* 1993. Systemic expression of HIV-1 tat gene in transgenic mice induces endothelial proliferation and tumors of different histotypes. Cancer Res. **53**: 5569–5575.

36. BARBANTI-BRODANO, G., R. SAMPAOLESI, D. CAMPIONI, *et al.* 1994. HIV-1 tat acts as a growth factor and induces angiogenic activity in BK virus/tat transgenic mice. Antibiot. Chemother. **46:** 88–101.
37. ALTAVILLA, G., C. TRABANELLI, M. MERLIN, *et al.* 1999. Morphological, histochemical, immunohistochemical, and ultrastructural characterization of tumors and dysplastic and non-neoplastic lesions arising in BK virus/tat transgenic mice. Am. J. Pathol. **154:** 1231–1244.
38. KUNDU, R.K., F. SANGIORGI, L.Y. WU, *et al.* 1999. Expression of the human immunodeficiency virus-Tat gene in lymphoid tissues of transgenic mice is associated with B-cell lymphoma. Blood **94:** 275–282.
39. PRAKASH, O., S. TENG, M. ALI, *et al.* 1997. The human immunodeficiency virus type 1 Tat protein potentiates zidovudine-induced cellular toxicity in transgenic mice. Arch. Biochem. Biophys. **343:** 173–180.
40. CHOI, J., R.M. LIU, R.K. KUNDU, *et al.* 2000. Molecular mechanism of decreased glutathione content in human immunodeficiency virus type 1 Tat-transgenic mice. J. Biol. Chem. **275:** 3693–3698.
41. MACHO, A., M.A. CALZADO, L. JIMENEZ-REINA, *et al.* 1999. Susceptibility of HIV-1-TAT transfected cells to undergo apoptosis. Biochemical mechanisms. Oncogene **18:** 7543–7551.
42. KRUMAN, I.I., A. NATH & M.P. MATTSON. 1998. HIV-1 protein Tat induces apoptosis of hippocampal neurons by a mechanism involving caspase activation, calcium overload, and oxidative stress. Exp. Neurol. **154:** 276–288.
43. LOCARDI, C., P. PUDDU, M. FERRANTINI, *et al.* 1992. Persistent infection of normal mice with human immunodeficiency virus. J. Virol. **66:** 1649–1654.
44. BOOTH, W. 1988. Of mice, oncogenes, and Rifkin [news]. Science **239:** 341–343.
45. LUSSO, P., P.D. MARKHAM, A. RANKI, *et al.* 1988. Cell-mediated immune response toward viral envelope and core antigens in gibbon apes (*Hylobates lar*) chronically infected with human immunodeficiency virus-1. J. Immunol. **141:** 2467–2473.
46. SPECTOR, D.H., E. WADE, D.A. WRIGHT, *et al.* 1990. Human immunodeficiency virus pseudotypes with expanded cellular and species tropism. J. Virol. **64:** 2298–2308.
47. LINIAL, M. & D. BLAIR. 1982. Genetics of retroviruses. *In* RNA Tumor Viruses: Molecular Biology of Tumor Viruses. R. Weiss, N. Teich, H. Varmus & J. Coffin, Eds.: 649–783. Cold Spring Harbor Laboratory. Cold Spring Harbor, NY.

Pathogenesis of HIV-Associated Cardiomyopathy

GIUSEPPE BARBARO[a] AND STEVEN E. LIPSHULTZ[b,c,d,e]

[a]*Department of Emergency Medicine, University "La Sapienza,"Rome Italy*

[b]*Department of Cardiology, Children's Hospital, Boston, Massachusetts, USA*

[c]*Department of Pediatrics, Harvard Medical School, Division of Pediatric Cardiology Boston, Massachusetts, USA*

[d]*Division of Pediatric Cardiology, University of Rochester Medical Center and Strong Children's Hospital, Rochester, New York, USA*

[e]*Department of Pediatrics, University of Rochester School of Medicine and Dentistry, Rochester, New York, USA*

ABSTRACT: Reviews and studies published before the introduction of highly active antiretroviral therapy (HAART) regimens have tracked the incidence and course of human immunodeficiency virus (HIV) infection in relation to cardiac illness in both children and adults. HAART regimens have significantly modified the course of HIV disease, with longer survival rates and improvement of life quality in HIV+ subjects expected. However, early data raised concerns about HAART's being associated with an increase in both peripheral and coronary arterial diseases. A variety of potential etiologies have been postulated in HIV-related heart disease, including myocardial infection with HIV itself, opportunistic infections, viral infections, autoimmune response to viral infection, drug-related cardiotoxicity, nutritional deficiencies, and prolonged immunosuppression. In this review article we discuss HIV-associated cardiovascular complications, focusing on pathogenetic mechanisms that may play a role in diagnosis, management, and therapy of these complications.

KEYWORDS: HIV; HIV-associated cardiomyopathy; pathogenesis; immunopathogenesis; myocarditis; viral myocardial infection; coxsackievirus; cytomegalovirus; Epstein-Barr virus; adenovirus; autoimmunity; chemokines; cytokines; HIV-associated pulmonary hypertension; nutritional disorders; drug cardiotoxicity; risk groups

The acquired immunodeficiency syndrome (AIDS) represents a unique opportunity to review the vulnerability of the heart to infections and the relation between myocarditis and dilated cardiomyopathy.[1] Several hypotheses have been proposed, although the pathogenesis of the heart muscle disease in AIDS is still unclear and subject of clinical and biological investigations.[2]

Address for correspondence: Giuseppe Barbaro, M.D., Viale Anicio Gallo 63, 00174 Rome, Italy. Voice/fax: +39-6-710-28-89.
g.barbaro@tin.it

PATHOGENESIS AND IMMUNOPATHOGENESIS OF HIV-ASSOCIATED CARDIOMYOPATHY

Myocarditis

The Dallas criteria define myocarditis as "*a process characterized by a lymphocytic infiltrate of the myocardium with necrosis and/or degeneration of adjacent myocytes not typical of the ischemic damage associated with coronary artery disease*"[3] (see FIGURES 1 and 2).

Myocarditis is documented at autopsy in 40% to 52% of patients who died of AIDS.[4-6] In more than 80% of these patients no specific etiologic factor is found for myocarditis. The remaining cases may be attributable to opportunistic pathogens such as *Toxoplasma gondii, Cryptococcus neoformans,* herpes simplex virus type 2, *Mycobacterium tuberculosis,* and *Mycobacterium avium intracellulare.*[6]

In the Gruppo Italiano per lo Studio Cardiologico dei pazienti affetti da AIDS (GISCA) series, a histologic diagnosis of myocarditis was made in 63 of the 76 patients with dilated cardiomyopathy who underwent endomyocardial biopsy.[7] Histologic diagnosis of myocarditis was made in 30 of 82 autopsy patients (37%) with cardiac involvement. Coxsackievirus B3 was identified in 10 of the 30 patients (8 with active and 2 with borderline myocarditis), Epstein-Barr virus in 7 (6 with active and 1 with borderline myocarditis), *Toxoplasma gondii* in 2 (both with borderline myocarditis), and *Mycobacterium avium intracellulare* in 1 patient with borderline myocarditis.[5] Of 12 autopsy patients with dilated cardiomyopathy, 10 (83%) had

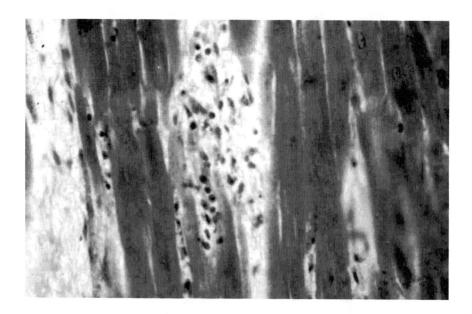

FIGURE 1. Myocarditis in an HIV+ patient with dilated cardiomyopathy (endomyocardial biopsy). Note the lymphocyte infiltrate with necrosis of adjacent myocytes (hematoxylin-eosin; magnification ×400).

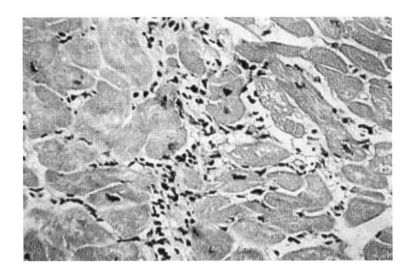

FIGURE 2. Lymphocytic myocarditis with interstitial inflammatory infiltrates and focal myocyte necrosis (hematoxylin-eosin; magnification ×40) (Courtesy of Dr. G. D'Amati, Department of Experimental Medicine and Pathology, University of Rome "La Sapienza").

active myocarditis at histological examination. Among them coxsackievirus B3 was identified in three of the patients, cytomegalovirus in two, and Epstein-Barr in one. The other two patients had extensive areas of interstitial and perivascular fibrosis, particularly involving the left ventricular subendocardium without inflammatory cell infiltrates. In one patient with dilated cardiomyopathy, active myocarditis was associated with a dense lymphocytic inflammatory infiltrate within the endocardium (lymphocytic endomyocarditis).

Viral Myocardial Infection and Autoimmunity

HIV can be detected in cardiac tissue by cell culture, Southern blot, or *in situ* hybridization.[5,7–11] Grody *et al.* detected HIV nucleic acid sequences in cardiac tissue sections from 27% of patients who died of AIDS.[9] Herskowitz *et al.* detected a positive hybridization signal for HIV-1 in endomyocardial biopsy specimens from 15 of 37 patients with left ventricular dysfunction. Histologic and immunohistologic techniques documented that most of these patients had myocarditis.[10]

HIV nucleic acid sequences were detected at autopsy by *in situ* DNA hybridization in 35% of the GISCA patients with cardiac involvement; 86% of them had active myocarditis at histological examination. Among patients with myocarditis, coinfection with coxsackievirus B3 was documented in 32%, with Epstein-Barr virus in 8%, and with cytomegalovirus (see FIGURES 3 and 4) in 4%.[5] Of the patients with dilated cardiomyopathy who underwent endomyocardial biopsy, a positive hybridization signal was detected in 76%; 62% of them had active myocarditis at histological examination. Coinfection with coxsackievirus B3, cytomegalovirus, or Epstein-Barr

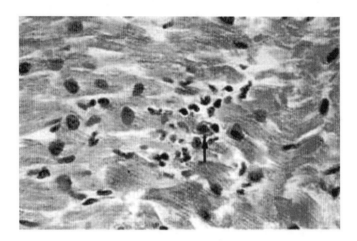

FIGURE 3. Cytomegalovirus myocarditis in HIV-infected patients with a typical viral inclusion (*arrow*) surrounded by scarce inflammatory infiltrate (hematoxylin-eosin; ×40) (Courtesy of Dr. G. D'Amati, Department of Experimental Medicine and Pathology, University of Rome "La Sapienza").

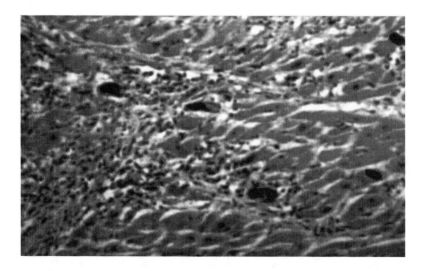

FIGURE 4. *In situ* hybridization of a cytomegalovirus (CMV)-specific probe in a section of autopsy myocardial tissue from a patient with dilated cardiomyopathy and HIV-1/CMV myocarditis. The intensely stained myocytes appear swollen and surrounded by inflammatory cells (hematoxylin-eosin; magnification ×20).

virus was documented in 17%, 6%, and 3% of them, respectively.[7] In both autopsy and endomyocardial biopsy samples, myocytes with a positive hybridization signal were sparse, usually only 1 to 4 cells per section (see FIGURE 5).[5,7]

Although about 70% of patients with positive hybridization signals had active myocarditis at histological examination, most myocytes with positive hybridization signal were not surrounded by inflammatory cells.[5,7] This finding is in agreement with results reported by Grody et al.[9] and by Bowles et al.[11,12]

In the GISCA autopsy subjects, HIV was documented by in situ hybridization in 83% of patients with myocarditis and in 62% of patients with dilated cardiomyopathy who underwent endomyocardial biopsy.[5,13] However, no hybridization signal was detected in the remaining 17% of autopsy patients with myocarditis. In 17% of autopsy patients with dilated cardiomyopathy, myocarditis was not documented during histologic examination.[5] Similarly, in 38% of the patients with myocarditis at histological examination, the in situ hybridization test was negative for HIV and for cardiotropic viruses, and in 18% of the cases, myocarditis was not documented at histological examination of endomyocardial biopsy specimens.[13]

It is possible that the HIV nucleic acid sequences documented by in situ hybridization are not within the lymphocytes infiltrating the myocardium, but within the myocardial cells themselves. However, it is unclear how the virus would enter CD4-receptor-negative cells such as myocytes.[2,14] It is possible that myocardial dendritic cells play a key role in the interaction between HIV and the myocyte and in the activation of cytotoxic cytokines.[13]

Coinfection with other viruses seems to have an important pathogenic role. The GISCA autopsy records show that 83% of patients with myocarditis and 50% of

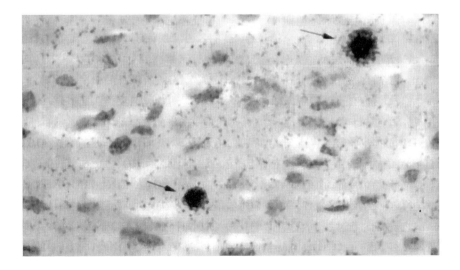

FIGURE 5. In situ hybridization of an HIV-1 RNA probe in a section of myocardial tissue obtained by endomyocardial biopsy from a patient with dilated cardiomyopathy. The 2 intensely stained myocytes (black arrows) are not surrounded by inflammatory cells (hematoxylin-eosin; ×350).

those with dilated cardiomyopathy were coinfected with cardiotropic viruses (usually coxsackievirus B3 and cytomegalovirus).[5,7] Among the patients with an echocardiographic diagnosis of dilated cardiomyopathy, a histologic diagnosis of myocarditis, and myocardial HIV-1 confirmed by *in situ* hybridization, 20% were coinfected with coxsackievirus B3, 7% with cytomegalovirus, and 5% with Epstein-Barr virus.[13]

Herskowitz *et al.* used *in situ* hybridization to detect myocardial cytomegalovirus infection in 48% of HIV-positive patients with left ventricular dysfunction who underwent endomyocardial biopsy.[10] Bowles *et al.* used polymerase chain reaction (PCR) and found that 42% of HIV-positive patients with cardiomyopathy had cytomegalovirus or adenovirus in the myocardial tissue.[11,12] Some patients with adenovirus coinfection had congestive heart failure but not myocarditis, suggesting that the virus may be virulent without associated inflammatory response.[11,12]

We may theorize that cardiac disease is related either to direct action of HIV on the myocardial tissue or to an autoimmune process induced by HIV, possibly in association with other cardiotropic viruses (particularly, coxsackievirus B3 and cytomegalovirus).[5,7] Additional pathogenic factors may include apoptosis and other adverse effects induced by viral proteins and the virus-induced transcriptional activation of various cellular genes.[2,14]

As HIV disease progresses, immunodeficiency may enhance the pathogenic action of both HIV and cardiotropic viruses and influence the clinical evolution of

TABLE 1. Immunopathological findings in patients with a histological diagnosis of myocarditis[13]

Lymphocytes or membrane antigens	n (%)	
	HIV-associated cardiomyopathy (n = 67)	Idiopathic dilated cardiomyopathy (n = 18)
T lymphocytes		
CD2 (OKT11)	22 (33)	7 (39)
CD3 (OKT3)	38 (57)	7 (39)
CD4 (OKT4)	5 (8)	15 (83)*
CD8 (OKT8)	57 (85)	6 (33)*
CD25 (IL2-R)	2 (3)	9 (50)*
B lymphocytes (MB1)	2 (3)	12 (67)*
NK cells, CD16 (Leu1 1B)	2 (3)	8 (44)*
Monocytes, CD11B (OKM1)	2 (3)	7 (39)*
CD57 (Leu7)	25 (37)	12 (67)
Increased MHC class I staining	47 (70)	12 (67)
Increased MHC class II staining	20 (30)	6 (33)

IL2-R: interleukin 2-receptor. NK: natural killer. MHC: major histocompatibility complex.
*$p < 0.001$ for the comparison with patients with HIV-associated cardiomyopathy.

cardiomyopathy. In fact, both cell-mediated and humoral immunity have been postulated to have an important pathogenic role in the development and progression of the viral cardiomyopathic process itself.[1]

TABLE 1 lists the immunopathologic findings in a group of patients with an echocardiographic diagnosis of dilated cardiomyopathy and a histological diagnosis of myocarditis. Compared to patients with idiopathic dilated cardiomyopathy who have predominantly CD4 and B lymphocytes, the inflammatory-cell infiltrates in HIV$^+$ patients were predominantly CD3 and CD8 lymphocytes, possibly reflecting the number of circulating lymphocytes in these patients in relation to the state of immunodeficiency. In about 70% of both HIV-associated and idiopathic dilated cardiomyopathy patients, increased staining was limited to major histocompatibility complex (MHC) class I molecules.[13]

These immunopathologic findings are in agreement with those reported either by Beschorner et al.[15] in the immunopathogical examination of endomyocardial biopsy specimens from 9 of 18 HIV-positive patients with active myocarditis and by Barbaro et al. in the examination of myocardial specimens from 30 HIV-positive autopsy patients with a histological diagnosis of lymphocytic myocarditis.[5]

The combination of viral hybridization and increased myocardial expression of MHC class I strongly suggests an active immune process in the myocardium.[5,7] Findings above are in agreement with those reported by Herskowitz et al. in the immunohistological examination of endomyocardial biopsy samples from AIDS patients with severe left ventricular dysfunction.[10] In a previous study, the same authors used indirect immunofluorescence and detected IgG anti-myosin antibodies in four of six AIDS patients with cardiomyopathy. These antibodies were not detected in HIV-positive patients without cardiomyopathy.[16] Similar findings have been reported also by Currie et al., who measured the frequency of circulating cardiac-specific autoantibodies (anti-alpha myosin autoantibodies) in HIV$^+$ patients.[17] They reported that HIV$^+$ patients were more likely to have specific cardiac autoantibodies than were controls (15% vs. 3.5%). Those with echocardiographic evidence of left ventricular dysfunction were particularly likely to have cardiac autoantibodies (43%), supporting the theory that cardiac autoimmunity plays a role in the pathogenesis of HIV-related heart disease and suggesting that cardiac autoantibodies may be markers of left ventricular dysfunction in HIV-positive patients with previously normal echocardiographic findings.[17]

Superantigens play an important role in the pathogenesis of many diseases by forming a trimolecular complex with MHC class II molecules on the antigen-presenting cells and the *Vb*-specific region on the T lymphocyte receptor.[18] The binding results in a massive stimulation of T lymphocytes. In HIV infection, the HIV regulatory protein (*Nef*) binds with MHC class II on antigen-presenting cells, and the T lymphocytes become activated. This stimulates the release of cytokines, such as tumor necrosis factor (TNF)-α, interferon-γ, and interleukin (IL)-2. Proliferation of B cells may result in hypergammaglobulinemia. An autoimmune response may occur as a result of B cell differentiation into immunoglobulin-secreting cells and the activation of T lymphocytes.[6,18]

Chemokines

HIV-1 entry into target cells and HIV-1 disease progression have recently been shown to depend upon chemokines which inhibit HIV-1 entry into cells and chemokine receptors which permit HIV-1 entry into cells, as regulated by genes and gene promoters.[19, 20] Binding of HIV to the macrophage or CD4+ T-cell lymphocyte takes place through cognate binding of the HIV glycoprotein 120 to 2 receptors: the CD4 molecule and a chemokine receptor.[20]

Evidence is accumulating that the macrophage/monocyte is the first cell to be infected by HIV by the binding of the virion gp 120 to the CCR5 chemokine receptor.[20] Certain chemokines can prevent HIV infection *in vitro.* The β-chemokines (MIP-1α, MIP-1β, RANTES) and the α-chemokine (SDF-1α) bind to chemokine receptors CCR5 and CXCR4 and competitively inhibit the binding of HIV glycoprotein 120 to the respective chemokine receptor.[20]

A role for chemokine receptors in HIV infection has been demonstrated by a mutant CCR5 receptor that is unable to properly bind to the HIV virion glycoprotein 120 *in vitro,* either preventing HIV infection (double allele) or slowing the progress of infection (single allele). Other chemokine receptors, mutant chemokine receptors, and a mutant chemokine itself have been shown to alter HIV-1 infection and disease progression.[21] An allelic variant of a chemokine receptor (CCR2) leads to slow HIV disease progression in animal models; this variant may be linked to the CCR5 promoter.[20] It is possible that chemokine expression is down-regulated and chemokine receptor expression is up-regulated allowing more HIV entry into cardiac myocytes in rapidly progressing infants and children with HIV infection. Further study is needed to elucidate these mechanisms.

Cytokines

Cytokines are regulatory proteins that rarely have constitutive production and act by autocrine, paracrine, and endocrine mechanisms at the cellular level to orchestrate the tissue response to a stimulus.[22] Cytokines have been shown to have key roles in the pathogenesis of congestive heart failure in general populations. Complex interactions suggest that profound disturbances exist in patients with chronic congestive heart failure where inflammatory cytokines are markedly elevated (TNF-α, IL-6, glycoprotein 130, soluble TNF receptors, soluble IL-6 receptor, enhanced IL-6 bioactivity in serum). Anti-inflammatory cytokine levels of IL-10 and transforming growth factor beta 1 were reduced. IL-10 was found to elevate insufficiently in response to elevated TNF-α. Markers of inflammation such as erythrocyte sedimentation rate, and TNF-α have been shown to correlate with prognosis and with similar markers.[22]

Tinkle *et al.* recently reported that cytokines play a role in the development of cardiomyopathy.[23] In this study, transgenic mice bearing a portion of the genome of a proviral, non-infectious HIV developed ventricular dysfunction and, in some cases, myocarditis, arteritis, and vasculitis. PCR detected no HIV, suggesting that the cardiac abnormalities were due to circulating factors or cytokines.[23]

In HIV disease, dendritic cells can initiate the primary immunologic response and present the antigen to T-lymphocytes. The interaction between dendritic cells and T lymphocytes, particularly CD8 cells, could promote a local elevation in the multifunctional cytokine TNF-α, which can also be produced and secreted by infected macrophages.[19] TNF-α produces a negative inotropic effect by altering intracellular calcium homeostasis, possibly by inducing nitric oxide (NO) synthesis, which also reduces myocyte contractility.[24,25]

NO, synthesized from L-arginine by three NO synthase enzymes, is a biological mediator with multiple actions.[26] Two of the NO enzymes are constitutive in neuronal and endothelial cells, respectively; the third form is inducible in many cells by endotoxin and cytokines, such as IL-1, interferon-γ and TNF-α.[26] The plasma concentration of acid-labile nitroso compounds (the end-products of NO metabolism) is correlated with the TNF-α level, suggesting that there may be a relationship between TNF-α and the inducible form of NO synthase (iNOS).[27]

Lowenstein et al. demonstrated that iNOS is induced in mice infected with coxsackievirus B3[28,29] and that NO inhibits coxsackievirus B3 replication by inactivating the virus's protease 3C.[29] Therefore, in murine myocarditis, iNOS is crucial for the host response to coxsackievirus B3.[30] However, when iNOS is chronically activated by cytokines in ventricular myocytes, their contractile function is altered[31] and they are less responsive to β-adrenergic agonists.[32]

The elevated levels of iNOS observed in patients with both HIV-associated cardiomyopathy and idiopathic dilated cardiomyopathy coincide with an abundant local source of TNF-α that is not present in controls.[13] The source is predominantly vascular, although the cytokine was also found in cardiac myocytes (see FIGURE 6).[13,33] Thus, it is possible that TNF-α diffuses from vessels to stimulate the myocytes or that both paracrine stimulation and intracellular stimulation by TNF-α occurs.

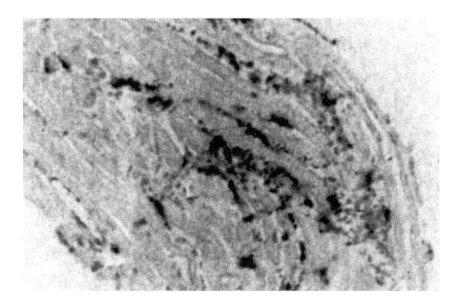

FIGURE 6. Endomyocardial biopsy specimen from an HIV-positive patient with dilated cardiomyopathy, showing strong immunostaining (optical density, 1.3 units) for iNOS in cardiac myocytes (avidin-biotin complex method; ×100).

TNF-α may also be affecting the vessels themselves.[33] Vascular production of NO could lead to vasodilation but, conversely, TNF-α could also be down-regulating the isoform of iNOS in the endothelium, since TNF-α reduces the stability of endothelial NOS-RNA.[34]

Compared to patients with idiopathic dilated cardiomyopathy, a greater intensity of both TNF-α and iNOS staining has been reported in patients with HIV-associated cardiomyopathy, specifically in those with a myocardial viral infection[13] (see FIGURE 7). Interestingly, among patients with HIV-associated cardiomyopathy, those with coinfection from coxsackievirus B3, cytomegalovirus, or other viruses have samples that stain more intensely for both TNF-α and iNOS. Moreover, patients coinfected with HIV and coxackievirus B3 have specimens that stain more intensely for iNOS than do patients with idiopathic dilated cardiomyopathy and myocardial infection with coxackievirus B3 or adenovirus alone.[13]

The intensity of both TNF-α and iNOS staining was inversely correlated to CD4 count and was not influenced by antiretroviral treatment, since it was similar among patients with equal CD4 counts who received different antiretroviral treatments.[13] Moreover, in both patients with HIV-associated cardiomyopathy and those with idiopathic dilated cardiomyopathy, the intensity of TNF-α and iNOS staining was inversely correlated with ejection fraction and with left ventricular end-diastolic volume index assessed by echocardiography. Other variables, such as age and duration of documented cardiomyopathy, did not correlate significantly with the intensity of TNF-α and iNOS staining or with echocardiographic functional findings.[13]

Considering these results, it seems possible that more severe immunodeficiency may favor the selection of more pathogenic viral variants or enhance the cardio-virulence of viral strains. In the GISCA records, mortality from congestive heart failure was higher in patients with HIV-associated cardiomyopathy (median survival, 11 months) than in those with idiopathic dilated cardiomyopathy (19 months; hazard ratio, 2.27 [95% confidence interval:1.15 to 4.41]).[13] In the patients with

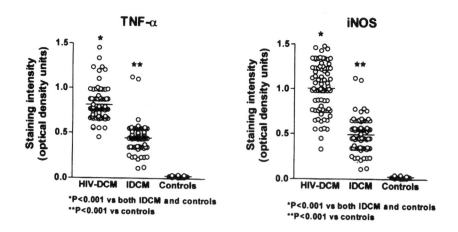

FIGURE 7. Mean optical density of staining of TNF-α and iNOS in patients with HIV-associated cardiomyopathy (HIV-DCM), with idiopatic dilated cardiomyopathy (IDCM) and controls. *Horizontal bars* represent mean values.

HIV-associated dilated cardiomyopathy, the survival rate was significantly lower in patients with more intense iNOS staining: those whose samples stained more than one optical density unit had a hazard ratio of mortality of 2.57 (95% confidence interval: 1.11 to 5.43). Survival in patients with less intense staining was not significantly different from survival in patients with idiopathic dilated cardiomyopathy.[13]

All patients with HIV-associated cardiomyopathy and with samples that stained stained more than 1 optical density unit had myocardial infection with coxsackievirus B3 or cytomegalovirus. Patients with idiopathic dilated cardiomyopathy and with myocardial coxsackievirus B3 or adenovirus alone had samples that stained less deeply than 1 optical density unit. Therefore, a value of 1 optical density unit may be useful as a cut-off value in patients with HIV-associated dilated cardiomyopathy.[13] In HIV-associated cardiomyopathy, the HIV myocardial infection, the interaction between HIV and cardiotropic viruses, and the immunodeficiency may all enhance the inflammatory response and increase both the expression and the cytotoxic activity of specific cytokines, such as TNF-α and iNOS.[31]

Relationship between Cardiomyopathy and Encephalopathy

Studies of HIV[+] children show that HIV-associated encephalopathy is associated with dilated cardiomyopathy.[35] In the multicenter Pulmonary and Cardiac Complications of HIV (P^2C^2 HIV) study, HIV[+] children who developed encephalopathy during follow-up had lower baseline fractional shortening; fractional shortening continued to decline during 2–3 years of follow-up, correlating with overall survival.[36] In the Women and Infants Transmission Study, dilated cardiomyopathy was present in 30% of the children with encephalopathy and in 2% of those without encephalopathy.[37]

In a trial performed by GISCA on a selected population of HIV-positive adults with dilated cardiomyopathy, the echocardiographic functional parameters were more abnormal in patients with encephalopathy at enrollment and worsened during the follow-up period. These patients were more likely to die of congestive heart failure than were patients without encephalopathy.[38]

Cardiac and central nervous system disease in HIV infection may each have multiple causes.[36,37] Neuronal loss may represent the result of a highly productive infection with intense macrophage activation. Both inflammatory mediators and HIV viral proteins may serve as neurotoxins, eventually causing neuronal death by apoptosis rather than cellular necrosis.[37]

Some manifestations of HIV-associated cardiomyopathy and encephalopathy may be the direct effect of HIV on the central nervous system and on the myocardial tissue. In the GISCA trial, 79% of patients with encephalopathy who died of congestive heart failure had HIV nucleic acid sequences within the multinucleated giant cells of cerebral cortex, whereas no hybridization signals were detected in autopsy cerebral tissue of patients without encephalopathy (see FIGURE 8). Moreover, 82% of the patients with encephalopathy had positive hybridization signals within myocardial cells compared to 70% of the patients without encephalopathy.[38]

However, other clinical manifestations should be attributed to immune mediators. Immunologic factors and cytokines, which have cardiotoxic and neurotoxic action, may play an important role in the development and progression of dilated cardiomyopathy and encephalopathy as well.[14,37] Proinflammatory cytokines activate iNOS,

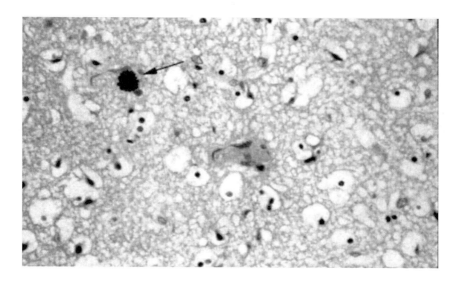

FIGURE 8. *In situ* hybridization of an HIV-1 RNA probe in a section of autopsy cerebral tissue in a patients with dilated cardiomyopathy showing an intense staining within a multinucleated giant cell (*arrow*). Note also the extensive area of demyelination along with another multinucleated giant cell with overlapping nuclei (hematoxylin-eosin; ×400).

thus stimulating production of NO, a sequence of events that may be contribute to the relationship between dilated cardiomyopathy and encephalopathy in HIV disease.[38]

The neurotoxic effects of *gp120* viral protein and *tat* seem to be mediated by cytokines such as TNF-α, IL-6, and endothelin-1.[39,40] These diffusible factors are released by activated or infected microglia and astrocytes, and the cytokines can produce NO in human brain culture by activating iNOS.[40,41] Activated oligodendrocytes produce NO by activating a gene encoding iNOS.[42] Furthermore, the activation of TNF-receptor 1 or Fas may induce myocyte apoptosis.[43] It is possible also that TNF-α-Fas-mediated cytotoxicity induces the release of mitochondrial pro-apoptotic factors, such as cytochrome C and apoptosis-inducing factor.[38]

In the GISCA study, the intensity of both TNF-α and iNOS immunostaining was greater in patients with encephalopathy and was inversely correlated to CD4 count, to HIV-1 viral load, to Folstein's mini mental status score, and to echocardiographic functional findings.[38] The overall mortality rate from congestive heart failure was 73% in patients with encephalopathy and 12% in patients without encephalopathy (hazard ratio, 3.39; 95% confidence interval: 1.68 to 6.73)[38] (see FIGURE 9). This observation could suggest that in HIV-associated cardiomyopathy and encephalopathy, the TNF-α activation of iNOS plays a significant pathogenic role. It may also suggest that immunodeficiency favors cellular damage by enhancing the inflammatory process induced by this cytokine.[41] Similar roles may also be played by other cytokines, such as IL-1, IL-6, endothelin-1, or IL-10.[39,40]

HIV-1 persists in reservoir cells in the myocardium and the cerebral cortex even after antiretroviral treatment, and these cells seem to play an important role in the

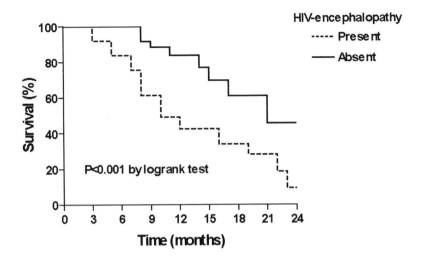

FIGURE 9. Kaplan-Meier curves comparing the survival rate during follow-up in patients with HIV-associated cardiomyopathy with and without encephalopathy.

development and progression of cardiomyopathy and encephalopathy.[44] The reservoir cells may hold HIV-1 on their surfaces for long periods and cause progressive tissue damage by chronic release of cytotoxic cytokines.[44]

FIGURE 10 portrays the possible mechanisms involved in the development of HIV-associated cardiomyopathy and encephalopathy. These mechanisms are speculative but may warrant further controlled clinical and experimental investigations.

HIV-associated Pulmonary Hypertension and Right Ventricular Dysfunction

The incidence of HIV-associated pulmonary hypertension is estimated to be 1/200, much higher than 1/200,000 found in the general population.[6] Primary pulmonary hypertension is estimated to occur in about 0.5% of hospitalized AIDS patients and is cause of severe cardiac impairment with cor pulmonale and death.[6,45,46] It has been reported in HIV+ patients without a history of thromboembolic disease, intravenous drug use, or pulmonary infections associated with HIV. The pathogenesis is multifactorial and poorly understood. HIV may cause endothelial damage and mediator-related vasoconstriction through stimulation by the envelope glycoprotein 120, including direct release and effects of endothelin-1 (vasoconstrictor), IL-6 and TNF-α, in the pulmonary arteries.[47] HIV is frequently identified in alveolar macrophages on histology.[6,48] These macrophages release TNF-α, oxide anions, and proteolytic enzymes in response to infection. Lymphokines may have a role in the etiology of endothelial proliferation seen in pulmonary hypertension by promoting leukocyte adhesion to the endothelium.[6] Activation of α1-receptors and genetic factors (increased frequency of HLA DR6 and DR52) have been also hypothesized in the pathogenesis of HIV-associated pulmonary hypertension.[6,46]

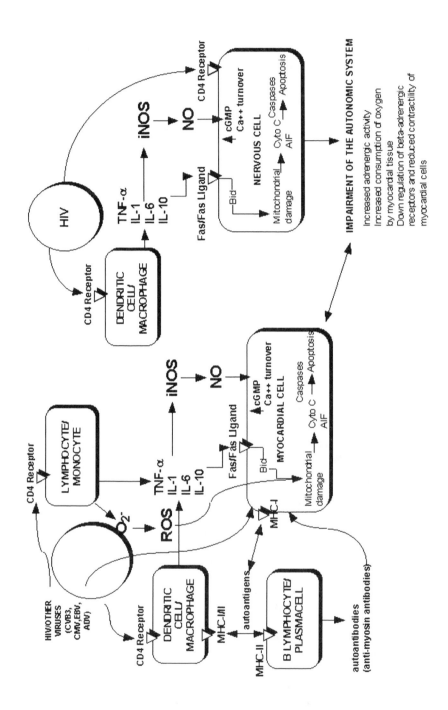

FACTORS INFLUENCING THE PREVALENCE OF
CARDIAC LESIONS IN AIDS

Nutritional Disorders

Micronutrient deficiencies are common in HIV[+] patients.[49] In particular, deficiencies of selenium, carnitine, and thiamine can impair ventricular function.[14,50,51]

Selenium, as a component of glutathione peroxidase, is involved in the antioxidant response in cells and tissues. Selenium deficiency is associated with congestive cardiomyopathy and skeletal-muscle disorders. Furthermore, low levels of selenium or other micronutients may be responsible for the cardiotoxic effects of coxsackievirus group B and for the ability of these viruses to enhance the toxic effects of zidovudine on skeletal muscle; both findings may be relevant to selenium-related ventricular dysfunction.[51–53]

The role of selenium deficiency in HIV-associated dilated cardiomyopathy is controversial, because most patients with HIV-associated cardiomyopathy do not have micronutrient deficiencies.[49] Moreover, studies in selenium-deficient mice have not found a relationship between selenium deficiency and cardiomyopathy.[52] However, selenium deficiency is common in HIV[+] children and is correlated with body weight, albumin levels, and CD4 count.[51,53]

In one study of 19 HIV[+] children, selenium levels and ventricular function were correlated, but the relationship was not statistically significant.[51] The same authors prospectively measured serum micronutrient levels in 64 HIV[+] children and 26 control children as part of a large study of nutrition and AIDS (the Nutrition for Healthy Living Study).[50] Preliminary data show that children with HIV infection have adequate intake of all major macronutrients and micronutrients, with the exception of zinc, vitamin E, and vitamin D. However, the HIV[+] and control groups consumed different amounts of riboflavin, vitamin D, vitamin K, calcium, folate, niacin, and thiamine, regardless of nutritional status.[50]

Chariot et al. measured selenium and vitamin E levels in eight HIV[+] patients with an echocardiographic diagnosis of dilated cardiomyopathy, and compared the results

---

FIGURE 10. The possible pathogenic mechanisms involved in the development of HIV-associated cardiomyopathy and encephalopathy and in their relationship. The infection of dendritic cells, of CD4 lymphocytes, and of myocardial or neuronal cell by HIV-1 or by other viruses may be responsible for release of specific cytokines (TNF-α, IL-1, IL-6, IL-10) which activate the inducible form of nitric oxide synthase (iNOS). The interaction between cytotoxic T lymphocytes and the receptoral complex Fas/Fas ligand located on the surface of the target cell may cause mitochondrial damage with release of mitochondrial pro-apoptosis factors (cytochome c, AIF). Similar mitochondrial damage may be caused by reactive oxygen species (ROS) released by activated lympho-monocytes. The interaction between autoantigens and major histocompatibility complex (MHC) molecules on the surface of dendritic cells/macrophages, of myocardial cells (MHC-I), and of B lymphocytes (MHC-II) determine the production of autoantibodies (e.g., α-antimyosin) which are responsible for direct cellular damage. The neuronal damage, specifically the impairment of the autonomic system, may enhance the functional damage to myocardial cells because of increased adrenergic activity and down-regulation of β-adrenergic receptors. CVB3: coxsackievirus B3. CMV: cytomegalovirus. EBV: Epstein-Barr virus. ADV: adenovirus. Bid: a protein of the BCL2 family involved in apoptosis.

to those from 8 HIV$^+$ patients with normal echocardiographic findings who were matched by gender, age, Karnofsky Performance Score, and CD4 count.[54] Antioxidant deficiency was more frequent in the subjects with dilated cardiomyopathy than in the matched controls. Two of the three patients with selenium deficiency showed clinical and echocardiographic improvement after three months of selenium supplementation (200 μg per day).[54] Generalizability is, however, limited by the small sample size.

Selenium deficiency may be involved in the increased production of free radicals in HIV disease.[55] In a clinical trial, asymptomatic HIV-positive subjects had impairments of the cardiac vagal system (assessed by corrected coefficients of variation of electrocardiographic R-R intervals)^f that were correlated significantly with lipoperoxidation markers.[55] The impairment of the autonomic nervous system may contribute in the progression of HIV-associated cardiomyopathy, and an increased lipoperoxidation rate may be involved in this impairment. However, the role of selenium deficiency in this lipoperoxidation process is still to be determined.

All of these data suggest that HIV-positive patients, particularly children, may be at risk for micronutrient deficiencies independent of nutritional status, which may affect organs such as the heart.[50,51,53] Therefore, when HIV$^+$ children and adults are evaluated for ventricular dysfunction, micronutrient status should be assessed because a deficiency is treatable.[51,53] However, controlled prospective studies are needed to better assess the importance of micronutrients.[4,6]

Drugs

An association between zidovudine and dilated cardiomyopathy has been reported in both adult and pediatric patients.[56,57] One study suggests that zidovudine is associated with diffuse destruction of cardiac mitochondrial ultrastructures and inhibition of mitochondrial DNA replication.[58] However, in a study of selected HIV$^+$ children, zidovudine neither worsened nor ameliorated cardiac function in patients with cardiomyopathy.[59] Infants born to HIV-positive mothers were followed from birth to age 5 years with serial echocardiographic studies every 4–6 months. No association with acute or chronic abnormalities in left ventricular structure or function was found with perinatal exposure to zidovudine.[60]

Other antiretroviral drugs, such as didanosine and zalcitabine, do not seem either to promote or to prevent dilated cardiomyopathy.[7] More recently, highly active antiretroviral therapy (HAART) regimens, which combine two nucleoside-transcriptase inhibitors and one protease inhibitor (PI), have been associated with an increased risk of cardiovascular complications.[6,61] Complications such as lipodystrophy, insulin resistance, high levels of low-density lipoprotein, and high triglyceride levels develop in up to 60% of patients treated with HAART regimens. In up to 10% to 20% of patients, these complications may be severe (unstable angina, acute myocardial

---

^{f}As heart rate and aging are major factors affecting R-R interval variations, the coefficient of variation (CV), to correct for heart rate, and the correct CV (CVc) were used in the analysis, in which:

CV = standard deviation R-R interval/mean R-R interval × 100;

CVc = CV/(−0.066) × age + 6.480.

The CVc value is a useful mean of interpreting the results without the need for age-matched controls.

infarction, stroke).[62–66] The metabolic alterations induced by PI may enhance the pathogenic action of pre-existing cardiovascular risk factors with an increase of acute coronary syndromes, even in young individuals, generally related to the duration of PI treatment and the type of PI used[62–66] (see FIGURE 11). A better understanding of PI effects on lipid and metabolic pathways will lead to a new generation of drug therapies without metabolic alterations. This understanding may also lead to new therapies for dyslipidemias and alterations of metabolism unrelated to HIV infection.

In AIDS patients with Kaposi's sarcoma, reversible cardiac dysfunction was associated with prolonged, high-dose therapy with interferon-α.[6,67] High-dose interferon-α treatment is not associated with myocardial dysfunction in other patient populations, so it has been proposed that it may have a synergistic effect with HIV infection.[68]

Doxorubicin (adriamycin) used to treat AIDS-related Kaposi's sarcoma and non-Hodgkin's lymphoma has a dose-related effect on dilated cardiomyopathy,[69] as does foscarnet sodium when used to treat cytomegalovirus disease.[70] The prevalence of hypertension associated with erythropoietin therapy is 47%; the effect may be related to the increase in hematocrit and blood viscosity.[71]

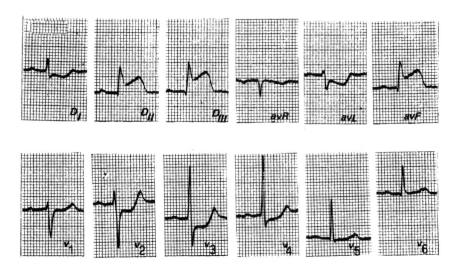

FIGURE 11. Inferior acute myocardial infarction in a 37-year-old HIV+ homosexual male who was receiving therapy with protease inhibitor (saquinavir) for three years [electrocardiographic recording performed at admission of the patient to Emergency Room (ER) two hours after the onset of acute chest pain]. He was a heavy smoker (40 cigarettes per day) and had a family history of hypertension. Treatment with saquinavir was associated with a 35% increase of total serum cholesterol along with a 20% reduction of HDL cholesterol. He was successfully treated in ER with i.v. rTPA and heparin and discharged 9 days after admission with enalapril, aspirin and pravastatin. Treatment with protease inhibitors was stopped and the patient continued antiretroviral treatment with non-nucleoside transcriptase inhibitors.

Cardiac arrhythmias [ventricular tachycardia or ventricular fibrillation, torsade de pointes (related to prolongation of electrocardiographic QT interval), atrioventricular conduction abnormalities] have been described with the administration of amphotericin B,[72] ganciclovir,[73] trimethoprim-sulfamethoxazole,[74] and pentamidine.[14] The principal actions/interactions of common HIV therapies are reported in TABLE 2.

Risk Groups

Infective endocarditis is more frequent in users of intravenous drugs (especially heroin). There is conflicting data about whether intravenous drug abuse is a risk factor for myocarditis or myocardial dysfunction among patients with AIDS.[49] The GISCA autopsy records showed no significant differences between drug addicts, homosexuals, and heterosexuals in the prevalence of dilated cardiomyopathy. However, intravenous drug users were more likely to have involvement of the right ventricle with secondary pulmonary hypertension related either to pulmonary infections or pulmonary microemboli.[5] Cocaine abuse has been associated with myocarditis and dilated cardiomyopathy in HIV-negative cocaine users, possibly because of intermittent microvascular spasms resulting from catecholamine surges.[75]

Homosexual HIV patients are more likely to have cardiac Kaposi's sarcoma and non-Hodgkin's lymphoma than are heterosexuals.[49] In the GISCA series, 2 of 3 homosexual patients with Kaposi's sarcoma had myocardial Kaposi's sarcoma lesions. Furthermore, 1 homosexual patient had cardiac B-cell immunoblastic lymphoma.[5] In a review of 21 cases, Duong et al. observed that all patients with HIV-associated non-Hodgkin's lymphoma of the heart were homosexuals.[76] The higher prevalence of cardiac lesions in homosexual patients may be related to their higher risk for human herpes virus 8 and Epstein-Barr virus infection, both of which have been associated with the development of Kaposi's sarcoma and with lymphoproliferative processes in AIDS.[49]

CONCLUSIONS

The increasing prevalence of HIV-associated cardiomyopathy strongly suggests that HIV-positive subjects should be given careful cardiologic evaluations early in the course of disease.[1] Early screening will detect cardiac abnormalities, and treatment based on these findings may be helpful. Serial echocardiographic screening non-invasively and accurately aids diagnosis during any change in clinical status and directs therapy. Patients will usually respond to early therapy for left ventricular dysfunction and increased left ventricular mass. Treatment based on these findings may prolong the quality and duration of life, and direct further patient evaluation.

The role of the cardiologist in the evaluation and treatment of patients with HIV infection should therefore be expanded to include asymptomatic patients for serial echocardiographic evaluation, and patients who are being evaluated for or who are receiving HAART therapy, especially those with underlying cardiovascular risk. It may be important to consider traditional coronary risk profiles and to alter those that can be modified in the evaluation and continued therapy of patients for HAART. Careful clinical and echocardiographic evaluation is required also for HIV+ patients who receive drugs with recognized cardiotoxic action (doxorubicin, interferon

TABLE 2. Cardiovascular actions/interactions of common HIV therapies (table continued next two pages)

Class	Drugs	Cardiac Drug Interactions	Cardiac Side Effects
Anti-retroviral A) Nucleoside Reverse Transcriptase Inhibitors	i) Abacavir (Ziagen) ii) Zidovudine (AZT, Retrovir)	ii) Dipyridamole	Rare: Lactic acidosis i) Hypotension ii) Skeletal muscle myopathy, (mitochondrial dysfunction hypothesized, but not seen clinically)
B) Non-Nucleoside Reverse Transcriptase Inhibitors	i) Delavirdine (Rescriptor) ii) Efavirenz (Sustiva) iii) Nevirapine (Viramune)	Warfarin (class interaction) i) Calcium channel blockers iii) Beta blockers, nifedipine, quinidine, steroids, theophylline.	
C) Protease Inhibitors	i) Amprenavir (Agenerase) ii) Indinavir (Crixivan) iii) Nelfinavir (Viracept) iv) Ritonavir (Norvir) v) Saquinavir (Invirase, Fortovase)	All are metabolized by cytochrome p-450 and interact with: sildenafil, amiodarone, lidocaine, quinadine, warfarin, "statins" iv) Calcium channel blockers, prednisone, quinine, Increases beta blocker levels 1.5–3×	Implicated in premature atherosclerosis, dyslipidemia, insulin resistance, fat wasting and redistribution (lipodystrophy).

TABLE 2/continued.

Class	Drugs	Cardiac Drug Interactions	Cardiac Side Effects
Anti-infective A) Antibiotics	i) Erythromycin	i) Cytochrome p-450 metabolism and drug interactions	Orthostatic hypotension, ventricular tachycardia, bradycardia, torsades (drug interactions)
	ii) Trimethoprim/ sulfamethoxazole (Bactrim)	ii) increases warfarin effects	Orthostatic hypotension, anaphylaxis, QT prolongation
B) Antifungal agents	i) Amphotericin B ii) Ketoconazole iii) Itraconazole (Sporanox)	Digoxin toxicity ii) & iii) Cytochrome p-450 metabolism and drug interactions- increases levels of sildenafil, warfarin, "statins," nifedipine, digoxin	i) Hypertension, arrhythmia, renal failure, hypokalemia, thrombophlebitis, bradycardia, angioedema, dilated cardiomyopathy
C) Antiviral agents	i) Foscarnet ii) Ganciclovir	ii) Zidovudine	i) Reversible cardiac failure, electrolyte abnormalities ii) Ventricular tachycardia, hypotension
D) Anti-parasitic	i) Pentamidine (IV)		Hypotension, arrhythmias (torsade de pointes, VT), hyperglycemia, hypoglycemia, sudden death Note: Contraindicated if baseline QTc > 0.48

TABLE 2/continued.

Class	Drugs	Cardiac Drug Interactions	Cardiac Side Effects
Chemotherapy agents	i) Vincristine	i) Decreases digoxin level	i) Arrhythmia, myocardial Infarction, cardiomyopathy
	ii) Interferon-α		ii) Orthostatic hypotension, myocardial infarction, cardiomyopathy, ventricular and supraventricular arrhythmias, sudden death, Atrioventricular block
	iii) IL-2		iii) Hypotension, arrhythmia, sudden death, myocardial infarction, cardiac failure, capillary leak, thyroid alterations
	iv) Doxorubicin (Adriamycin)	iv) Decreases digoxin level	iv) Myocarditis, cardiomyopathy, cardiac failure

alpha, pentamidine), for those whose CD4 count is below 400/mm,[3] and for those with HIV-associated encephalopathy.[1,2]

In addition to its clinical implications, HIV-associated heart disease may be an important model for the mechanisms behind dilated cardiomyopathy.[1] Virus-induced activation of specific proinflammatory cytokines induces iNOS, reduces myocyte contractility, and decreases responsiveness to β-adrenergic agonists.[13,38] The study of these immunologic factors may provide useful information about testable therapies for HIV-associated cardiomyopathy. Such findings would also have important implications for non-HIV-related cardiovascular diseases.[1] The role of infection and inflammation in many other cardiovascular diseases is beginning to be recognized, and discovering the molecular mechanisms of HIV-related heart disease may provide the basis for rational therapeutic strategies and improved care for a broader range of patients.[1,2]

REFERENCES

1. BARBARO, G. 1999. Dilated cardiomyopathy in the acquired immunodeficiency syndrome. Eur. Heart J. **20:** 629–630 (Editorial).
2. LIPSHULTZ, S.E. 1998. Dilated cardiomyopathy in HIV-infected patients. N. Engl. J. Med. **339:** 1153–1155 (Editorial).
3. ARETZ, H.T. 1987. Myocarditis: the Dallas criteria. Hum. Pathol. **18:** 619–624.
4. YUNIS, N.A. & V.E. STONE. 1998. Cardiac manifestations of HIV/AIDS: a review of disease spectrum and clinical management. J. AIDS Hum. Retrovirol. **18:** 145–154.
5. BARBARO, G., G. DI LORENZO, B. GRISORIO, et al. 1998. Cardiac involvement in the acquired immunodeficiency syndrome. A multicenter clinical-pathological study. AIDS Res. Hum. Retroviruses **14:** 1071–1077.
6. RERKPATTANAPIPAT, P., N. WONGPRAPARUT, L.E. JACOBS, et al. 2000. Cardiac manifestations of acquired immunodeficiency syndrome. Arch. Intern. Med. **160:** 602–608.
7. BARBARO, G., G. DI LORENZO, B. GRISORIO, et al. 1998. Incidence of dilated cardiomyopathy and detection of HIV in myocardial cells of HIV positive patients. N. Engl. J. Med. **339:** 1093–1099.
8. FLOMENBAUN, M., R. SORIERO, S.A. UDEM, et al. 1989. Proliferative membranopathy and human immunodeficiency virus in AIDS heart. J. AIDS **2:** 129–135.
9. GRODY, W., L. CHENG & W. LEWIS. 1990. Infection of the heart by the human immunodeficiency virus. Am. J. Cardiol. **66:** 203–206.
10. HERSKOWITZ, A., W. TZYY-CHOOU, S.B. WILLOUGHBY, et al. 1994. Myocarditis and cardiotropic viral infection associated with severe left ventricular dysfunction in late-stage infection with human immunodeficiency virus. J. Am. Coll. Cardiol. **24:** 1025–1032.
11. BOWLES, N.E., D.L. KEARNEY, J. NI, et al. 1999. The detection of viral genomes by polymerase chain reaction in the myocardium of pediatric patients with advanced HIV disease. J. Am. Coll. Cardiol. **34:** 857–865.
12. BOWLES, N.E., N. JIYUAN, D. KEARNEY, et al. 1997. Identification of viral causes of cardiac complications associated with HIV infection in children. Pediatrics **100:** 429–430.
13. BARBARO, G., G. DI LORENZO, M. SOLDINI, et al. 1999. The intensity of myocardial expression of inducible nitric oxide synthase influences the clinical course of human immunodeficiency virus-associated cardiomyopathy. Circulation **100:** 633–639.
14. KASTEN-SPORTES, C. & C. WEINSTEIN. 1998. Molecular mechanisms of HIV cardiovascular disease. In Cardiology in AIDS. S.E. Lipshultz, Ed.: 265–282. Chapman & Hall. New York.
15. BESCHORNER, W.E., K.L. BAUGHMAN, R.P. TURNICKY, et al. 1990. HIV-associated myocarditis. Pathology and immunopathology. Am. J. Pathol. **137:** 1365–1371.

16. HERSKOWITZ, A., S.B. WILLOUGHBY, T.C. WU, *et al.* 1993. Immunopathogenesis of HIV-1 associated cardiomyopathy. Clin. Immunol. Immunopathol. **68:** 234–241.
17. CURRIE, P.F., J.H. GOLDMAN, A.L. CAFORIO, *et al.* 1998. Cardiac autoimmunity in HIV related heart muscle disease. Heart **79:** 599–604.
18. JOHNSON, H.M., B.A. TORRES & J.M. SOOS. 1996. Superantigens: structure and relevance to human disease. Proc. Soc. Exp. Biol. Med. **212:** 99–109.
19. LUSTER, A.D. 1998. Chemokines-chemotactic cytokines that mediate inflammation. N. Engl. J. Med. **338:** 445.
20. GARZINO-DEMO, A., A.L. DEVICO & R.C. GALLO. 1998. Chemokine receptors and chemokines in HIV infection. J. Clin. Immunol. **18:** 243–255.
21. WINKLER, C., W. MODI & M.W. SMITH. 1998. Genetic restiction of AIDS pathogenesis by an SDF-1 chemokine gene variant. Science **279:** 389–393.
22. TRACEY, K.J. & A. CERAMI. 1993. Tumor necrosis factor, other cytokines and disease. Annu. Rev. Cell Biol. **9:** 317–343.
23. TINKLE, B.T., L. NGO, P.A. LUCIW, *et al.* 1997. Human immunodeficiency virus-associated vasculopathy in transgenic mice. J. Virol. **71:** 4809–4814.
24. FINKEL, M.S., C.V. ODDIS, T.D. JACOB, *et al.* 1992. Negative inotropic effects of cytokines on the heart mediated by nitric oxide. Science **257:** 387–389.
25. YOKOHAMA, T., L. VACA, R.D. ROSSEN, *et al.* 1993. Cellular basis for the negative inotropic effect of tumor necrosis factor-alpha in the adult mammalian heart. J. Clin. Invest. **92:** 2303–2312.
26. MONCADA, S., R.M. PALMER & E.A. HIGGS. 1991. Nitric oxide: physiology, pathology and pharmacology. Pharmacol. Rev. **43:** 109–142.
27. TORRE-ARMIONE, G., S. KAPADIA, J. LEE, *et al.* 1995. Expression and functional significance of tumor necrosis factor receptors in human myocardium. Circulation **92:** 1487–1493.
28. LOWENSTEIN, C.J., S.L. HILL, A. LAFOND-WALKER, *et al.* 1996. Nitric oxide inhibits viral replication in murine myocarditis. J. Clin. Invest. **97:** 1837–1843.
29. SAURA, M., C. ZARAGOZA, A. MCMILLAN, *et al.* 1999. An antiviral mechanism of nitric oxide: inhibition of a viral protease. Immunity **10:** 21–28.
30. ZARAGOZA, C., C. OCAMPO, M. SAURA, *et al.* 1998. The role of inducible nitric oxide synthase in the host response to coxsackievirus myocarditis. Proc. Natl. Acad. Sci. USA **95:** 2469–2474.
31. FREEMAN, G.L., J.T. COLSTON, M. ZABALGOITIA, *et al.* 1998. Contractile depression and expression of proinflammatory cytokines and iNOS in viral myocarditis. Am. J. Physiol. **274:** 249–258.
32. UNGUREANU-LONGROIS, D., J.L. BALLIGAND, W.W. SIMMONS, *et al.* 1995. Induction of nitric oxide synthase activity by cytokines in ventricular myocytes is necessary but not sufficient to decrease contractile responsiveness to beta-adrenergic agonists. Circ. Res. **77:** 494–502.
33. HABIB, F.M., D.R. SPRINGALL, G.J. DAVIES, *et al.* 1996. Tumor necrosis factor and inducible nitric oxide synthase in dilated cardiomyopathy. Lancet **347:** 1151–1155.
34. YOSHIZUMI, M., M.A. PERRELLA, J.C. BURNETT JR., *et al.* 1993. Tumor necrosis factor downregulates an endothelial nitric oxide synthase mRNA by shortening its half-life. Circ Res **73:** 205–209.
35. LUGINBUHL, L.M., E.J. ORAV, K. MCINTOSH, *et al.* 1993. Cardiac morbidity and related mortality in children with HIV infection. JAMA **269:** 2869–2875.
36. LIPSHULTZ, S.E., K.A. EASLEY, E.J. ORAV, *et al.* 1998. Left ventricular structure and function in children infected with human immunodeficiency virus. The prospective P^2C^2 HIV multicenter study. Circulation **97:** 1246–1256.
37. COOPER, E.R., C. HANSON, C. DIAZ, *et al.* 1998. Encephalopathy and progression of human immunodeficiency virus disease in a cohort of children with perinatally acquired human immunodeficiency virus infection. J. Pediatr. **132:** 808–812.
38. BARBARO, G., G. DI LORENZO, M. SOLDINI, *et al.* 2000. Clinical course of cardiomyopathy in HIV-infected patients with or without encephalopathy related to the myocardial expression of TNF-α and iNOS. AIDS **14:** 827–838.
39. PHILIPPON, V. 1994. The basic domain of the lentivirus protein is responsible for damage in mouse brain: involvement of cytokines. Virology **205:** 519–529.

40. YEUNG, M.C., L. PULLIAM & A. LAU. 1995. The HIV envelope protein gp120 is toxic to human brain culture through the induction of interleukin-6 and tumor necrosis factor-α. AIDS 9: 137–143.
41. BUKRINSKY, M.I., H.S. NOTTET, H. SCHMIDTMAYEROVA, et al. 1995. Regulation of nitric oxide synthase activity in human immunodeficiency virus type 1 (HIV-1)-infected monocytes: implications for HIV-associated neurological disease. J. Exp. Med. 181: 735–745.
42. MERRILL, J.E., S.P. MURPHY, B. MITROVIC, et al. 1997. Inducible nitric oxide synthase and nitric oxide production by oligodendrocytes. J. Neurosci. Res. 48: 372–384.
43. MELDRUM, D.R. 1998. Tumor necrosis factor in the heart. Am. J. Physiol. 274: 577–595.
44. SCHRAGER, L.K. & M.P. D'SOUZA. 1998. Cellular and anatomical reservoirs of HIV-1 in patients receiving potent antiretroviral combination therapy. JAMA 280: 67–71.
45. HIMELMAN, R.B., M. DOHRMANN, P. GOODMAN, et al. 1989. Severe pulmonary hypertension and cor pulmonale in acquired immunodeficiency syndrome. Am. J. Cardiol. 64: 1396–1399.
46. MESA, R.A., E.S. EDELL, W.F. DUNN, et al. 1998. Human immunodeficiency virus infection and pulmonary hypertension. Mayo Clin. Proc. 73: 37–44.
47. EHRENREICH, H., P. RIECKMANN, F. SINOWATZ, et al. 1993. Potent stimulation of monocytic endothelin-1 production by HIV-1 glycoprotein. J. Immunol. 150: 4601–4609.
48. PELLICELLI, A.M., F. PALMIERI, C. D'AMBROSIO, et al. 1998. Role of human immunodeficiency virus in primary pulmonary hypertension: case reports. Angiology 49: 1005–1011.
49. BARBARO, G. & G. BARBARINI. 1999. Cardiac manifestations of the acquired immunodeficiency syndrome. In AIDS und HIV-infektionen. H. Jager, Ed.: 1–16; Ecomed Verlagsgesellschaft AG & Co. KG. Landsberg.
50. MILLER, T.L., E.J. ORAV, S.D. COLAN, et al. 1997. Nutritional status and cardiac mass and function in children infected with the human immunodeficiency virus. Am. J. Clin. Nutr. 66: 660–664.
51. MILLER, T.L. 1998. Cardiac complications of nutritional disorders. In Cardiology in AIDS. S.E. Lipshultz, Ed.: 307-316. Chapman & Hall. New York.
52. BECK, M.A., P.C. KOLBECK, Q. SHI, et al. 1994. Increased virulence of a human enterovirus (coxackievirus B3) in selenium-deficient mice. J. Infect. Dis. 170: 351–357.
53. HOFFMAN, M., S.E. LIPSHULTZ & T.L. MILLER. 1999. Malnutrition and cardiac abnormalities in the HIV-infected patients. In Nutritional Aspects of HIV Infection. T.L. Miller & S. Gorbach, Eds.: 33–39. Arnold. London.
54. CHARIOT, P., H. PERCHET & I. MONNET. 1999. Dilated cardiomyopathy in HIV-infected patients. N. Engl. J. Med. 340: 732 (letter).
55. BARBARO, G., G. DI LORENZO, M. SOLDINI, et al. 1997. Vagal system impairment in human immunodeficiency virus-positive patients with chronic hepatitis C: does glutathione deficiency have a pathogenetic role? Scand. J. Gastroenterol. 32: 1261–1266.
56. HERSKOWITZ, A., S.B. WILLOUGHBY, K.L. BAUGHMAN, et al. 1992. Cardiomyopathy associated with anti-retroviral therapy in patients with HIV infection: a report of six cases. Ann. Intern. Med. 116: 311–313.
57. DOMANSKI, M.J., M.M. SLOAS, D.A. FOLLMAN, et al. 1995. Effect of zidovudine and didanosine treatment on heart function in children infected with human immunodeficiency virus. Pediatrics 127: 137–146.
58. LEWIS, W., J.F. SIMPSON & R.R. MEYER. 1994. Cardiac mitochondrial DNA polymerase gamma is inhibited competitively and noncompetitively by phosphorylated zidovudine. Circ. Res. 74: 344–348.
59. LIPSHULTZ, S.E., E.J. ORAV, S.P. SANDERS, et al. 1992. Cardiac structure and function in children with human immunodeficiency virus infection treated with zidovudine. N. Engl. J. Med. 327: 1260–1265.
60. LIPSHULTZ, S.E., K.A. EASLEY, E.J. ORAV, et al. 2000. Absence of cardiac toxicity of zidovudine in infants. N. Engl. J. Med. 343: 759–766.

61. SORELLE, R. 1998. Vascular and lipid syndromes in selected HIV-infected patients. Circulation 9: 829–830.
62. SULLIVAN, A.K., M.R. NELSON, G.J. MOYLE, et al. 1998. Coronary artery disease occuring with protease inhibitor therapy. Int. J. STD AIDS 9: 711–-712.
63. HENRY, K., H. MELROW, J. HUEBSCH, et al. 1998. Severe coronary heart disease with protease inhibitors. Lancet 351: 1328 (letter).
64. BEHRENS, G., H. SCHMIDT, D. MEYER, et al. 1998. Vascular complications associated with use of HIV protease inhibitors. Lancet 351: 1958 (letter).
65. JUTTE, A., A. SCHWENK, C. FRANZEN, et al. 1999. Increasing morbidity from myocardial infarction during HIV protease inhibitor treatment? AIDS 13: 1796–1797 (letter).
66. FLYNN, T.E. & L.A. BRICKER. 1999. Myocardial infarction in HIV-infected men receiving protease inhibitors. Ann. Intern. Med. 131: 548 (letter).
67. SONNENBLICK, E.H. & A. ROSIN. 1991. Cardiotoxicity of interferon: a review of 44 cases. Chest 99: 557–561.
68. DEYTON, L., R. WALKER, J. KOVACS, et al. 1989. Reversible cardiac dysfunction associated with interferon alpha therapy in AIDS patients with Kaposi's sarcoma. N. Engl. J. Med. 321: 1246–1249.
69. BRISTOW, M.R., J.W. MASON, M.E. BILLINGHAM, et al. 1978. Doxorubicin cardiomyopathy: evaluation by phonocardiography, endomyocardial biopsy and cardiac catheterization. Ann. Intern. Med. 88: 168–175.
70. BROWN, D.L., S. SATHER & M.D. CHEITLIN. 1993. Reversible cardiac dysfunction associated with foscarnet therapy for cytomegalovirus esophagitis in an AIDS patient. Am. Heart J. 125: 1439–1441.
71. RAINE, A.E. 1988. Hypertension, blood viscosity and cardiovascular morbidity in renal failure: implication of erythropoietin therapy. Lancet 1: 97–100.
72. ARSURA, E.L., Y. ISMAIL, S. FREEMAN, et al. 1994. Amphotericin B-induced dilated cardiomyopathy. Am. J. Med. 97: 560–562.
73. COHEN, A.J., B. WEISER, Q. AFZAL, et al. 1990. Ventricular tachycardia in two patients with AIDS receiving ganciclovir (DHPG). AIDS 4: 807–809.
74. LOPEZ, J.A., J.G. HAROLD, M.C. ROSENTHAL, et al. 1987. QT prolongation and torsade de pointes after administration of thrimethoprim-sulfamethoxazole. Am. J. Cardiol. 59: 376–377.
75. FACTOR, S.M. & E.H. SONNENBLICK. 1985. The pathogenesis of clinical and experimental congestive cardiomyopathies and recent concepts. Prog. Cardiovasc. Dis. 27: 395–420.
76. DUONG, M., C. DUBOIS, M. BUISSON, et al. 1997. Non-Hodgkin's lymphoma of the heart in patients infected with human immunodeficiency virus. Clin. Cardiol. 20: 497–502.

Pathogenesis of HIV-Related Pulmonary Hypertension

ADRIANO M. PELLICELLI, FABRIZIO PALMIERI,
STEFANIA CICALINI, AND NICOLA PETROSILLO

*Istituto Nazionale per le Malattie Infettive, "Lazzaro Spallanzani,"
IRCCS, 00149 Rome, Italy*

ABSTRACT: Human immunodeficiency virus (HIV)–related pulmonary hypertension (HRPR) is a cardiovascular complication of HIV infection that has been recognized in the last years with increasing frequency. The etiology of HRPH is unknown. All the attempts to isolate HIV on pulmonary vessels in HRPH patients failed, and an indirect role for HIV in this disease has been hypothesized. Current theories on the pathogenesis focus on abnormalities of endothelial and smooth muscle cells of pulmonary vasculature. Endothelial and smooth muscle cell injury could be due to a high production or to a reduced clearance of cytokines in these patients. In fact, in several studies high levels of ET-1, IL-1α, IL-6 and PDGF in primary pulmonary hypertension (PPH) and in HRPH have been found. HIV gp 120 could induce the production of these cytokines by a stimulation of monocytes/macrophages. A high α_1-adrenoreceptors stimulation of pulmonary vessels could be also implicated in the pathogenesis of HRPH. Chronic hypoxia is observed with increased frequency in HIV patients, and this could induce a chronic stimulation of α_1-receptors of pulmonary vasculature with typical pathological changes. However, only a small percentage of HIV⁻ patients develop HRPH. This observation suggests the existence of an idiosyncratic susceptibility to the development of vascular disease. This susceptibility could have a genetic basis, and might be determined by particular major histocompatibility complex alleles.

KEYWORDS: HIV-related pulmonary hypertension; cytokines; HIV; α_1-adrenergic-receptors

INTRODUCTION

With the highly active antiretroviral treatment (HAART), and the increased time of survival, over the past few years non-infectious conditions associated with human immunodeficiency virus (HIV) infection have been recognized with increasing frequency. HIV-related pulmonary hypertension (HRPH) is one such condition, and more than 131 cases have now been documented.[1]

HRPH is a disease of unclear etiology, and different factors could induce a remodeling of pulmonary vasculature leading to elevations of vascular resistance.

Address for correspondence: Dr. Adriano M. Pellicelli, Istituto Nazionale per le Malattie Infettive, "Lazzaro Spallanzanir,"—IRCCS, Via Portuense, 292, 00149 Rome, Italy.
Voice: +39 06 55170449; fax: +39 06 5594224.
adriapel@tin.it

As in primary pulmonary hypertension (PPH), HRPH is characterized pathologically by three distinct subsets: plexogenic arteriopathy, veno-occlusive disease, and thrombotic pulmonary arteriopathy. Thrombosis *in situ* and pulmonary medial hypertrophy can also co-exist with plexogenic arteriopathy and veno-occlusive disease.

This article discusses the different factors that could be responsible for pathophysiologic modifications of pulmonary vasculature, such as smooth muscle and endothelial cells proliferation and migration and excessive pulmonary vascular vasoconstriction leading to occlusive arterial lesions (see FIGURE 1).

HISTOPATHOLOGY OF HRPH

Before describing the pathogenic mechanisms that could be at the basis of HRPH, the most common histopathologic alterations of pulmonary artery vessels of this disease will be discussed. The histopathology of HRPH is similar to that of PPH. The most common changes are: plexogenic pulmonary arteriopathy, thrombotic pulmonary arteriopathy, and pulmonary veno-occlusive disease.

Plexiform lesions are to be regarded as characteristic of severe vasoconstrictive pulmonary hypertension (PH). As a rule these rather complicated vascular alterations can be easily recognized in histological sections. These vessel alterations have been described only in HRPH, in PH due to congenital heart disease with shunt, in pulmonary schistosomiasis, and in PPH.

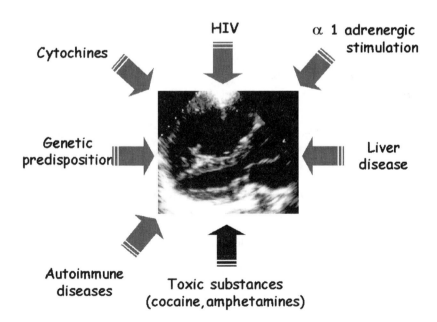

FIGURE 1. Different factors that could be implicated in the pathogenesis of HRPH.

Plexogenic lesions are present in 70% of patients with PPH and are the most common histopathologic findings in HRPH. These alterations are characterized by medial hypertrophy with concentric intimal proliferation. Moreover, in the late phases of PPH these alterations are characterized by severe intimal proliferation with little medial hypertrophy and near complete luminal obstruction with formation of channels.

In some cases of HRPH, medial hypertrophy is the only present lesion; this could be due to the initial phase of the disease and is the expression of a vasoconstrictive mechanism, which is at the basis of this disease. Pulmonary veno-occlusive disease has been reported in only three HRPH cases.[2,3] The changes in pulmonary vasculature were characterized by eccentric intimal fibrosis, predominantly involving pulmonary veins, obliteration of the lumen by intravascular fibrous septa and formation of several small channels.

ROLE OF HIV IN HRPH

Direct Role

In the majority of HRPH cases, the development of PH was solely related to HIV infection. [1,4,5] Therefore, it was hypothesized that HIV could be directly implicated in the pathogenesis of PH. In 1992, Mette *et al.* described three cases of HRPH and attempted to isolate HIV-1 nucleic acid in the endothelial cells of affected pulmonary vessels, using *in situ* hybridization with a full-length HIV-DNA and polymerase chain reaction (PCR).[6] They could not detect HIV-1 sequences in the patient's abnormal pulmonary vessels, although HIV infection has been previously found in other not CD4[+] cells.[7,8]

In a study by Humbert *et al.*, the presence of HIV-1 p24 antigen and HIV-1 gag RNA was analyzed in lung samples of a patient displaying HRPH by immunochemistry and *in situ* hybridization, respectively. Furthermore, in this case HIV was not identified in the pulmonary artery vessels.[9]

Electron microscopy was also used in an attempt to locate virus particles in vascular endothelium, but no evidence of direct HIV infection was found. Although no viral particles were identified, the affected vascular endothelium contained numerous tubuloreticular structures. Similar alterations have been found in systemic lupus erythematosus and other inflammatory diseases, as well as in patients known to be infected with HIV-1 without PH.[6]

It is possible that these structures are the result of an endothelial cell alteration induced by lymphokines released in response to HIV infection and not by the direct effect of the virus.

In the absence of evidence of direct pulmonary endothelium cell infection by HIV-1, an indirect role of the virus mediated by cytokines can be hypothesized.[6]

Indirect Role

Endothelin-1 (ET-1) is a potent vasoconstrictor, which has inotropic and mitogenic properties and stimulates the renin-angiotensin-aldosterone and the sympathetic nervous system. Thus, the overall effect of ET-1 is to increase vascular tone and blood pressure. The major site of the generation of ET-1, assessed in terms of the expression of m-RNA for preproendothelin-1 and the presence of intracellular converting enzyme, is found in the endothelial cells.[10–12] However, ET-1 is also produced by macrophages. In fact, in HIV infection, Ehrenreich *et al.* demonstrated that macrophages are a source of multifunctional cytokines; in particular, HIV-1 gp120 seems to stimulate the secretion of a large amount of ET-1 from macrophages.[13]

ET-1 action is mediated by the interaction between ET-1 and ET_A-ET_B endothelin receptors, localized respectively on vascular smooth and endothelial cells.[14] While activation of ET_A receptor causes vasoconstriction and tends to elevate blood pressure, activation of vascular endothelial ET_B receptor promotes vasodilatation, natriuresis, and decreases blood pressure. The overall cardiovascular effect of endogenous ET-1 will depend on the balance between ET_A-mediated and ET_B-mediated effects.

However, hypotensive effects of combined $ET_{A/B}$ receptor antagonists on healthy subjects, suggest that the overall physiological effect of ET-1 is to increase blood pressure. Another ET-1 effect is an increase of intracellular expression of mRNA for the growth-promoting proto-oncogenes c-*for* and c-*myc,* and subsequently migration and proliferation of smooth muscle cells.[15] ET-1 is rapidly cleared from the circulation, and a substantial proportion of clearance appears to occur through receptor binding and then internalization.

Animal studies have established the lungs as a major site for ET-1 removal. Furthermore, Dupuis *et al.* found that the normal human lungs can extract 47% ± 7 of ^{125}I-ET-1.[16] Pulmonary clearance of radio-labeled ET-1 can be blocked by pretreatment with a large dose of unlabeled ET-1, supporting the hypothesis that its clearance is receptor mediated.[17]

It could be hypothesized, that an increased pulmonary concentration or a reduced clearance of ET-1 is implicated in the pathogenesis of PH. Several studies have demonstrated in PPH an increased plasma concentration of ET-1 and the pulmonary circulation seems to generate more ET-1 than the systemic circulation.[18,19] In fact, the arterial:venous concentration ratio is significantly greater than unity.[18] This is not the case for healthy controls, who have an arterial:venous ratio substantially less than unity.

A study by Giaid *et al.* demonstrated a high expression of ET-1 mRNA and ET-1-like immunoreactivity in endothelial cells of pulmonary arteries that were most affected by the morphologic abnormalities of pulmonary hypertension.[20] Furthermore, there was a strong correlation between the intensity of ET-1 immunoreactivity and pulmonary vascular resistance,[20] which could suggest that PPH is associated with an increased expression of ET-1 in vascular endothelial cells.

Several studies have found an increased expression of ET-1 in vascular endothelial cells, suggesting that local production of ET-1, may contribute to the vascular abnormalities typical of PPH.[16,21,22] In a study by Cacoub *et al.*, ET-1-like immunoreactivity was measured in lung tissue specimens from patients with severe PH.[22] This study found that there was a significant increase in ET-1-like immunoreactivity pulmonary concentration, that correlated with pulmonary vascular resistance.

Dupuis *et al.* have shown that in PPH there was a reduced clearance of ET-1, which may possibly contribute to the increase in circulating ET-1, whereas the pulmonary release of ET-1 into circulation was unchanged.[16]

Interleukin-1β (IL-1β), Interleukin-6 (IL-6) and tumor necrosis factor α (TNFα) are pro-inflammatory cytokines produced by monocytes/macrophages, endothelial cells, and other cell types.[23–25] The activation of these cells is required to trigger the synthesis of these mediators, which should be regarded as markers of inflammation and immune reaction.

In PPH, inflammatory infiltrates with T and B lymphocytes and macrophages have been described in plexiform lesions and may participate in the production of these cytokines. Cytokines are potent growth factors for smooth muscle cells, fibroblasts, and endothelial cells and may be involved in the anatomic damage leading to PH.

In particular, the involvement of IL-1β in the development of PPH may not be restricted only to the induction of cell proliferation but may also involve the inflammatory cell migration and the local imbalance between pro-coagulant and anticoagulant factors.

In fact, IL-1β stimulates the induction of a pro-coagulant activity by endothelial cells. This ability to promote thrombosis[26,27] may thus contribute to development of the microthrombotic pulmonary lesions frequently observed in patients with severe PPH. Furthermore, IL-1β increases the expression of adhesion molecules by

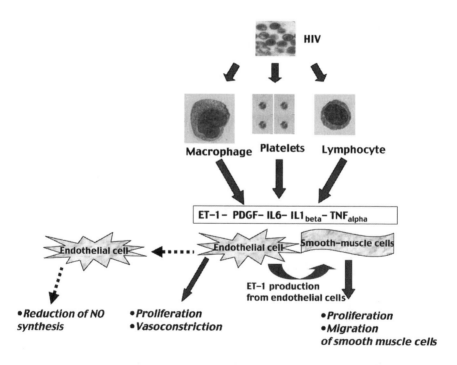

FIGURE 2. HIV-1 stimulates macrophages/monocytes, platelets and lymphocytes to produce cytokines. Note: In particular endothelin-1, interleukin-1β, interleukin-6 and PDGF can interact with endothelial and smooth muscle cells. The final effects will be a reduction of vascular nitric oxide production, arterial vasoconstriction, proliferation and migration of smooth muscle cells, and an antiapoptotic effect.

endothelial cells and the production by these latter cells of cytokines with chemotactic properties.[23]

Humbert *et al.* have demonstrated an increase of IL-1β and IL-6 serum concentration in 29 patients with severe PPH, and they were the first to suggest the important role of these cytokines in the pathogenesis of PPH.[28] The effects of these cytokines on pulmonary vascular vessels could be direct or partly indirect and mediated by platelet-derived growth factor (PDGF). PDGF production is upregulated by IL-1β; furthermore, PDGF appears capable of promoting IL-1β synthesis by macrophages, suggesting a self-perpetuating loop between these two cytokines.

While no studies have evaluated circulating cytokines in HRPH patients, a study by Humbert *et al.* found an elevated PDGF expression in lung biopsies from patients displaying PPH and in one patient with HRPH.[9] In particular PDGF-A chain mRNA was detected by semi-quantitative RT-PCR in the accumulation of perivascular inflammatory cells. It is probably that HRPH is not due to a direct action of the virus itself but to effects of second mediators such as ET-1, IL-1β, IL-6 and growth factors including PDGF.[9]

Interestingly, only a minority of HIV+ patients develop HRPH, suggesting that the development of PH in the context of HIV infection requires some predisposition.

A study, which will be discussed later in this paper, found that HRPH could reflect a particular host response to HIV-1 determined by one or more human leukocyte antigen (HLA) DR alleles.[29] FIGURE 2 describes the effects of cytokines on endothelial and smooth muscle cells in HRPH.

α_1-ADRENERGIC HYPOTHESIS

The pulmonary vasculature expresses α-adrenoreceptors and β-adrenoreceptors, both of which help to regulate pulmonary vascular tone by producing vasoconstriction or vasodilatation.[30] The stimulation of α_1-adrenoreceptors increases DNA and protein synthesis in vascular smooth muscle cells, and the activation of β-adrenoreceptors inhibits the process described above. In normal pulmonary circulation, there is a balance that favors vasodilatation and the inhibition of proliferation of smooth muscle cells, which is maintained by a predominantly β-adrenergic effect.

In HIV+ patients different factors can induce a chronic stimulation of α_1-adrenoreceptors of pulmonary vasculature, which include: chronic hypoxia, high circulating levels of norepinephrine (NE), use of appetite-suppressant agents or cocaine, and pulmonary pressure or volume overload, commonly associated with HIV-correlated cardiac disease.

Chronic pulmonary alveolar hypoxia could be present in HIV+ patients owing to a high incidence of chronic obstructive pulmonary disease and pulmonary infections.[31,32] Several studies have demonstrated that HIV infection accelerates the onset of smoking-induced emphysema.[33] The results of these studies support the emerging concept that cytotoxic lymphocytes may have an important role in emphysema pathogenesis.

As a matter of fact, it was found that in HIV+ patients there was an unexplained reduction in pulmonary diffusing capacities prior to the development of HIV-related pulmonary complications.[33] Chronic hypoxia can upregulate α_1-adrenoreceptors by

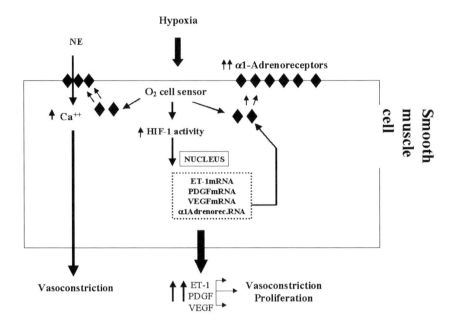

FIGURE 3. Effect of chronic hypoxia on pulmonary artery smooth muscle cells. Chronic hypoxia stimulates intracellular production of HIF-1 (hypoxia-inducible factor) which induces the transcription of various genes such as ET-1, PDGF, VEGF. Furthermore, HIF-1 enhances the production of α_1-adrenoreceptors and a reduction of β-adrenoreceptors on the smooth muscle cell surface. Hypoxia can also increase NE (norepinephrine) plasmatic levels. NE, in the presence of an increased number of α_1-adrenoreceptors, will induce an increase of intracellular free calcium levels and have a vasocostrictor effect. On the other hand, an increased production of cytokines will enhance vasoconstriction and produce cell proliferation.

activation of a hypoxia-inducible factor-1 (HIF-1) localized in smooth muscle cells of pulmonary circulation.[34]

Furthermore, HIF-1 induces the transcription of various genes with a high production of vascular endothelial growth factor (VEGF), ET-1, and PDGF.[35] These cytokines stimulate the growth of new pulmonary capillaries in order to improve local oxygen delivery, induce vasoconstriction of resistance-sized pulmonary arteries, and have an anti-apoptosis effect.[3] The final result is an excessive proliferation of smooth muscle cells and fibroblasts, pulmonary vascular hypertrophy, and excessive vasoconstriction of pulmonary vascular medium-sized arteries.[36–38] These alterations will lead to the development of PH (see FIGURE 3).

TOXIC SUBSTANCES

Patients with a history of chronic intravenous drug use may develop PH. Pulmonary artery thrombosis is the main pathological finding in such conditions, and it is believed to be due to foreign particle pulmonary emboli, following injections of solutions derived from ordinary heroin. However, ordinary heroin does not seem to contain enough crystalline debris to induce extensive pulmonary angiothrombosis.

In 1970, Tomashefski and Hirsh reported the results of autoptic examinations from 70 intravenous drug users (IVDUs). They concluded that, unless the individual was injecting crushed oral medications in which talc was a frequent component, there would be no risk of developing foreign-body granulomas, which could eventually lead to PH.[39]

In our study, in HIV[+] patients who were IVDUs, the mean systolic pulmonary artery pressure value (SPAP) was similar to that of patients with other risk factors for HIV infection.[40] Consequently, the risk factors associated with intravenous drug use do not coincide with increased mean SPAP, any more than other risk categories do.

Cocaine

The use of cocaine has been associated with PH and various contractile vascular responses.[41] The action of cocaine is primarily dependent on stimulation of α_1-adrenoreceptors,[42] suggesting that PH associated with cocaine could be due to stimulation of the α_1-adrenergic receptors in the pulmonary artery. In HIV[+] patients who are IVDUs, the use of heroin is often concurrent with the use of cocaine, which could predispose them to the development of PH.

Appetite Suppressant Agents

Appetite suppressant agents are associated with a sixfold greater risk for the development of PH. A multicenter prospective case control study reported that the use of appetite suppressant agents increased by 23-fold, the risk of developing PH when these drugs were used for more than 3 months.[43]

α_1-Adrenoreceptors are present in high density in the paraventricular nucleus of the hypothalamus, the area associated with the regulation of food intake. It has been demonstrated that appetite suppressant agents stimulate the α_1-adrenoreceptors localized in the paraventricular hypothalamic nucleus and in this way suppress food intake.

Dexfenfluramine, a new appetite suppressant agent, has also been associated with the development of PH. It acts mainly by releasing NE by blocking its re-uptakes or by directly stimulating the α_1-adrenoreceptors in the hypothalamus.[44] α_1-Adrenoreceptors present in the brain and those of pulmonary artery smooth muscle cells may be of similar subtypes and possess similar agonist affinities. The final effect will be a release of a large amount of serotonin in the brain, pulmonary circulation with vasoconstriction, and proliferation of smooth muscle cells.

HIV[+] patients seldom use appetite suppressant agents; these agents must be excluded when diagnosing HRPH.

LIVER DISEASE AND PH

The term hepatopulmonary syndrome (HPS) was first described by Snell in the 1930s to explain arterial hypoxemia with vascular dilatations in patients with chronic liver disease without significant pulmonary and cardiac disease.[45]

More than 70% of patients with cirrhosis have been reported to have hypoxemia.[46] Hypoxemia is associated with an increased alveolar to arterial oxygen gradient and has been attributed to shunting and intrapulmonary vascular dilatations. In HPS there is low pulmonary vascular resistance, whereas in PH associated to portal hypertension, there is high pulmonary vascular resistance.

PH may occur in liver cirrhosis, with the presence or absence of arterial hypoxemia. The prevalence of PH ranges from 0.25% to 0.73%, although a higher percentage has been found when patients with PH were studied by cardiac catheterization.[47] In fact, Hadengue et al. found that in 507 patients hospitalized with portal hypertension, but without known cardiac disease, there was a 2% prevalence of PH assessed by cardiac catheterization.[48] They concluded that the risk of developing PH might increase with the duration of portal hypertension. Furthermore, PH was not related to the degree of portal hypertension, hepatic failure, or to the amount of blood shunted.

The hypertensive pulmonary vascular disease that occurs in patients with liver disease appears similar to that found in patients with PPH. Although hypoxemia can contribute to the histologic alterations of pulmonary vessels (as reported above), it seems that increases in the circulating humoral factors rather than mechanical agents, could produce modifications of pulmonary vasculature.

Various studies have demonstrated that enhanced synthesis and reduced metabolism of ET-1 in cirrhotic hepatocytes could be an important mechanism associated with elevated ET-1 plasma concentration in cirrhotic patients.[49,50]

We recently found high values of SPAP in HRPH patients with cirrhosis due to HCV or HBV infection, compared to HRPH patients without cirrhosis.[40] It is possible that high circulating cytokine levels in liver diseases could contribute to the development of PH. Furthermore, it was hypothesized that in some cirrhotic patients with PH, the use of β-blockers could have contributed to the development of PH.[51]

AUTOIMMUNE DISEASE AND HRPH

PPH has been associated with the presence of various autoantibodies, including antinuclear antibodies (ANA) or antibodies against smooth muscle cells and cardiolipin.[52–54] However, there have been no generally accepted pathogenic links between these abnormalities and PPH itself.

In a study by Opravil et al.,[55] the rheumatoid factor or antibodies against native DNA, cardiolipin IgG and IgM, and glomerular basal membrane were frequently detected in low titers in HIV+ patients with and without HRPH. It was hypothesized that probably their presence was not a direct effect of HIV infection but was due to an aspecific stimulation of B lymphocytes induced indirectly by HIV itself.

Only anticardiolipin IgM and anti-SS-B were significantly more frequent in HRPH cases, in comparison with the control subjects. These findings could also be accidental and without pathogenic significance. Anticardiolipin antibodies were found to increase with age and the number of vascular risk factors in a stroke population and seem to be non-specific for vascular disease.[56]

Nevertheless, the indirect viral role in the pathogenesis of pulmonary hypertension in HIV+ patients should be considered, while the role of an autoimmune phenomenon in the pathogenesis remains undetermined.

HLA AND HRPH

Interestingly, HRPH develops in very few individuals, suggesting that some predisposition is required to display HRPH in the context of HIV infection. In a study by Morse and co-workers, it was found that in 10 racially mixed HIV+ patients with HRPH, there was a significant increase in the frequency of human leukocyte antigen (HLA) class II DR52 and DR6, and of the linked alleles HLA-DRB1 1301/2, DRB3 0301, DQB1 0603/4, compared with the frequencies of the same alleles in normal Caucasian control subjects.[29]

HLA DR6 and its DRB1 1301/2 subtypes were also significantly increased in HRPH patients compared with the respective frequencies in racially diverse HIV+ control subjects.[29] These data could suggest that susceptibility to HRPH in the HIV+ population is determined by different major histocompatibility complex alleles, in comparison to the non-HIV population. Furthermore, HLA-DR6 and the DRB1-1301 subtype have also been reported to increase in HIV+ patients who develop diffuse infiltrative lymphocytosis syndrome (DILS).[57,58]

The immunogenetic similarities between HRPH patients and HIV+ patients with DILS prompted us to examine whether these entities may have clinical similarities, despite the different organs involved. Since lymphocytic pulmonary infiltrates are a prominent feature of DILS, some reported patients with co-existent plexogenic arteriopathy and lymphocytic interstitial pneumonitis may illustrate a clinical overlap between HRPH and DILS. It is possible that both entities represent a different spectrum of a common HLA-DR determined host response to HIV-1.

REFERENCES

1. METHA, N.J. *et al.* 2000. HIV-related pulmonary hypertension. Analytic review of 131 cases. Chest **118:** 1133–1141.
2. RUCHELLI, E.D. *et al.* 1994. Pulmonary venoocclusive disease: another vascular disorder associated with human immunodeficiency virus infection. Arch. Pathol. Lab. Med. **118:** 664–666.
3. ESCAMILLA, R. *et al.* 1995. Pulmonary venoocclusive disease in a HIV-infected intravenous drug abuser. Eur. Respir. J. **8:** 1982–1984.
4. PELLICELLI, A.M. *et al.* 1998. Role of human immunodeficiency virus in primary pulmonary hypertension-case reports. Angiology **49:** 1005–1011.
5. MESA, R.A. *et al.* 1998. Human immunodeficiency virus infection and pulmonary hypertension: two new cases and a review of 86 reported cases. Mayo Clin. Proc. **73:** 37–45.
6. METTE, S.A. *et al.* 1992. Primary pulmonary hypertension in association with human immunodeficiency virus infection: a possible viral etiology for some forms of hypertensive pulmonary arteriopathy. Am. Rev. Respir. Dis. **145:** 1196–1200.

7. TATENO, M., F. GONZALES-SCARANO & J.A. LEVY. 1989. Human immunodeficiency virus can infect CD4 negative human fibroblastoid cells. Proc. Natl. Acad. Sci USA **86:** 4287–4290.

8. BARBARO, G. *et al.* 1998. Incidence of dilated cardiomyopathy and detection of HIV in myocardial cells of HIV positive patients. N. Engl. J. Med. **339:** 1093–1099.

9. HUMBERT, M. *et al.* 1998. Platelet-derived growth factor expression in primary pulmonary hypertension: comparison of HIV seropositive and HIV seronegative patients. Eur. Respir. J. **11:** 554–559.

10. INOUE, A. *et al.* 1989. The human endothelin family: three structurally and pharmacologically distinct isopeptides predicted by three separate genes. Proc. Natl. Acad. Sci. USA **86:** 2863–2867.

11. INOUE, A. *et al.* 1989. The human preproendothelin-1 gene: complete nucleotide sequence and regulation of expression. J. Biol. Chem. **264:** 14954–14959.

12. LEE, M.E. *et al.* 1990. Functional analysis of the endothelin-1 release by angiotensin and vasopressin. Hypertension **265:** 10446–10450.

13. EHRENREICH, H. *et al.* 1993. Potent stimulation of monocytic endothelin-1 production by HIV-1 glycoprotein. J. Immunol. **150:** 4601–4609.

14. HAYNES, W.G., F.E. STRACHAN & D.J. WEBB. 1995. Endothelin ET_A and ET_B receptors mediate vascocostriction of human resistance and capacitance vessels in vivo. Circulation **92:** 357–363.

15. KOMURO, I. *et al.* 1998. Endothelin stimulates c fos and c myc expression and proliferation of vascular smooth muscle cells. FEBS Lett **238:** 249–252.

16. DUPUIS, J. *et al.* 1998. Reduced pulmonary clearance of endothelin-1 in pulmonary hypertension. Am. Heart J. **135:** 614–620.

17. SIRVIO, M.L. *et al.* 1990. Tissue distribution and half-life of 125 I endothelin in the rats: importance of pulmonary clearance. Biochem. Biophys. Res. Commun. **167:** 1191–1195.

18. STEWARD, D.J. *et al.* 1991. Increased plasma endothelin-1 in pulmonary hypertension: marker or mediator of disease? Ann. Int. Med. **114:** 464–469.

19. CACOUB, P. *et al.* 1993. Endothelin-1 in primary pulmonary hypertension and the Eisenmenger syndrome. Am. J. Cardiol. **71:** 448–450.

20. GIAID, A., M. YANAGISAWA & D. LANGLEBEN. 1993. Expression of endothelin-1 in the lungs of patients with pulmonary hypertension. N. Engl. J. Med. **328:** 1732–1739.

21. GIAID, A. 1998. Nitric oxide and endothelin-1 in pulmonary hypertension. Chest **114:** 208S–212S.

22. CACOUB, P. *et al.* 1997. Endothelin-1 in the lungs of patients with pulmonary hypertension. Cardiovasc. Res. **33:** 196–200.

23. DINARELLO, C.A. 1991. Interleukin-1 and interleukin-1 antagonism. Blood **77:** 1627–1652.

24. AKIRA, S. & T. KISHIMOTO. 1992. IL-6 and NF-IL-6 in acute-phase response and viral infection. Immunol. Rev. **127:** 25–50.

25. JAATTELA, M. 1991. Biologic activities and mechanisms of action of tumor necrosis factor-α/cachectin. Lab. Invest. **64:** 724–742.

26. BEVILACQUA, M.P. *et al.* 1984. Interleukin 1 induces biosynthesis and cell surface expression of procoagulant activity in human vascular endothelial cells. J. Exp. Med. **160:** 618–624.

27. BEVILACQUA, M.P. *et al.* 1986. Recombinant tumor necrosis factor induces procoagulant activity in cultured human vascular endothelium: characterization and comparison with the actions of interleukin 1. Proc. Natl. Acad. Sci. USA **83:** 4533–4537.

28. HUMBERT, M. *et al.* 1995. Increased interleukin-1 and interleukin-6 serum concentrations in severe primary pulmonary hypertension. Am. J. Respir. Crit. Care Med. **151:** 1628–1631.

29. MORSE, J.H. *et al.* 1996. Primary pulmonary hypertension in HIV infection. An outcome determined by particular HLA class II alleles. Am. J. Respir. Crit. Care Med. **153:** 1299–1301.

30. BEVAN, R.D. Influence of adrenergic innervation on vascular growth and mature characteristics. 1989. Am. Rev. Respir. Dis. **140:** 1478–1482.

31. DIAZ P.T., T.L. CLANTON & E.R. PACHT. 1992. Emphysema-like pulmonary disease associated with human immunodeficiency virus infection. Ann. Intern. Med. **116:** 124–128.
32. DIAZ, P.T *et al.* 1999. The pathophysiology of pulmonary diffusion impairment in human immunodeficiency virus infection. Am. J. Respir. Crit. Care Med. **160:** 272–277.
33. DIAZ, P.T. *et al.* 2000. Increased susceptibility to pulmonary emphysema among HIV-seropositive smokers. Ann. Intern. Med. **132:** 369–372.
34. SEMENZA, G.L. 1996. Transcriptional regulation by hypoxia-inducible factor-1: molecular mechanisms of oxygen homeostasis. Trends Cardiovasc. Med. **6:** 151–157.
35. GUILLEMIN, K. & M.A. KRASNOW. 1997. The hypoxic response: huffing or HIFing. Cell **89:** 9–12.
36. YU, S.M. *et al.* 1996. Mechanism of catecholamine-induced proliferation of vascular smooth muscle cells. Circulation **94:** 547–554.
37. CHEN, L.Q. *et al.* 1995. Regulation of vascular smooth muscle growth by α_1-adrenoreceptor subtypes in vitro and in situ. J. Biol. Chem. **270:** 30980–30988.
38. DEBLOIS, D. *et al.* 1996. Chronic α_1-adrenoreceptor stimulation increases DNA synthesis in rat arterial wall: modulation of responsiveness after vascular injury. Arterioscler. Thromb. Vasc. Biol. **16:** 1122–1129.
39. TOMASHEFSKI, J.F. & C.S. HIRSCH. 1980. The pulmonary vascular lesions of intravenous drug abuse. Hum. Pathol. **11:** 133–145.
40. PELLICELLI, A.M. *et al.* 2001. Primary pulmonary hypertension in HIV patients: a systematic review. Angiology **52:** 31–41.
41. SCHAIBERGER, P.H. *et al.* 1993. Pulmonary hypertension associated with the long term inhalation of crank methamphetamine. Chest **104:** 614–616.
42. BRANCH, C.A. & M.M. KNUEPFER. 1992. Adrenergic mechanisms underlying cardiac and vascular responses to cocaine in conscious rats. J. Pharmacol. Exp. Ther. **263:** 742–751.
43. ABENHEIM, L. *et al.* 1996. Appetite suppressant drugs and the risk of primary pulmonary hypertension. N. Engl. J. Med. **335:** 609–616.
44. ATKINSON, R.L. *et al.* 1995. Combined drug treatment of obesity. Obesity Res. **3:** S497–S500.
45. KEYS, A. & A.M. SNELL. 1938. Respiratory properties of arterial blood in normal man and in patients with disease of the liver: position of the oxygen dissociation curve. J. Clin. Invest. **107:** 167–174.
46. NAEIJE, R. *et al.* 1981. Hypoxic pulmonary vasoconstriction in liver cirrhosis. Chest **80:** 570–574.
47. MCDONNELL, P.J. P.A. TOYE & G.M. HUTCHINS. 1983. Primary pulmonary hypertension and cirrhosis: are they related? Am. Rev. Respir. Dis. **127:** 437–441.
48. HADENGUE, A. *et al.* 1991. Pulmonary hypertension complicating portal hypertension: prevalence and relation to splanchnic hemodynamics. Gastroenterology **100:** 520–528.
49. KUDDUS, R.H. *et al.* 2000.Enhanced synthesis and reduced metabolism of endothelin-1 (ET-1) by hepatocytes—an important mechanism of increased endogenous levels of ET-1 in liver cirrhosis. J. Hepatol. **33:** 725–732.
50. GANDHI, C.R. *et al.* 1996. Altered endothelin homeostasis in patients undergoing liver transplantation. Liver Transplant. Surg. **2:** 362–369.
51. MAL, H. *et al.* 1999. Pulmonary hypertension following hepatopulmonary syndrome in a patient with cirrhosis. J. Hepatol. **31:** 360–364.
52. ISERN, R.A. *et al.* 1992. Autoantibodies in patients with primary pulmonary hypertension: association with anti-Ku. Am. J. Med. **93:** 307–312.
53. YANAI LANDAU, H.H. *et al.* 1995. Autoimmune aspects of primary pulmonary hypertension. Pathobiology **63:** 71–75.
54. BADESH, D.B. *et al.* 1993. Hypothyroidism and primary pulmonary hypertension: an autoimmune pathogenetic link? Ann. Intern. Med. **119:** 44–46.
55. OPRAVIL, M. *et al.* 1997. HIV-associated primary pulmonary hypertension. Am. J. Respir. Crit. Care Med. **155:** 990–995.

56. MUIR, K.W. *et al.* 1994. Anticardiolipin antibodies in an unselected stroke population. Lancet **344:** 452–456.
57. ITESCU, S. *et al.* 1993. Tissue infiltration in a CD8 lymphocytosis syndrome associated with human immunodeficiency virus-1 infection has the phenotypic appearance of an antigenically driven response. J. Clin. Invest. **91:** 2216–2225.
58. ITESCU, S., L.J. BRANCATO & W. WINCHESTER. 1989. A sicca syndrome in HIV infection: association with HLA-DR5 and CD8 lymphocytosis. Lancet **2:** 466–468.

Cell Death in HIV Pathogenesis and Its Modulation by Retinoids

ZSUZSA SZONDY,[a] RÉKA TÓTH,[a] ÉVA SZEGEZDI,[a] UWE REICHERT,[b] PHILIPPE ANCIAN,[b] AND LÁSZLÓ FÉSÜS[a]

[a]*Department of Biochemistry and Molecular Biology, Medical and Health Science Center, University of Debrecen, H-4012 Debrecen, Hungary*

[b]*Galderma Research and Development, Sophia Antipolis, F-06902 Sophia Antipolis, France*

KEYWORDS: **Patients infected with the human immunodeficiency virus exhibit a progressive decline in the CD4 T-cell number, resulting in immunodeficiency and increased susceptibility to opportunistic infections and malignancies. Although CD4 T cell production is impaired in patients infected with HIV, there is now increasing evidence that the primary basis of T cell depletion is accelerated apoptosis of CD4 and CD8 T cells. The rate of lymphocyte apoptosis in HIV infection correlates inversely with the progression of the disease: it is low in long-term progressors and in patients undergoing highly active anti-retroviral therapy. Interestingly, only a minor fraction of apoptotic lymphocytes are infected by HIV, indicating that the enhanced apoptosis does not necessarily always serve to remove the HIV$^+$ cells and results from mechanisms other than direct infection. Thus, understanding and influencing the mechanisms of HIV-associated lymphocyte apoptosis may lead to new therapies for HIV disease. In this paper the potential effects of retinoids on CD4 T cell apoptosis is discussed.**

KEYWORDS: **apoptosis; CD4$^+$ T cells; CD95 ligand; retinoic acid; nur77; HIV**

PHYSIOLOGICAL APOPTOSIS OF T LYMPHOCYTES

Apoptosis or active cell death plays an essential role in shaping the T lymphocyte repertoire. Lymphocytes differentiating in the thymus randomly generate their T cell receptors (TCR) and become selected in the CD4$^+$CD8$^+$ stage. The selection is based on the quality of the TCR. The majority of T cells express TCRs that cannot interact with self-MHC; these cells enter the apoptotic program because of neglect. Those cells, which express potentially autoreactive TCRs undergo apoptosis after interacting with the antigen-presenting cells.[1] Only those cells which express TCRs that recognize self-MHC but have low or no affinity for self-antigens become positively selected and differentiate into mature CD4$^+$ or CD8$^+$ single positive thymocytes.[2] In

Address for correspondence: Dr. László Fésüs, Department of Biochemistry and Molecular Biology, Medical and Health Science Center, University of Debrecen, Nagyerdei krt. 98, H-4012 Debrecen, Hungary. Voice/fax:36 52 416432.

fesus@indi.dote.hu

these cells bcl-2, an apoptosis inhibitory protein[3] becomes upregulated and protects cells against death.[4]

Mature T lymphocytes entering the periphery are relatively resistant to various apoptosis-inducing signals owing to the constant expression of bcl-2.[5] After mitogenic stimulation, however, their proliferation and survival depends on interleukin-2 (IL-2) production,[6] which upregulates bcl-X_L, another apoptosis inhibitory protein.[5] After clearance of antigen, in the absence of further antigenic stimulation IL-2 production declines and many of the lymphocyte clones die from the lack of a survival signal (mechanism of immune down-regulation).

In case of chronic activation, on the other hand, the limitation of the immune response occurs by a different mechanism. TCR-stimulation leads to the production of Fas ligand (FasL), tumor necrosis factor (TNFα) or TNF-related apoptosis-inducing ligand (TRAIL). These cytokines initiate the apoptotic program in the apoptosis-sensitive peripheral CD4^{+} [7] and CD8^{+} T cells[8,9] (mechanism of feedback control of T cell proliferation). The apoptotic sensitivity of activated T cells is regulated by the amount of IL-2, which thus harmonizes the rate of apoptosis with the intensity of lymphocyte proliferation.[10] The apoptotic sensitivity may be partially related to the downregulation of c-FLIP, a protein, which inhibits Fas-mediated apoptosis in T cells.[11]

Besides controlling the T cell repertoire, T cells also use the program of apoptosis to remove unwanted (virally infected or malignant cells) cells from the body. To kill these cells cytotoxic T cells either synthesize FasL[12] or release the granzyme B enzyme.[13]

MAIN PATHWAYS OF APOPTOSIS

Up to now two main pathways of apoptosis have been described. One is initiated via cell death receptors belonging to the TNF receptor family, such as TNFR, TRAIL receptor and Fas.[14] Besides ligand binding, the activity of these receptors is regulated by various proteins that can bind to the ligand-receptor complex, such as c-FLIP,[11] SADS[15] or FAP.[16] The second cell death pathway affects mitochondrial permeability leading to release of various mitochondrial proteins, such as cytochrome c,[17] apoptosis-inducing factor[18] or Smac/Diablo,[19] into the cytosol. This latter pathway is regulated by interaction between various pro- and antiapoptotic members of the bcl-2 family of proteins. Their biological activity and capability to interact is regulated by their amount, phosphorylation state or proteolysis which is regulated by the balance of cell death–inducing and survival signals.[20]

No matter, however, how apoptosis is initiated, intracellular caspases that cleave proteins at aspartate residues will be activated. Hence inhibition of caspases can delay or inhibit most forms of apoptosis.[21] Caspases are synthesized as inactive zymogens and become activated after proteolytic removal of a terminal prodomain. Activated caspases catalyze the cleavage of other caspases, which in turn, activate various cellular proteases and endonucleases that cleave host cell structural and regulatory proteins as well as host nuclear DNA, leading to cell death. Though caspase activation can occur by two separate pathways, caspases activated via cell death receptors can cleave members of the bcl-2 family in this way activating the mito-chondrial pathway as well.[22]

The importance of the death receptor pathway is seen in *lpr* (Fas-deficient) or *gld* (FasL-deficient) mice, which develop splenomegaly and SLE-like autoimmune disease.[23] The importance of the mitochondrial pathway in the immune homeostasis is seen in the bax/bak (proapoptotic bcl-2 family members) double knock out mice, which develop huge thymus, lymph nodes, and spleen owing to the severely dis-turbed lymphocyte apoptosis.[24]

T CELL APOPTOSIS IN HIV INFECTION

Apoptosis during HIV Disease Progression

When lymphocytes from HIV[+] patients were analyzed, it was found that they are highly sensitive to apoptosis. As compared to non-infected individuals, a much high-er proportion of the isolated cells are Annexin V positive. Additionally, a higher per-centage of lymphocytes die spontaneously or following TCR, Fas stimulation, or calcium ionophore treatment in a 24h culture.[25] T lymphocytes from HIV-infected individuals express higher level of Fas, and FasL is also elevated in peripheral blood mononuclear cells.[26] Additionally, the plasma level of FasL is also increased and the increase correlates with HIV burden.[27] In addition to FasL, the serum level of TNF is also elevated in symptomatic but not in asymptomatic patients.[28]

The magnitude of apoptosis observed in HIV[+] patients correlates well with the stage of HIV disease in longitudinal and cross-sectional analyses. Spontaneous or induced apoptosis is greater in HIV[+] patients with progressive disease than uninfect-ed patients.[25] In addition, spontaneous apoptosis in patients with long-term nonpro-gressive HIV infection is similar to that of HIV[-] patients.[29] Thus the rate of apoptosis correlates inversely with CD4 depletion.

Interestingly, only a minor fraction of apoptotic lymphocytes are infected by HIV, indicating that the enhanced apoptosis does not necessarily serve to remove HIV-infected cells and results from mechanisms other than direct infection. These obser-vations strongly indicate that the enhanced apoptosis of lymphocytes observed in HIV[+] individuals may strongly contribute to the pathomechanism of progressive HIV disease and CD4 cell depletion. During the past years of intensive research, var-ious mechanisms were discovered that may contribute to the observed increase in the T lymphocyte apoptosis (see TABLE 1).

Apoptosis Related to Killing of Viral Infected CD4 T Cells

Although numerous pathogenic viruses have developed mechanisms to prevent apoptosis of host cells, no such antiapoptotic machinery is present in HIV. HIV, thus, induces apoptosis in infected host cells. The mechanism of virus-induced apoptosis is p53 dependent and is independent of Fas.[30] Additionally, virus-infected cells can be recognized and killed by various defense mechanisms of the host immune system.[31] Both forms of cell death lead to the deletion of mature peripheral and immature thymic cells, but provide an important mechanism for inhibiting viral rep-lication using the cell death program of infected host cells (beneficial apoptosis).[31]

TABLE 1. **Proposed mechanisms for apoptosis induced by HIV infection**

Effector	Proposed Mechanism	Target Cell
Virus infection	p53 dependent Fas independent killing	Infected cell
HIV protease	Cleavage of cellular proteins	Infected cell
CD8-mediated cytotoxicity	FasL and granzyme B-mediated	Infected cell
Activation-induced death	FasL, TRAIL and TNF-mediated	Uninfected cells
HIV Tat	Enhanced Fas sensitivity Enhanced FasL production	Infected and uninfected cells
HIV Nef	Enhanced FasL production Fas independent	Infected cells Uninfected cells
Gp120	Enhanced Fas sensitivity Enhanced FasL production	Uninfected cells
Autologous cell-mediated	Cytotoxic ligands released from killing or expressed by infected cells including FasL, gp120, Tat, Nef	Uninfected cells

Apoptosis Related to Chronic Immune Activation

Chronic uncontrolled infections provide continuous antigenic stimulation that causes persistent immune activation and consequent apoptosis. This is the mechanism by which infectious diseases, such as cytomegalovirus, cause enhanced apoptosis and lymphopenia. Similarly, as we have shown, chronic immune activation in systemic autoimmune diseases also leads to enhanced apoptosis and lymphopenia.[32] In accordance with these observations, 50 to 60% of the apoptotic cells of HIV-infected individuals exhibit an activated phenotype. Additionally, a positive correlation was found between the TCR- or Fas-mediated apoptosis in both CD4 and CD8 T cells, the progression of the disease, and their *in vivo* expression of molecules characteristic for activated T cells. These findings indicate that the chronic activation of the immune system occurring throughout HIV infection is an important mechanism for the cell deletion process.[25] Since administration of Fas, TRAIL or TNF antagonists reduces activation-induced death in cells from patients infected with HIV, all these three cell death receptors seem to be involved in the signaling.[33,34]

Physiological activators of T lymphocytes are antigens, which are recognized, in the context of MHC molecules, through their interaction with the variable V portions of the TCR α and β chains.[35] HIV-encoded antigens, present in high amount, alone can be responsible for inducing a chronic immune activation. However, T cells recognize another category of ligands, the superantigens, on the basis of the Vβ alone, independently of other variable TCR segments. The superantigens bind to MHC proteins and this complex, by engaging Vβ, can stimulate many T-cells (1/30 to 1/3 compared to 1/1000–1/10 000 for conventional peptides). If HIV can code a protein, which acts as superantigen for the T cells of HIV$^+$ individuals, this protein could additionally be responsible for the increased activation and the consequent deletion of T cells. In addition, superantigens can also induce apoptosis of immature thymocytes. Such a mechanism was reported in the pathogenesis of a murine acquired-immunodeficiency syndrome, where a truncated gag protein of a retrovirus acted as superantigen.[36] In accordance with this model, a more restricted Vβ repertoire (Vβ 14 through Vβ 20 appeared deleted) was found in HIV[+] patients with advanced disease.[37]

Apoptosis Related to the Effects of Various Viral Proteins Encoded by HIV

Besides inducing death by providing a chronic immune stimulus, HIV is unique in its ability to induce lymphocyte apoptosis through additional mechanisms as well; for example, it can encode proteins which alone are able to induce apoptosis of infected and/or uninfected cells.

Gp120 is an HIV envelope glycoprotein that can bind to and cross-link the CD4 receptor and the chemokine coreceptors. Cross-linking of CD4 T cells by gp120 causes the induction of enhanced susceptibility to Fas-mediated killing[38] and initiates apoptosis in previously activated T cells.[39] The effect of gp120 does not depend on the presence of viable virions: gp120 alone, in circulating immune complexes, in replication-incompetent viruses, or on the surface of virally infected cells can induce death in a similar manner.

Transfection experiments have shown that Tat can also induce apoptosis in lymphocytes and CD4 T cell lines. Tat is a transcriptional regulator protein that is readily secreted by transfected cells and can be taken up and transported into the nucleus of intact cells. It enhances the transcription of both caspase-8[40] and FasL,[41] and facilitates Fas-mediated killing. This way it can affect the death of both infected and uninfected cells.

HIV-encoded Nef has also been suggested to mediate apoptosis in both infected and uninfected cells. In infected cells Nef induces the synthesis of FasL perhaps by interacting with the CD4 receptor,[42] while in a broad spectrum of uninfected cells it initiates a Fas-independent death by binding to an as-yet-unidentified receptor.[43]

It has been shown that the expression of HIV protease correlates with apoptosis *in vivo*. The enzyme directly cleaves caspase-8[44] and can modify cellular susceptibility to apoptosis by proteolytic degradation of the antiapoptotic protein bcl-2.[45] These observations suggest that HIV protease may also play a role in the death of infected cells.

Autologous Infected Cell-mediated Killing

Macrophages,[46] monocytes,[47] CD4[48] and CD8[49] T cells derived from HIV[+] patients all can induce the death of uninfected CD4 T lymphocytes in *in vitro* experiments. Autologous infected cell-mediated killing may involve both gp120 interactions and the Fas/FasL system. Evidence that autologous infected cell-mediated killing may play a role *in vivo* was provided by the observation that macrophages and monocytes from HIV[+] individuals have significantly elevated FasL expression and that the levels of tissue apoptosis directly correlate with the levels of macrophage-associated FasL.[50]

Cellular Damage in Other Tissues

However, cell damage occurs in HIV[+] patients not only in the immune system, but in many other tissues, including heart.[51,52] The death characteristics of these cells resemble those of apoptosis. Since cardiomiocytes are sensitive to FasL,[53] one possibility is that their damage is mediated by soluble FasL or by cells expressing high levels of FasL. Consequently, any therapeutic approach which decreases the production of FasL in HIV disease may have therapeutic potential to prevent tissue damage and heart complications. Additionally cytotoxic compounds, such as Nef, released from infected cells may also be responsible for the observed damage.

Apoptosis following Antiretroviral Therapy

While during progression of HIV disease an increased rate of lymphocyte apoptosis is observed, apoptosis of lymphocytes is dramatically decreased in response to protease inhibitor-based HIV therapy.[54] This decrease in the rate of apoptosis has been suggested to be a strong contributor to the reconstitution of the immune system following therapy. The decrease in apoptosis, however, is rapid and is seen as early as four days after protease therapy is initiated. Because the decrease precedes significant changes in viral replication, it has been suggested that protease inhibitors may be antiapoptotic possibly by inhibiting caspases involved in apoptosis.[55]

In line with these suggestions, an inhibited apoptosis and accumulation of preapoptotic cells following HAART therapy was found in our study, when cells expressing tissue transglutaminase (tTG) was investigated. tTG is an apoptosis-related enzyme, the expression of which is induced in many forms of *in vivo* apoptosis[56] including HIV disease, where an increased number of tTG[+] lymphocytes were found.[57] Unexpectedly, an increased number of tTG[+] cells can be detected in patients undergoing antiretroviral therapy as well, and the percentage of tTG[+] cells is inversely correlated with the rate of apoptosis of tTG[+] cells (see TABLE 2). Such an accumulation of tTG[+] preapoptotic cells was reported in lpr mice as well,[58] where lymphocytes cannot die in the absence of functional Fas. Our preliminary data indicate a block in the apoptotic program following HAART, which may be partially responsible for the accumulation of TNFα-producing apoptosis-resistant CD8 cells observed in treated patients.[59]

Modulation of Apoptosis as a Therapeutic Approach in HIV Infection

If CD4 T cell depletion by apoptosis is the main cause of the CD4 T cell loss in HIV disease, it may be expected that inhibition of apoptosis may delay the progression of the disease. To investigate this hypothesis, the effect of a broad-spectrum caspase inhibitor (z-VAD-fmk) was tested *in vitro* on peripheral blood cells of HIV[+] individuals.[60] z-VAD-fmk in these experiments, however, rendered individual cells more permissive to productive viral replication, presumably by inhibiting the virus cytopathic effect or by preventing caspases from degrading the virus. These observations underlined that part of the apoptosis observed in HIV[+] individuals is beneficial since it contributes to the removal of virally infected cells and limits the replication of the virus. Consequently, an alternative approach that does not affect beneficial apoptosis should be used to inhibit harmful apoptosis. This approach could be inhibition of FasL production, since FasL-mediated apoptosis has been suggested to be the mechanism in most forms of the apoptosis induced by HIV proteins (TABLE 1) but not that of virally infected cells.

Various compounds have been shown to inhibit FasL production of T cells, including glucocorticoids and cyclosporin A. However, these compounds are also inhibitors of lymphocyte proliferation and induce lymphocyte cell depletion in the long term. Retinoic acids (RAs), a third group of compounds known to inhibit FasL production, however, do not inhibit T-cell proliferation.[61] That is why they could be considered as apoptosis modulators.

Retinoids

RAs are physiological ligands for retinoic acid (RARs) and retinoid X receptors (RXRs) that belong to the steroid/thyroid/retinoid nuclear receptor family and regulate transcription of various genes.[62] All-*trans* and 9-*cis* RAs are equipotent in

TABLE 2. Effect of HAART on the number of tissue transglutaminase-expressing apoptotic and non-apoptotic cells within the CD4 and CD8 T cell population

Patient	CD4+	tTG/CD4+	Ap/tTG+ CD4+ %	CD8+	tTG/CD8+	Ap/tTG+ CD8+
Healthy donors						
1	44.6	1.1	50.1	23.2	0.9	29.1
2	37.9	1.9	45.2	26.6	0.9	27.1
3	47.7	0.6	47.1	27.7	0.7	28.7
Nontreated						
1	17.3	63.9	49.8	52.9	14.5	23.7
2	33.7	72.1	45.9	44.2	14.6	21.4
3	8.8	73.5	43.9	46.3	13.3	26.4
Treated						
1	18.2	4.4	26.1	58.5	6.9	12.1
2	12.7	6.2	30.7	28.3	7.7	9.7
3	26.7	3.4	36.5	30.5	9.2	12.9
4	42.9	3.3	5.9	24.7	17.8	1.9
5	23.1	8.1	2.8	29.9	17.9	2.8
6	15.7	9.4	2.6	40.2	30.7	1.8
7	27.3	53.6	2.3	50.7	61.0	0.9
8	4.6	67.6	1.7	60.3	89.1	0.5

NOTE: Peripheral blood mononuclear cells were freshly isolated from patients and healthy donors and stained for CD4, CD8 or tissue transglutaminase expression and apoptosis (detected by 7-aminoactinomycin D). Percentage of cells were determined by a Becton Dickinson flow cytometer. Please note that the apoptosis sensitivity of tTG positive cells is similar in healthy donors and non-treated patients, while it is greatly decreased in patients undergoing antiretroviral therapy.

activating RAR, whereas activation of RXR by all-*trans* RA is 50-fold less than that by 9-*cis* RA.[63] Though all-*trans* RA does not bind to RXRs, the observed activation at high concentrations is explained by conversion of all-*trans* RA to 9-*cis* RA within the cells by unknown mechanisms.[64] RA receptors function in the form of RAR/RXR heterodimers or RXR/RXR homodimers in the presence of RAs.[65] In addition, RXR can form heterodimers with various other members of the steroid/thyroid/retinoid receptor family including nur77.[66] The presence of RXR in most of the heterodimers is needed to enhance the cooperative binding of these receptors to DNA; activation requires only the presence of the cognate ligand, but can be modulated by the simultaneous binding of the RXR ligand.[67] These complex interactions and the existence of multiple RARs (RARα, RARβ, and RARγ) as well as RXRs (RXRα, RXRβ, and RXRγ), differentially expressed in various tissues and cell types, account for the pleiotropic effects of retinoids in practically all type of cells.

Effect of Retinoids on the Apoptosis of HIV-infected Individuals

It was first shown by Ashwell's group that retinoic acids inhibit TCR-mediated death of T lymphocytes and the inhibition is based on blocking TCR-induced FasL production.[68] On the basis of observation they administered all-*trans* RA orally to six HIV⁺ patients and they observed a reduction in *ex vivo* activation-induced apoptosis of peripheral blood mononuclear cells from treated patients compared to non-treated ones.[69] We have extended these studies and have shown that high concentrations (10 μM) of all-*trans* RA can inhibit both activation-induced FasL release observed at day 1 and activation-induced increase in FasL protein level observed at day 2 in *ex vivo* T lymphocyte cultures of HIV⁺ individuals.[34] What is more, only CD4 apoptosis was affected; the CD8 apoptosis, which controls the size of the activated CD8 T-cell pool, was not. These results strongly indicate that retinoids should be considered as apoptosis modulators in HIV disease. The limitation is, however, that a high concentration of *trans*-RA should be used to get a therapeutic effect.

Mechanism of Retinoid Action

To investigate the mechanism of retinoid action we used various retinoid receptor agonists and antagonists and Jurkat T cells.[70] These studies have revealed, that the effect of retinoic acids are mediated via RARα since RARα agonists were able to block both TCR-mediated apoptosis and FasL expression. (see FIGURE 1) Interestingly, RARγ analogues had the opposite effect. Since the two receptors compete in their effect, this explains why a physiological concentration of all-*trans* RA, which activates both receptors, cannot inhibit death. Interestingly, 9-*cis* RA, which also binds to both receptors, was able to inhibit FasL synthesis at much lower concentrations. We found that the reason for this is that 9-*cis* RA additionally binds to the RXR receptor, and ligand-bound RXR promotes the RARα pathway.[71]

Up to now no retinoid-response element has been found in the FasL promoter, suggesting that retinoids do not directly affect FasL synthesis. However, another transcription factor, *nur77*,[72] was shown to transduce TCR-mediated signaling on the synthesis of FasL. While RARα-specific retinoids did not significantly affect the TCR-induced synthesis of *nur77* (FIG. 1), they strongly inhibited *nur77*-mediated

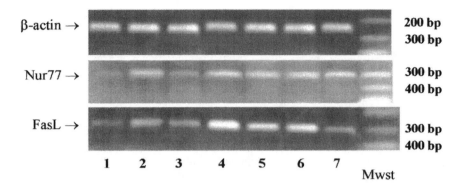

FIGURE 1. Effect of various retinoids on the activation-induced mRNA levels of nur77 orFasL determined by RT-PCR in human Jurkat T cells. *nur77* and FasL mRNA were measured in Jurkat T cells at 6 h in culture in medium (*lane 1*), in the presence of 0.3 μM CD437 (*lane 2*), 10 μM of CD2019 (*lane 3*) RARγ agonists, or after anti-CD3 stimulation with 0.3 μM CD437 (*lane 4*) alone (*lane 5*), with 10 μM of CD2019 (*lane 6*), or 0.3 μM CD336, an RARα agonist (*lane 7*). β–Actin was used as an internal control. Expected sizes for PCR products are 286, 301, and 247 bp for FasL, *nur77*, and β-actin, respectively. Please, note that RARγ specific agonists increase, whereas RARα specific agonists decrease TCR-mediated induced production FasL.

transcription when tested in a transient transfection experiment using a reporter construct containing NBRE in the promoter.[70] Our findings are supported by other investigations, which have shown that transfection of RARα into Jurkat cells provides protection against TCR-mediated cells. Additionally, a direct interaction between RARα and *nur77* was shown using a two-hybrid yeast system.[73]

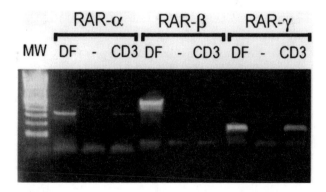

FIGURE 2. Retinoid acid receptor expression in purified CD3 + human peripheral T cells. RAR expression was detected by RT-PCR. Expected sizes for the PCR products are 332, 596, and 150 bp for RARα, RARβ, and RARγ, respectively. From the negative controls (–) the reverse transcriptase step was omitted from the PCR reaction. DF, retinoic acid treated human dermal fibroblast in culture (positive control); CD3, purified CD3+ human peripheral T cells. Please, note that RARα and RARγ are expressed by these cells.

Because RARα is also expressed in peripheral T cells (see FIGURE 2) it is very likely that retinoids mediate their effect via RARα in those cells as well. Since RARα agonists are strong inhibitors of FasL synthesis, they are able to get a therapeutic effect in much lower concentrations than all-*trans* RA. Though 9-*cis* RA is also very effective in inhibiting FasL production, *in vivo* it has many side affects[74] because it activates RXR in addition to RAR. Since RXR is the common binding partner for members of the steroid/thyroid/retinoid nuclear family,[67] stimulation of it affects many nuclear signaling pathways. Our investigations indicate that RARα-specific retinoids should be considered as potential therapeutic compounds to down-regulate harmful FasL production instead of 9-*cis* RA. Lower levels of FasL would be expected to prevent damage of both Fas-sensitive T cells and other Fas-sensitive tissues, which were shown to be affected during HIV infection.

ACKNOWLEDGMENTS

The authors thank Marie-Lise Gougeon for allowing us to carry out the retinoid-related HIV studies in her laboratory at the Pasteur Institut, France.

The research presented in this paper was supported by grants from Hungarian National Research Fund OTKA (T 022 705, T029528, F33051), Hungarian Health Research Program T (48/2000), and the Copernicus program PL 966118.

REFERENCES

1. JENKINSON, E.J., R. KINGSTON, *et al.* 1989. Antigen-induced apoptosis in T cells: a mechanism for negative selection of T cell receptor repertoire. Eur. J. Immunol. **19:** 2175–2177.
2. GROETTRUP, M. & H. VON BOEHMER. 1993. A role for a pre-T-cell receptor in T-cell development. Immunol. Today **14:** 610–617.
3. HOCKENBERY, D.J., M. ZUTTER, *et al.* 1991. BCL2 protein is topographically restricted in tissues characterized by apoptotic cell death. Proc. Natl. Acad. Sci. USA **88:** 6961–6965.
4. SENTMAN, C.L., J.R. SHUTTER, *et al.* 1991. Bcl-2 inhibits multiple form of apoptosis but not negative selection of thymocytes. Cell **67:** 879–888.
5. YANG, E. & S.J. KORSMEYER. 1996. Molecular thanatopsis: a discourse on the bcl-2 family and cell death. Blood **88:** 386–401.
6. DUKE, R.C. & J.J. COHEN. 1986. IL-2 addiction: withdrawal of growth factor activates a suicide program in dependent T Cells. Lymphokine Res. **5:** 289–298.
7. DHEIN, J., H. WALCZAK, *et al.* 1995. Autocrine T-cell suicide mediated by APO-1/(Fas/CD95) Nature **373:** 438–441.
8. ZHENG, L., G. FISHER, *et al.* 1995. Induction of apoptosis in mature T cells by tumor necrosis factor. Nature **377:** 348–351.
9. BODMER, J.L., N. HOLLER, *et al.* 2000. TRAIL receptor-2 signals apoptosis through FADD and caspase-8. Nat. Cell Biol. **2:** 241–243.
10. LENARDO, M. 1991. Interleukin-2 programs mouse alpha beta T lymphocytes for apoptosis. Nature **353:** 858–861.
11. SCAFFIDI, C., I. SCHMITZ, *et al.* 1999. The role of c-FLIP in modulation of CD95-induced apoptosis. J. Biol. Chem. **274:** 1541–1548.
12. GOLSTEIN P. & S. NAGATA. 1995. The Fas death factor. Science **267:** 1449–1456.
13. NAKAJIMA, H., P. GOLSTEIN & P.A. HENKART. 1995. The target cell nucleus is not required for cell-mediated granzyme- or Fas-based cytotoxicity. J. Exp. Med. **181:** 1905–1909.

14. SCHNEIDER, P. & J. TSCHOPP. 2000. Apoptosis induced by death receptors. Pharm. Acta Helv. **74:** 281–286.
15. SUZUKI, A., S. OBATA, *et al.* 2001. SADS: A new component of Fas-DISC is the accelerator for cell death signalling and is downregulated in patients with colon carcinoma. Nature Med. **7:** 88–93.
16. SATO, T., S. IRIE, *et al.* 1995. FAP-1: a protein tyrosine phosphatase that associates with Fas. Science **268:** 411–415.
17. KLUCK, R.M., E. BOSSY-VETZEL, *et al.* 1997. The release of cytochrome c from mitochondria: a primary site for Bcl-2 regulation of apoptosis. Science **275:** 1132–1136.
18. SUSIN, S.A., H.K. LORENZO, *et al.* 1999. Molecular characterization of mitochondrial apoptosis-inducing factor. Nature **397:** 441–446.
19. CHAI, J., C. DU, *et al.* 2000. Structural and biochemical basis of apoptotic activation by Smac/DIABLO. Nature **406:** 855–862.
20. REED, J.C. 1998. Bcl-2 family proteins. Oncogene **17:** 3225–3236.
21. TALANIAN, R.V., K.D. BRADY & V.L. CRYNS. 2000. Caspases as targets for anti-inflammatory and anti-apoptotic drug discovery. J. Med. Chem. **43:** 3351–3371.
22. YIN, X.M. 2000. Bid, a critical mediator for apoptosis induced by the activation of Fas/TNF-R1 death receptors in hepatocytes J. Mol. Med. **78:** 203–211.
23. NAGATA, S. 1998. Human autoimmune lymphoproliferative syndrome, a defect in the apoptosis-inducing Fas receptor: a lesson from the mouse model. J. Hum. Genet. **43:** 2–8.
24. LINDSTEN, T., A.J. ROSS, *et al.* 2000. The combined functions of proapoptotic Bcl-2 family members Bak and Bax are essential for normal development of multiple tissues. Mol. Cell. **6:** 1389–1399.
25. GOUGEON, M.L., H. LECOEUR, *et al.* 1996. Programmed cell death in peripheral lymphocytes from HIV-infected persons. J. Immunol. **156:** 3509–3520.
26. SLOAND, E.M., N.S. YOUNG, *et al.* 1997. Role of Fas ligand and receptor in the mechanism of T-cell depletion in acquired immunodeficiency syndrome: effect of CD4$^+$ T cell depletion and human immunodeficiency virus replication. Blood **89:** 1357–1363.
27. HOSAKA, N., N. OYAIZU, *et al.* 1998. Membrane and soluble forms of Fas (CD95) and Fas ligand in peripheral blood mononuclear cells and in plasma fom human immunodeficiency virus–infected persons. J. Infect. Dis. **178:** 1030–1039.
28. ZANGERLE, R., H. GALLATI, *et al.* 1994. Tumor necrosis factor alpha and soluble tumor necrosis factor receptors in individuals with human immunodeficiency virus infection. Immunol. Lett. **41:** 229–234.
29. LIEGLER, T.J., W. YONEMOTO, *et al.* 1998. Diminished spontaneous apoptosis in lymphocytes from human immunodeficiency virus-infected long-term progressors. J. Infect. Dis. **178:** 669–679.
30. GENINI, D., D. SHEETER, *et al.* 2001. HIV induces lymphocyte apoptosis by a p53-initiated mitochondrial-mediated mechanism. FASEB J. **15:** 5–6.
31. GRAZIOZI, C., K.R. GANTT, *et al.* 1996. Kinetics of HIV DNA RNA synthesis during primary HIV infection. Proc. Natl. Acad. Sci. USA **93:** 6505–6509.
32. ZEHER, M., P. SZODORAY, *et al.* 1999. Correlation of increased susceptibility to apoptosis of CD4$^+$ T cells correlates with lymphocyte activation and activity of disease in patients with primary Sjögren's syndrome. Arthritis Rheum. **42:** 1673–1681.
33. KATSIKIS, P.D., M.E GARCIA-OJEDA, *et al.* 1997. Interleukin-1 converting enzyme-like protease involvement in Fas-induced and activation-induced peripheral T-cell apoptosis in HIV infection: TNF-related apoptosis-inducing ligand can mediate activation-induced T-cell death in HIV infection. J. Exp. Med. **186:** 1365–1372.
34. SZONDY, Z., H. LECOEUR, *et al.* 1998. All-trans retinoic acid inhibition of anti-CD3 induced T cell apoptosis in HIV-infection mostly concerns CD4 T lymphocytes and is mediated via regulation of FAS-L expression. J. Infect. Dis. **178:** 1288–1298.
35. DAVIS, M.M. & P.J. BJORLMAN. 1988. T cell antigen receptor genes and T cell recognition. Nature **334:** 395–402.
36. HUGIN, A., M. VACCHIO & H. MORSE. 1991. A virus-encoded superantigen in a retrovirus-induced immunodeficiency syndrome of mice. Science **252:** 424.

37. IMBERTI, L., A. SOTTINI, et al. Selective depletion in HIV infection of T cells that bear specific T cell receptor V beta sequences. Science **254:** 860.
38. BANDA, N.K., J. BERNIER, et al. 1992. Crosslinking CD4 by human immunodeficiency virus gp120 primes T cells for activation-induced apoptosis. J. Exp. Med. **76:** 1099–1106.
39. OYAIZU, N., T.W. MCCLOSKEY, et al. 1994. Crosslinking of CD4 molecules upregulates Fas expression in lymphocytes by inducing interferon-γ and tumor necrosis-α secretion. Blood **84:** 2622–2631.
40. BARTZ, S.R. & M. EMERMAN. 1999. Human immunodeficiency virus type tat induces apoptosis and increases sensitivity to apoptotic signals by upregulating FLICE/caspase-8. J. Virol. **73:** 1956–1963.
41. LI-WEBER, M., O. LAUR, et al. 2000. T cell activation-induced and HIV tat-enhanced CD95 (Apo1/Fas) ligand transcription involves NFκB. Eur. J. Immunol. **30:** 661–670.
42. ZAULI, G., D. GIBELINI, et al. 1999. Human immunodeficiency virus type 1 Nef protein sensitizes CD4$^+$ T lymphoid to apoptosis via functional upregulation of the CD95/CD95 ligand pathway. Blood **93:** 1000–1010.
43. OKADA, H., R. TAKEI & M. TASHIRO. 1997. HIV-1 Nef protein-induced apoptotic cytolysis of a broad spectrum of uninfected human blood cells independently of CD95(Fas). FEBS Lett. **414:** 603–606.
44. PHENIX, B.N., B. BECKETT, et al. 1999. HIV protease induces apoptosis in HIV infected T cells through activation of caspase 8. Eight Annual Canadian Conference of HIV/AIDS Research. Victoria British Columbia Abstract 409.
45. STRACK, P.R., M. WEST FREY, et al. 1996. Apoptosis mediated by HIV protease is preceded by cleavage of bcl-2. Proc. Natl. Acad. Sci. USA **93:** 9571–9576.
46. BADLEY A.D., J.A. MCELHINNY, et al. 1996. Upregulation of Fas ligand expression by human immunodeficiency virus in human macrophages mediates apoptosis of uninfected T lymphocytes. J. Virol. **70:** 199–206.
47. COTTREZ, F., F. MANCA, et al. 1997. Priming of human CD4$^+$ antigen-specific T cells to undergo apoptosis by HIV-infected monocytes. J. Clin. Invest. **99:** 257–266.
48. KAMEOKA, M., S. SUZUKI, et al. 1997. Exposure of resting peripheral blood T cells to HIV-1 particles generates 25+ killer cells in a small subset, leading to induction of apoptosis of bystander cells. Int. Immunol. **9:** 1453–1462.
49. KOJIMA, H., K. ESHIMA, et al. Leukocyte function-associated antigen-1 dependent lysis of Fas$^+$ (CD95$^+$/APO-1$^+$) innocent bystanders by antigen-specific CD8$^+$ CTL. J. Immunol. **158:** 2728–2734.
50. DOCKRELL, D.H., A.D. BADLEY, et al. 1998. The expression of Fas ligand by macrophages and its upregulation by human immunodeficiency virus infection. J. Clin. Invest. **101:** 1105–1109.
51. STARC, T.J., S.E. LIPSHULTZ, et al. 1999. Cardiac complications in children with human immunodeficiency virus infection. Pediatric Pulmonary and Cardiac Complications of Vertically Transmitted HIV Infection (P^{2}C^2 HIV) Study Group, National Heart, Lung, and Blood Institute. Pediatrics **104:** e14.
52. MILEI, J., D. GRANA, et al. 1998. Cardiac involvement in acquired immunodeficiency syndrome—a review to push action. The Committee for the Study of Cardiac Involvement in AIDS. Clin. Cardiol. **7:** 465–472.
53. FEUERSTEIN, G.Z. & P.R.YOUNG. 2000. Apoptosis in cardiac diseases: stress- and mitogen-activated signaling pathways. Cardiovasc. Res. **45:** 560–569.
54. BÖHLER, T., J. WALCHER, et al. 1999. Early effects of combination antiretroviral therapy on activation, apoptosis and regeneration of T cells in HIV-1 infected children and adolescents. AIDS **13:** 779–789.
55. PHENIX, B.N., J.B. ANGEL, et al. 2000. Decreased HIV-associated T cell apoptosis by HIV protease inhibitors. AIDS Res. Hum. Retroviruses **16:** 559–567.
56. SZEGEZDI, E., Z. SZONDY, et al. 2000. Apoptosis linked in vivo regulation of the tissue transglutaminase gene promoter. Cell Death Differ. **7:** 1225–1233.
57. AMENDOLA, A., M.L. GOUGEON, et al. 1996. Induction of "tissue" transglutaminase in HIV pathogenesis: evidence for high rate of apoptosis of CD4$^+$ T lymphocytes and accessory cells in lymphoid tissues. Proc. Natl. Acad. Sci. USA **93:** 11057–11062.

58. D'AMATO, M., C. IANNICOLA, *et al.* 1999. Mapping and sequencing of the murine 'tissue' transglutaminase (Tgm2) gene: absence of mutations in MRLlpr/lpr mice. Cell Death Differ. **6:** 216–217.
59. LEDRU, E., N. CHIRSTEFF, *et al.* 2000. Alteration of tumor necrosis factor-α T cell homeostasis following potent antiretroviral therapy: contribution to the development of human immunodeficiency virus-associated lipodystrophy syndrome. Blood **95:** 3191–3198.
60. CHINNAIYAN, A.M., C. WOFFENDIN, *et al.* 1997. The inhibition of proapoptotic ICE-like proteases enhances HIV replication. Nat. Med. **3:** 333–337.
61. GARBE, A., J. BUCK, *et al.* 992. Retinoids are important cofactors in T cell activation. J. Exp. Med. **176:** 109–117.
62. CHAMBON, P. 1994. The retinoid signaling pathway: molecular and genetic analyses. Semin. Cell. Biol. **5:** 115–125.
63. HEYMAN, R.A., D.J. MANGELSDORF, *et al.* 1992. 9-*cis* retinoic acid is a high affinity ligand for the retinoic acid X receptor. Cell **68:** 397–406.
64. URBACH, J. & R.R. RANDO. 1994. Isomerization of all-*trans*-retinoic acid to 9-*cis*-retinoic acid. Biochem. J. **299:** 459–465.
65. ZHANG, X.K. & J. LEHMANN, *et al.* Homodimer formation of retinoid X receptor induced by 9-*cis* retinoic acid. Nature **358:** 587–591.
66. PERLMANN, T. & L. JANSSON. 1995. A novel pathway for vitamin A signalling mediated by RXR heterodimerisation with NGFI-B and NURR1. Genes Dev. **9:** 769–782.
67. YU, V.C., C. DELSERT, *et al.* 1991. RXR beta: a corregulator that enhances binding of retinoic acid, thyroid hormone, and vitamin D receptors to their cognate response element. Cell **67:** 1251–1266.
68. YANG, Y., V.S. VACCHIO, *et al.* 1993. 9-*cis* retinoic acid inhibits activation driven apoptosis: implications for retinoid X receptor involvement in thymocyte development. Proc. Natl. Acad. Sci. USA **90:** 6170–6174.
69. YANG, Y., J. BAILEY, *et al.* 1995. Retinoic acid inhibition of ex vivo human immunodeficiency virus-associated apoptosis of peripheral blood cells. Proc. Natl. Acad. Sci. USA **92:** 3051–3055.
70. TÓTH, R., E. SZEGEZDI, *et al.* 2001. Activation-induced apoptosis and cell surface expression of Fas (CD95) ligand are reciprocally regulated by retinoc acid receptor alpha and gamma and involve nur77 in T cells. Eur. J. Immunol. In press.
71. SZONDY, Z., U. REICHERT & L. FÉSÜS. 1998. Apoptosis regulation of T lymphocytes by retinoic acids: implications for interplay between RAR and RXR receptors in regulating T lymphocyte death. Cell Death Diffen. **5:** 4–10.
72. WORONICZ, J.D., B. CALNAN, *et al.* 1994. Requirement for the orphan steroid receptor *nur77* in apoptosis of T cell hybridomas. Nature **367:** 277–281.
73. KANG, H.J., M.R. SONG, *et al.* 2000. Retinoic acid and its receptors repress expression and transactivation function of nur77: a possible mechanism for the inhibition by retinoic acid. Exp. Cell. Res. **256:** 545–554.
74. YOUNES, A., M. CRISTOFANILI, *et al.* 2000. Evidence with 9-*cis* retinoic acid in patients with relapsed and refractory non-Hodgkin's lymphoma. Leukemia & Lymphoma **40:** 79–85.

"Tissue" Transglutaminase Expression in HIV-Infected Cells

An Enzyme with an Antiviral Effect?

ALESSANDRA AMENDOLA,[a,b] CARLO RODOLFO,[c] ANTONINO DI CARO,[a] FABIOLA CICCOSANTI,[b] LAURA FALASCA,[b] AND MAURO PIACENTINI[b,c]

[a]Laboratory of Virology, "Lazzaro Spallanzani"—IRCCS, Rome, Italy

[b]Laboratory of Cell Biology and Electronic Microscopy, "Lazzaro Spallanzani"—IRCCS, Rome, Italy

[c]Department of Biology, University of Rome "Tor Vergata," Rome, Italy

ABSTRACT: The cytopathic effect of HIV has been shown to be associated with the induction of apoptosis and the inhibition of proliferation of T cells. However, the cellular and molecular mechanisms at the basis of the dramatic immune cell loss caused by HIV in patients suffering from acquired immunodeficient syndrome (AIDS), are not yet fully established. We demonstrated that "tissue" transglutaminase (tTG) gene expression is induced in the immune system of seropositive individuals (peripheral blood mononuclear cells and lymph nodes). tTG is a multifunctional protein involved in a variety of fundamentally important cellular functions, in addition to cell death by apoptosis. The presence of high tTG levels in immune-competent cells of HIV+ persons might exert an important role in HIV-infection by influencing viral production. We propose that, in addition to its multiple functions, tTG might interfere with HIV replication by altering the viral mRNA trafficking between the nucleus and the cytoplasm. This effect might be due to its specific interaction with eIF5A, a cellular partner of HIV Rev protein, which is essential for HIV replication in immune-competent cells. Given the presence of high tTG levels in HIV+ individuals, it would be of interest to pursue the potential role of this multifunctional protein in the development of strategies aimed at the pharmacologic regulation of HIV production.

KEYWORDS: HIV replication; cell death; apoptosis; tTG; retinoic acid; tTG antisense

DIRECT AND INDIRECT MECHANISMS OF HIV-INDUCED T CELL DEPLETION

Infection with HIV leads to a progressive decline in immune functions in parallel with a concomitant depletion in CD4 T cells. The resulting progressive immune dysfunction renders infected persons susceptible to opportunistic infections and malignancies, ultimately leading to death. Despite years of investigation, the reason(s) for

Address for correspondence: Dr. Mauro Piacentini, Laboratory of Cell Biology and Electronic Microscopy, "Lazzaro Spallanzani"—IRCCS, Via Portuense, 292, 00149 Rome, Italy. Voice: (39) 6 55 170 429.
mauro.piacentini@uniroma2.it

108

the killing of CD4 T cells in HIV[+] patients remains controversial. *Direct* and *indirect* mechanisms have been suggested, but the relative contributions of each of these mechanisms leading to CD4 T cell depletion *in vivo* remain unknown.

Several lines of evidence indicate that in the AIDS pathogenesis the rate of CD4 T cell depletion directly correlates to the rate of HIV-1 production. Massive viral replication and budding of HIV may mediate the depletion of CD4 T lymphocytes by leading to disruption of the host cell membrane (cytopathic effects, CPE).[1] Furthermore, the accumulation of unintegrated HIV DNA, HIV virions or proteins can be directly cytotoxic or cytostatic, leading to impaired cellular homeostasis and death.[2,3] Another mechanism by which HIV may contribute to CD4 T cell decline is the formation of multinucleate giant cells (syncytia),[4,5] because of fusion of HIV[+] cells with other infected or uninfected CD4 cells. However, despite *in vitro* observations, infected multinucleated cells are observed infrequently in tissues during HIV disease, thus suggesting that cell-cell fusion may not be the predominant cytopathic mechanism *in vivo*.[1] Another type of HIV-induced cytopathology results in the death of single cells that is predominant in acutely infected peripheral blood mononuclear cells (PBMC).[6,7] The degenerative changes in HIV[+] cells undergoing lysis resemble the death process of necrosis[7]: generalized loss of membrane integrity and collapse of mitochondrial cristae.[8] HIV-specific immune responses may also directly account for CD4 T cell depletion. Antibodies directed against HIV-encoded gp41 and/or gp120 may bind the surface of infected cells expressing HIV proteins and elicit antibody-dependent cell-mediated cytotoxicity or complement-mediated direct destruction of the infected cell.[9] Similarly, cytotoxic T lymphocytes and/or NK cells may directly kill HIV[+] cells.[10]

In addition to *direct* mechanisms of CD4 T cell depletion, several *indirect* mechanisms have been proposed. HIV gp120 and gp41 share structural homology with the major histocompatibility complex (MHC) class II antigens.[11] Therefore, antibodies specific for gp41 or gp120 could cross-react with host HLA class II molecules to generate an inappropriate allogeneic immune response and indirectly cause depletion of MHC class II-bearing cells (including CD4 T cells). In fact, such cross-reacting antibodies were detected in the sera of patients infected with HIV.[11]

PROGRAMMED CELL DEATH (APOPTOSIS) IN AIDS

HIV-induced cell death has been shown to occur by apoptosis or programmed cell death (PCD).[12-15] Although the exact role of apoptosis in the pathogenesis of HIV infection remains to be defined, deregulated apoptosis is considered to be the major contributor to the depletion of immune-competent cells *in vivo*. In HIV[+] individuals, circulating CD4 and CD8 T cells are prone to apoptosis compared with T cells from uninfected donors;[14,15] activation of apoptosis has been demonstrated in lymph nodes of infected persons.[16,17] Apoptosis occurs in both HIV[+] and uninfected T cells,[18] but the mechanism(s) by which T cells are primed for apoptosis is not completely known. The perturbation of the CD4 T cell receptor, due to gp120-CD4 interaction, might be responsible for CD4[+] T cell anergy and/or the induction of apoptosis as a consequence of incomplete signal transduction.[19,20] Furthermore, following HIV infection, the predominance of an activated T cell phenotype, elevated expression of Fas/CD95 and TNF receptor, and increases in T cell-derived Fas ligand may contribute to the activation of induced cell death.[21] The abnormal expression of the CD95/CD95L system may also play an important role in the induction of apoptosis in immune-competent cells.[22,23]

A PRO-APOPTOTIC ENZYME: "TISSUE" TRANSGLUTAMINASE (tTG)

Physiological cell death is invariably associated with the induction and the activation of the Ca^{2+}-dependent enzyme "tissue" transglutaminase (tTG).[24–26] The tTG *gene* induction, followed by its Ca^{2+}-dependent activation, leads to the formation of highly cross-linked intracellular protein polymers, which play a fundamental role in the induction of the irreversible structural changes featuring cells dying by apoptosis.[26–29]

The transglutaminase family includes several intracellular and extracellular enzymes that catalyze Ca^{2+}-dependent reactions resulting in the post-translational modification of proteins at the level of glutamine and lysine residues.[26,30–32] This post-translational modification of proteins leads to the formation of the ε(γ-glutamyl)lysine cross-links and/or to the covalent incorporation of polyamines into proteins.[26,28,30–32] Di-amines and polyamines can also participate in crosslinking reactions through the formation of N,N-bis(γ-glutamyl)polyamine bonds.[26,28,30–32] The formation of these covalent cross-links leads to oligomerization of substrate proteins, which become highly resistant to mechanical and chemical attack.[33]

In vivo, the enzyme encoded by tTG gene is undetectable in the majority of cells, with the exception of a few cell types (endothelial cells, smooth muscle cells, and mesangial cells) in which this gene is constitutively expressed. It has been established in various experimental systems that tTG is one of the few genes specifically induced during apoptosis *in vivo.*[34–36] In fact, as a consequence of the onset of apoptosis, mRNA encoding for tTG and its protein are produced.[34] The accumulation of tTG protein inside the cell is not always associated with the activation of its cross-linking activity, since the intracellular tTG cross-linking activity is inhibited by GTP and nitric oxide.[26,37] The onset of the apoptotic program and tTG activation requires sustained high levels of calcium.[26] In viable cells, free cytosolic calcium is normally present at low levels and consequently the tTG protein is inactive in its G-protein configuration, with a further inhibition of the cross-linking activity.[38,39] During activation of programmed cell death, the increase of free cytosolic calcium from intracellular reservoir, induces Ca^{2+}-dependent activation of tTG.

Several lines of evidence indicate that tTG synthesis is not only associated with apoptosis, but in some cell types may also play an important role in the killing process.[28,35,40] Overexpression of tTG in human neuroblastoma SK-N-BE(2) cells, L929, and NIH 3T3 fibroblasts enhances their susceptibility to apoptosis.[28,40] Human neuroblastoma cells overexpressing tTG showed a large reduction in their growth capacity, not only *in vitro* but also when xenografted into SCID mice.[40,41] Consistent with this, transfection of these neuroblastoma cells or human promonocytic U937 cells with an expression vector containing a segment of the human tTG cDNA in the *antisense* orientation resulted in a decrease of both spontaneous and retinoic acid-induced apoptosis.[40,42] Despite these data, the precise position of the tTG in the cascade of events leading to establishment of the death phenotype has not yet been fully clarified.[37]

tTG IN HIV-INFECTED INDIVIDUALS

Previous studies indicate that both CD4 and CD8 T cells, obtained from HIV[+] individuals, undergo apoptosis when cultured *in vitro* in the absence of growth factors or when stimulated with bacteria superantigen, thus suggesting that a large number of preapoptotic T lymphocytes are present in the peripheral blood of HIV[+] individuals.[14,43,44] Resting T cells do not express tTG; however, upon cross-linking of the CD4 receptor by gp120 protein of HIV, human T cell clones synthesize the protein.[45] The induction of the enzyme precedes the appearance of the apoptotic phenotype, which occurs only when preapoptotic cells receive additional CD3-transduced signals and following a sustained increase in the intracellular free Ca^{2+} levels.[43–45] These findings are in line with the data showing increased tTG expression both in peripheral blood mononuclear cells (PBMCs) and in lymph nodes of a large cohort of HIV[+] individuals.[46] With respect to seronegative donors, the PBMCs from HIV[+] individuals show a drastic increase (7- to 8-fold) in the number of cells expressing the tTG gene. The percentage of tTG-positive mononuclear cells in asymptomatic and AIDS patients *in vivo* matches that of apoptotic cells detected by DNA fragmentation analysis, after 24 h of culturing PBMCs from HIV[+] individuals.[46] These findings confirmed that extensive priming for apoptosis takes place in PBMCs from seropositive individuals, and that tTG expression represent a good marker of the preapoptotic state *in vivo*.[46] The phenotype analysis of tTG-positive PBMCs from HIV[+] individuals demonstrated that both CD4 and CD8 T cells and monocytes express intense staining with specific antibody direct to tTG protein. It has been calculated that approximately 80% of the total tTG-positive cells detected in HIV[+] individuals were CD4 T cells, and about 10% of tTG-positive PBMCs were CD8 T cells and monocytes.[46]

The tTG expression observed in peripheral blood cells reflects a similar pattern in lymphoid tissues. The tTG antibody markedly stained the paracortical and interfollicular regions, as well as the apical light zone of the follicle of HIV-1 and HIV-1/HIV-2-coinfected lymph nodes. The accumulation of tTG protein was observed not only in T cells, but also in a large number of polymorphic cells, syncytia and, to a lower extent, in the germinal centers. By performing *in situ* staining with TUNEL technique, it was demonstrated that about 50% of tTG-positive cells in the HIV[+] lymph nodes were also positive for the DNA fragmentation.[46] The observation that tTG co-localized with DNA fragmentation in a large proportion of accessory cells of HIV[+] lymph nodes, confirmed that different types of immune-competent cells undergo apoptosis. In addition to macrophages, varying numbers of syncytia, lymphocytes, and follicular dendritic cells stained by the tTG antibody were detected in HIV[+] lymph nodes.[46]

A positive correlation between *tTG* expression and the state of activation of the immune system has been suggested. A threefold higher number of tTG-positive cells was detected in the HIV[+] lymph nodes showing histological signs of activation (follicular hyperplasia), thus indicating that the enzyme accumulates specifically in activated immune cells.[46] This implies that *tTG* expression, as proposed for the induction of apoptosis, does not correlate with the stage of the disease and viral burden, but is a consequence of the pathological activation of the immune system during infection.[16]

Macrophages play an important role in the pathogenesis and progression of the HIV-induced disease, representing the major reservoir of HIV in lymph nodes and extra-lymphoid tissues at all stages of the disease.[47] Despite various efforts, the characterization of the factor(s) allowing *in vivo* and *in vitro* persistently infected macrophages to overcome the cytopathic effect of HIV has been unsuccessful. It has been recently demonstrated that the neurotrophin *nerve growth factor* (NGF) is an autocrine factor actively produced by HIV+ macrophages. High levels of NGF in supernatants of HIV+ monocytes/macrophages are essential for their survival. In fact, exposure to neutralizing anti-NGF antibody activates the apoptotic signal in these cells.[48] Thus, it has been suggested that NGF is a survival factor that possesses the ability to rescue monocytes/macrophages from the cytopathic effects caused by HIV infection.[48] It is interesting to note that about 40–60% of tTG-positive cells detected in the HIV+ lymph nodes were macrophages.[46] Similarly to lymph nodes of HIV+ individuals, alveolar macrophages, obtained from the lavage of the lung from HIV+ patients with pulmonary tuberculosis (TB), display high levels of the tTG in their cytoplasm and DNA fragmentation.[49]

A NEW MARKER OF APOPTOTIC RATE

We and other groups have previously demonstrated that an increased apoptotic rate in any organ/tissue under physiological or pathological conditions, is followed by an elevation of the free circulation ε(γ-glutamyl)lysine isodipeptide.[50,51] The ε(γ-glutamyl)lysine isodipeptide results from the degradation of tTG-catalyzed protein cross-links polymers in protein, which are subsequently degraded to single aminoacids in phagolysosomes after engulfment of apoptotic bodies by neighboring cells.[26,34,52] However, the ε(γ-glutamyl)lysine bonds are resistant to proteases, and intact free isodipeptides are released from the phagocyte upon degradation of the apoptotic cells.[26,34,52]

During HIV-induced disease, plasma levels of ε(γ-glutamyl)lysine isodipeptide are significantly and progressively enhanced, as a consequence of the *in vivo* induction of tTG gene and the active participation of the enzyme in the biochemical pathway of apoptosis. The number of tTG-positive PBMCs reaches a plateau in the asymptomatic phase, whereas the plasma concentration of ε(γ-glutamyl)lysine isodipeptide continues to increase, reaching its maximal concentration in parallel with the massive disruption of tTG-positive cells observed in the lymphoid tissues in late stages of the disease.[46] Conversely, in human plasma of HIV-negative donors, a negligible amount of the physiological level of the isodipeptide is constantly present in the blood, deriving from the basal rate of apoptosis under physiological conditions and from the plasmin degradation of the XIIIa-catalyzed cross-linking of fibrin.[50,52] For these reasons, the ε(γ-glutamyl)lysine isodipeptide measurement in the plasma might be a useful marker to quantify the apoptotic rate *in vivo* in biological systems.

To our knowledge, the ε(γ-glutamyl)lysine isodipeptide detection is currently the only biological marker by which the total body apoptotic rate can be monitored.

THE POTENTIAL ANTIVIRAL ROLE OF tTG PROTEIN

The induction of tTG in HIV[+] immune-competent cells undergoing apoptosis[46,49] suggests that tTG may play a role in reducing the production and/or spreading of viral particles.[53,54]

Evidence supporting this role of tTG is provided by an *in vitro* model, in which HIV[+] human promonocytic U937 cell line is treated with all-*trans*-retinoic acid (RA). RA treated U937 cells are blocked in the G1 phase and undergo differentiation.[38,55] In parallel with these events, RA treatment induces tTG gene and synthesis of the enzyme (see FIGURE 1). Upon RA treatment, U937 cells beware "primed" to undergo apoptosis and are particularly susceptible to programmed cell death induced by different stimuli (calcium ionophore A23187, calphostin C, staurosporine and cyclo-heximide).[42] In chronically HIV-1 IIIB-infected U937 cell line, RA exerts a potent suppressive effects on HIV expression, as previously described.[56,57] Here we show

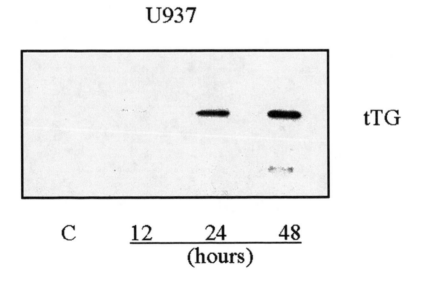

FIGURE 1. Induction of tTG by RA in U937 cells. Western blot analysis of tTG protein was performed in U937 cells cultured in 10% FCS, after exposure to 1μM RA (SIGMA Chemicals, USA) for 12 h, 24 h, and 48 h. After each treatment interval, aliquots of total protein extracts (50 μg), were run on 7.5% SDS-PAGE and electroblotted overnight at 4°C onto nitrocellulose membrane. tTG positive bands were revealed with monoclonal antibody specific for tTG (NeoMarkers, USA) and detection was achieved using the appropriate secondary antibody (goat anti-mouse; Bio-Rad, USA) conjugated horseradish peroxidase and by enhanced ECL chemiluminescence detection system (Amersham, UK). Upon RA treatment, U937 cells are particularly susceptible to programmed cell death.

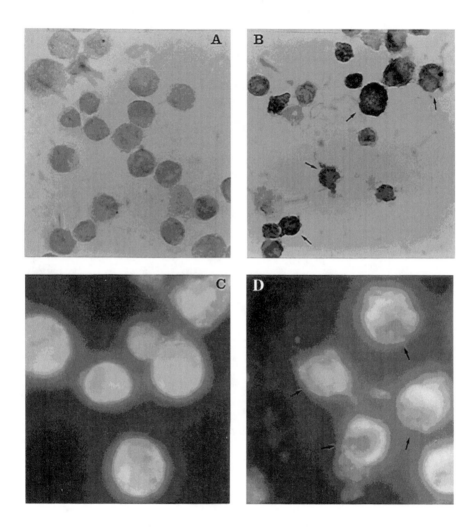

FIGURE 2. Characterization of tTG and HIV viral proteins in chronically HIV-1 IIIB-infected U937 cell line. Cells were grown in 10% FCS in the presence of RA 1μM (SIGMA Chemicals, USA) for 48 h and, after treatment, fixed in 2.5% paraformaldeyde. Cells were stained by using monoclonal antibody direct to tTG (NeoMarkers, USA) and revealed with AEC chromogen. Counterstaining was performed with hematoxylin. Normally, chronically HIV-1 IIIB-infected U937 cells do not synthesize tTG (**A**). After 48 h culture in the presence of 1μM RA (SIGMA Chemicals, USA), tTG protein accumulates in the cytoplasm of 90% of cells (**B**). The immunofluorescence staining of the chronically HIV-1 IIIB-infected U937 cells with anti-HIV human serum (**C**) showed a lower presence of viral proteins on the cell surface of all cells after 48 h of treatment with RA (**D**).

that the RA-mediated inhibition of viral replication strongly correlates with higher levels of tTG protein induced in the cells by RA treatment. After 48 h of culture in the presence of RA, chronically HIV-1 IIIB-infected U937 cells accumulate tTG protein in the cytoplasm (see FIGURE 2B) and the immunofluorescence staining of the cells with anti-HIV human serum showed the presence of lower levels of viral proteins on the cell surface of all cells, thus confirming a generalized reduction of HIV replication (FIG. 2D). The effect mediated by RA is time and dose dependent. Analysis of viral production, performed by quantitative detection of the p24 core antigen of HIV in cell culture supernatants, confirmed a dramatic decrease of viral protein production in treated cultures (see FIGURE 3).

These data seems to support the hypothesis that tTG may play an important role in cells infected by viruses; by reducing viral production, it might limit virus-specific protein synthesis. Consistent with this view, it has been recently demonstrated that there is a very efficient interaction between tTG and the eukaryotic initiation factor 5A *in vivo*.[58] The tTG-eIF5A interaction is promoted by RA, Ca^{2+} and Mg^{2+} treatment when tTG is in its cross-linking configuration and is not detected when tTG is

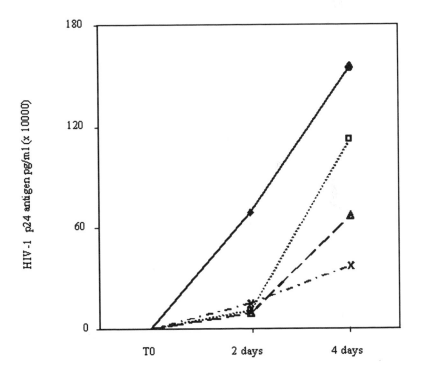

FIGURE 3. Effect of RA treatment upon HIV-1 production in chronically HIV-1 IIIB-infected U937 cells. A dramatic inhibition of virus production was detected in cells exposed to RA 0.2μM (□), 1μM (△), and 5μM (×) for 3 and 6 days. HIV-1 p24 gag antigen production was evaluated in supernatants by commercially available ELISA kit (Vironos-tika, Organon Technika, USA). The figure represents a typical experiment of three.

pre-loaded with GTP.[58] The eukaryotic initiation factor 5A (eIF5A) is an essential protein regulating cell viability through effects on protein synthesis and nuclear RNA export.[59] Furthermore, eIF5A is one cellular co-factor required for the nuclear RNA export, mediated by the HIV-1 *Rev* regulatory protein and HTLV-1 RNA *Rex* export factor.[59–61] HIV-1 *Rev* is an essential factor for the expression of viral structural proteins and HIV replication. HIV-1 *Rev* activity mediates the translocation of viral mRNAs from the nucleus to the cytoplasm by interacting with a *cis*-acting RNA target [the Rev response element (RRE)] present in all unspliced viral transcripts.[62] The incompletely spliced viral mRNAs accumulate in the cytoplasm to serve as templates for protein synthesis or as viral genomes.[59,60] To mediate the transport of viral mRNAs across the nuclear envelope, the *Rev* activation domain interacts with host cell proteins that are involved in nuclear-cytoplasmic translocation. Various cellular proteins which appear to be specific binding partners of the *Rev* activation domain have been described, including the eukaryotic initiation factor 5A,[61] the nucleoporin-like protein hRIP/Rab,[63,64] and nuclear export factor CRM1, which appears to be a general nuclear export signal receptor.[65,66] Distinct nonfunctional mutants of eIF5A, which inhibit the nuclear export of Rev protein and thereby HIV-1 replication in human T cells, have been described.[59,67] Moreover, microinjection studies have demonstrated that antibodies directed against eIF5A specifically block the nucleocytoplasmic viral mRNAs translocation mediated by HIV-1 *Rev* and HTLV-1 *Rex* in somatic cells, indicating that eIF5A is an essential element of a specific nucleocytoplasmic export pathway.[68,69]

Taken together, these data raise interesting questions about the mechanisms by which tTG might influence viral production in HIV$^+$ immune-competent cells. One interesting possibility is that tTG might regulate the HIV-specific protein synthesis and RNA trafficking by sequestering eIF5A. In fact, when tTG is in a GDP-bound state, it is able to bind eIF5A and maintain eIF5A in the cytoplasm. By this action, tTG could prevent the interaction of eIF5A with the other proteins involved in protein synthesis and RNA trafficking between the nucleus and the cytoplasm, thus consequently limiting viral production in HIV$^+$ cells. Therefore, the induction of the tTG gene may effectively be a natural and non-specific mechanism of host defense, aimed to reduce viral spreading from infected cells to neighboring cells and tissues. Preliminary results, obtained by using chronically HIV-1 IIIB-infected U937 cells in which tTG gene expression is limited by transfection with tTG antisense vector, show that, in absence of tTG, viral production is significantly higher with respect to the wild type chronically HIV-1 IIIB-infected U937 cells. Thus, our results seem to support the hypothesis that tTG induction may act as a self-limiting mechanism of the host to limit viral replication.

Defining the role of tTG in HIV-induced programmed cell death *in vivo* might be useful for developing anti-HIV strategies based on modulation of tTG activity. New protocols of anti-HIV gene therapy designed to block essential HIV co-factors of host cells could be powerful instruments in the fight to reduce the loss of the immune cells and prolong the life of AIDS sufferers.

ACKNOWLEDGMENTS

This work was partially supported by Ricerca Corrente e Finalizzato Project from Ministery of Health, Italian AIDS Program from ISS and EU Program.

REFERENCES

1. PANTALEO, G., C. GRAZIOSI & A.S. FAUCI. 1993. New concepts in the immunopathogenesis of human immunodeficiency virus infection. N. Engl. J. Med. **328:** 327–335.
2. ROSENBERG, Z. & A.S. FAUCI. 1991. Immunopathogenesis of HIV infection. FASEB J. **5:** 2382–2390.
3. FERMIN, C.D. & R.F. GARRY. 1992. Membrane alterations linked to early interactions of HIV with the cell surface. Virology **191:** 941–946.
4. SODROSKI, J., W.C. GOH, C. ROSEN, *et al.* 1986. Role of the HTLV-III/LAV envelope in syncytium formation and cytopathogenicity. Nature **322:** 470–474.
5. LIFSON J.D., G.R. REYES, M.S. MCGRATH, *et al.* 1986. AIDS retrovirus induced cytopathology: giant cell formation and involvement of CD4 antigen. Science **232:** 1123–1127.
6. SOMASUNDARAN, M. & H. ROBINSON. 1988. A major mechanism of HIV-induced cell killing does not involve cell fusion. J. Virol. **61:** 3114–3119.
7. PLYMALE, D.R., D.S. NG TANG, A.M. COMARDELLE, *et al.* 1999. Both necrosis and apoptosis contribute to HIV-1-induced killing of CD4 cells. AIDS **13:** 1827–1839.
8. CAO, J., I.W. PARK, *et al.* 1996. Molecular determinants of acute single-cell lysis by human immunodeficiency virus type 1. J. Virol. **70:** 1340–1354.
9. FAUCI, A.S., S.M. SCHNITTMAN, G. POLI, *et al.* 1991. NIH conference. Immunopathogenic mechanisms in human immunodeficiency virus (HIV) infection. Ann. Intern. Med. **114:** 678–693.
10. ROOS, M.T., J.M. LANGE, R.E. DE GOEDE, *et al.* 1992. Viral phenotype and immune response in primary human immunodeficiency virus type 1 infection. J. Infect. Dis. **165**(3): 427–432.
11. GOLDING, H., F.A. ROBEY, F.T. GATES, *et al.* 1988. Identification of homologous regions in human immunodeficiency virus I gp41 and human MHC class II beta 1 domain. I. Monoclonal antibodies against the gp41-derived peptide and patients' sera react with native HLA class II antigens, suggesting a role for autoimmunity in the pathogenesis of acquired immune deficiency syndrome. J. Exp. Med. **167:** 914–923.
12. LAURENT-CRAWFORF, A.G., B. KRUST, S. MULLER, *et al.* 1991. The cytopathic effect of HIV is associated with apoptosis. Virology **185:** 829–839.
13. TERAI, C., R.S. KORNBLUTH, C.D. PAUZA, *et al.* 1991. Apoptosis as a mechanism of cell death in cultured T lymphoblasts acutely infected with HIV-1. J. Clin. Invest. **87:** 1710–1715.
14. LEWIS, D.E., D.S. NG TANG, A. ADU-OPPONG, *et al.* 1994. Anergy and apoptosis in CD8$^+$ T cells from HIV-infected persons. J. Immunol. **153:** 412–420.
15. GOUGEON, M.L., H. LECOEUR, A. DULIOUST, *et al.* 1996. Programmed cell death in peripheral lymphocytes from HIV-infected persons. J. Immunol. **156:** 3509–3520.
16. MURO-CHACO, C.A., G. PANTALEO & A.S. FAUCI. 1995. Analysis of apoptosis in lymph nodes of HIV-infected persons. Intensity of apoptosis correlates with the general state of activation of the lymphoid tissue and not with stage of disease or viral burden. J. Immunol. **154:** 5555–5566.
17. FINKEL,T.H., G. TUDOR-WILLIAMS, N.K. BANDA, *et al.* 1995. Apoptosis occurs predominantly in bystander cells and not in productively infected cells of HIV- and SIV-infected lymph nodes. Nat. Med. **1:** 129–134.
18. FINKEL, T.H. & N.K. BANDA. 1994. Indirect mechanisms of HIV pathogenesis: how does HIV kill T cells? Curr. Opin. Immunol. **6:** 605–615.

19. AMEISEN, J.C., J. ESTAQUIER, T. IDZIOREK & F. DE BELS. 1995. Programmed cell death and AIDS pathogenesis: significance and potential mechanisms. Curr. Top. Microbiol. Immunol. **200:** 195–211.
20. GOUGEON, M.L. 1995. Chronic activation of the immune system in HIV infection: contribution to T cell apoptosis and V beta selective T cell anergy. Curr. Top. Microbiol. Immunol. **200:** 177–193.
21. BADLEY, A.D., D. DOCKRELL & C.V. PAYA. 1997. Apoptosis in AIDS. Adv. Pharmacol. **41:** 271–294.
22. WESTENDORP, M.O., R. FRANK, C. OCHSENBAUER, et al. 1995. Sensitization of T cells to CD95-mediated apoptosis by HIV-1 Tat and gp120. Nature **375:** 497–500.
23. KATSIKIS, P.D., E.S. WUNDERLICH, C.A. SMITH & L.A. HERZENBERG. 1995. Fas antigen stimulation induces marked apoptosis of T lymphocytes in human immunodeficiency virus-infected individuals. J. Exp. Med. **181:** 2029–2036.
24. PIACENTINI, M. 1995. Tissue transglutaminase: a candidate effector element of physiological cell death. Curr. Top. Microbiol. Immunol. **200:** 163–175.
25. WYLLIE, A.H. 1992. Apoptosis and the regulation of cell numbers in normal and neoplastic tissues: an overview. Cancer Metastasis Rev. **11:** 95–103.
26. FESUS, L., P.J.A. DAVIES & M. PIACENTINI. 1991. Apoptosis: molecular mechanism in programmed cell death. Eur. J. Cell Biol. **56:** 170–177.
27. PIACENTINI, M., L. FESUS, M.G. FARRACE, et al. 1991. The expression of "tissue" transglutaminase in two human cancer cell lines is related with the programmed cell death (apoptosis). Eur. J. Cell Biol. **54:** 246–254.
28. GENTILE, V., V. THOMAZY, M. PIACENTINI, et al. 1992. Expression of tissue transglutaminase in BALB-C 3T3 fibroblasts: effects on cellular morphology and adhesion. J. Cell Biol. **119:** 463–474.
29. KNIGHT, C.R.L., D. HAND, M. PIACENTINI & M. GRIFFIN. 1993. Characterization of the transglutaminase-mediated large molecular weight polymer from rat liver; its relationship to apoptosis. Eur. J. Cell Biol. **60:** 210–217.
30. GREENBERG, C.S., J. BIRCKBICHLER & R.H. RICE. 1992. Transglutaminases: multifunctional cross-linking enzymes that stabilize tissues. FASEB J. **5:** 3071–3077.
31. PIACENTINI, M., N. MARTINET, S. BENINATI & J.E. FOLK. 1988. Free and protein-conjugated polyamines in mouse epidermal cells. J. Biol. Chem. **263:** 3790–3794.
32. FOLK, J.E. 1980. Transglutaminases. Annu. Rev. Biochem. **49:** 517–531.
33. FESUS, L., V. THOMAZY, F. AUTUORI, et al. 1989. Apoptotic hepatocytes become insolubile in detergents and chaotropic agents as a result of transglutaminase action. FEBS Lett. **245:** 150–154.
34. PIACENTINI, M., P.J.A. DAVIES & L. FESUS. 1994. Tissue transglutaminase in cells undergoing apoptosis. In Apoptosis II: The Molecular Basis of Apoptosis in Disease. L.D. Tomei & F.O. Cope, Eds.: 143–165. Cold Spring Harbor Lab. Press. Cold Spring Harbor, NY.
35. PIREDDA, L., A. AMENDOLA, V. COLIZZI, et al. 1997. Lack of tissue transglutaminase protein cross-linking leads to leakage of macromolecules from dying cells: relationship to development of autoimmunity in MRLlpr/lpr mice. Cell Death Differ. **4:** 463–472.
36. NAGY, L., V.A. THOMAZY, R.A. HEYMAN & P.J.A. DAVIES. 1998. Retinoid-induced apoptosis in normal and neoplastic tissues. Cell Death Differ. **5:** 11–19.
37. MELINO, G. & M. PIACENTINI. 1998. 'Tissue' transglutaminase in cell death: a downstream or a multifunctional upstream effector? FEBS Lett. **430:** 59–63.
38. DEFACQUE, H., T. COMMES, V. CONTET, et al. 1995. Differentiation of U937 myelomonocytic cell line by all-trans retinoic acid and 1,25-dihydroxyvitamin D3: synergistic effects on tissue transglutaminase. Leukemia **9:** 1762–1767.
39. SINGH, U.S. & R.A. CERIONE. 1996. Biochemical effects of retinoic acid on GTP-binding protein/transglutaminases in HeLa cells. Stimulation of GTP-binding and transglutaminase activity, membrane association, and phosphatidylinositol lipid turnover. J. Biol. Chem. **271:** 27292–27298.
40. MELINO, G., M. ANNICHIARICO-PETRUZZELLI, L. PIREDDA, et al. 1994. Tissue transglutaminase and apoptosis: sense and antisense transfection studies in human neuroblastoma cells. Mol. Cell. Biol. **14:** 6584–6592.

41. PIACENTINI, M., L. PIREDDA, D. STORACE, *et al.* 1996. Differential growth of N- and S-type human neuroblastoma cells xenografted into SCID mice. Correlation with apoptosis. J. Pathol. **180:** 31–38.

42. OLIVERIO, S., A. AMENDOLA, C. RODOLFO, *et al.* 1999. Inhibition of tissue transglutaminase increases survival by preventing apoptosis. J. Biol. Chem. **274:** 34123–34128.

43. GOUGEON, M.L. & L. MONTAGNIER. 1993. Apoptosis in AIDS. Science **260:** 1269–1270.

44. MEYAARD, L., S.A. OTTO, R.R. JONKER, *et al.* 1992. Programmed death of T cells in HIV-1 infection. Science **257:** 217–219.

45. AMENDOLA, A., G. LOMBARDI, S. OLIVERIO, *et al.* 1994. HIV-1 gp120-dependent induction of apoptosis in antigen-specific human T cell clones is characterized by tissue transglutaminase expression and prevented by cyclosporin A. FEBS Lett. **339:** 258–264.

46. AMENDOLA, A., M.L. GOUGEON, F. POCCIA, *et al.* 1996. Induction of tissue transglutaminase in HIV pathogenesis: evidence for high rate of apoptosis of CD4+ T lymphocytes and accessory cells in lymphoid tissues. Proc. Natl. Acad. Sci. USA **93:** 11057–11062.

47. ORENSTEIN, J.M., C. FOX & S.M. WAHL. 1997. Macrophages as a source of HIV during opportunistic infections. Science **276:** 1857–1861.

48. GARACI, E., M.C. CAROLEO, L. ALOE, *et al.* 1999. Nerve growth factor is an autocrine factor essential for the survival of macrophages infected with HIV. Proc. Natl. Acad. Sci. USA **96:** 14013–14018.

49. PLACIDO, R., M. MANCINO, A. AMENDOLA, *et al.* 1997. Apoptosis of human monocytes/macrophages in *Mycobacterium tuberculosis* infection. J. Pathol. **181:** 31–38.

50. FESUS, L., E. TARCSA, N. KEDEI, *et al.* 1991. Degradation of cells dying by apoptosis leads to accumulation of ε(γ-glutamyl)lysine isopeptide in culture fluid and blood. FEBS Lett. **284:** 109–112.

51. HARSFALVI, J., E. TARCSA, M. UDVARDY, *et al.* 1992. Presence and possible origin of ε(γ-glutamyl)lysine isopeptide in human plasma. Thromb. Haemost. **67:** 60–62.

52. LORAND, L. & S.M. CONRAD. 1984. Transglutaminases. Mol. Cell. Biochem. **58:** 9–35.

53. BERGAMINI, A., M. CAPOZZI & M. PIACENTINI. 1994. Macrophage-colony stimulating factor (M-CSF) stimulation induces cell death in HIV-infected human monocytes. Immunol Lett. **42:** 35–40.

54. FRATAZZI, C., R.D. ARBEIT, C. CARINI & H.G. REMOLD. 1997. Programmed cell death of *Mycobacterium avium* serovar 4-infected human macrophages prevents the mycobacteria from spreading and induces mycobacterial growth inhibition by freshly added, uninfected macrophages. J. Immunol. **158:** 4320–4327.

55. HARRIS, P. & P. RALPH. 1985. Human leukemic models of myelomonocytic development: a review of the HL-60 and U937 cell lines. J. Leukoc. Biol. **37:** 407–422.

56. YAMAGUCHI, K., J.E. GROOPMAN & R.A. BYRN. 1994. The regulation of HIV by retinoic acid correlates with cellular expression of the retinoic acid receptors. AIDS **8:** 1675–1682.

57. TOWERS, G., J. HARRIS, G. LANG, *et al.* 1995. Retinoic acid inhibits both the basal activity and phorbol ester-mediated activation of the HIV long terminal repeat promoter. AIDS **9:** 129–136.

58. SINGH, U.S., Q. LI & R. CERIONE. 1998. Identification of the eukaryotic initiation factor 5A as a retinoic acid-stimulated cellular binding partner for tissue transglutaminase II. J. Biol. Chem. **273:** 1946–1950.

59. BEVEC, D., H. JAKSCHE, M. OFT, *et al.* 1996. Inhibition of HIV-1 replication in lymphocytes by mutants of the Rev cofactor eIF5A. Science **271:** 1858–1860.

60. THOMAS, S.L., M. OFT, H. JAKSCHE, *et al.* 1998. Functional analysis of the human immunodeficiency virus type 1 Rev protein oligomerization interface. J. Virol. **72:** 2935–2944.

61. RUHL, M., M. HIMMELSPACH, G.M. BAHR, *et al.* 1993. Eukaryotic initiation factor 5A is a cellular target of the human immunodeficiency virus type 1 Rev activation domain mediating trans-activation. J. Cell Biol. **123:** 1309–1320.

62. POLLARD V.W. & M.H. MALIM. 1988. The HIV-1 Rev protein. Annu. Rev. Microbiol. **52:** 491–532.

63. BOGERD, H.P., R.A. FRIDELL, S. MADORE & B.R. CULLEN. 1995. Identification of a novel cellular cofactor for Rev/Rex class of retroviral regulatory proteins. Cell **82:** 485–494.
64. FRITZ, C.C., M.L. ZAPP & M.R. GREEN. 1995. A human nucleoporin-like protein that specifically interacts with HIV Rev. Nature **376:** 530–533.
65. STADE, K., C.S. FORD, C. GUTHRIE & K. WEIS. 1997. Exportin 1 (Crm1p) is an essential nuclear export factor. Cell **90:** 1041–1050.
66. OSSAREH-NAZARI, B., F. BACHELERIE & C. DARGEMONT. 1997. Evidence for a role of CRM1 in signal-mediated nuclear protein export. Science **278:** 141–144.
67. JUNKER, U., D. BEVEC, C. BARSKE, *et al.* 1996. Intracellular expression of cellular eIF5A mutants inhibits HIV-1 replication in human T cells: a feasibility study. Hum. Gene Ther. **7:** 1861–1869.
68. SCHATZ, O., M. OFT, C. DASCHER, *et al.* 1998. Proc. Natl. Acad. Sci. USA **95:** 1607–1612.
69. ELFGANG, C., O. ROSORIUS, L. HOFER, *et al.* Evidence for specific nucleocytoplasmic transport pathways used by leucine-rich nuclear export signals. Proc. Natl. Acad. Sci. USA **96:** 6229–6234.

Cardiomyopathy and Encephalopathy in AIDS

ANDREA ANTINORI, MARIA LETIZIA GIANCOLA, LUCIA ALBA,
FABIO SOLDANI, AND SUSANNA GRISETTI

*National Institute for Infectious Diseases "Lazzaro Spallanzani"—IRCCS,
00149 Rome, Italy*

ABSTRACT: HIV encephalopathy has been in the past years the most typical
CNS disorder in patients with AIDS. Histologic abnormalities consist in astrocytosis, myelin pallor, infiltration by infected macrophages, resident microglia
and multinucleated giant cells, generally in absence of direct infection of neurons. Mononuclear phagocytes in the brain are the main target of HIV-1 infection and the site of productive viral replication, and viral stimulation leads to
the release of neurotoxic products causing neurologic damage. Subclinical cardiac abnormalities are common in HIV+ patients and several studies suggested
a role for cytokines and other inflammatory products as mediators of cardiac
abnormalities. The common pathway for neurologic and cardiac manifestations supports the relationship between neurologic disease and cardiac dysfunction in HIV infection. Clinical observations suggest that cardiomyopathy
could be associated with encephalopathy in HIV+ patients and that it may
affect survival. Antiretroviral therapy may reduce impact of neurologic and
cardiac abnormalities by suppressing plasma HIV-1 viral load.

KEYWORDS: HIV; cardiomyopathy; HIV-dementia; TNF-α; inducible nitric
oxide synthase; antiretroviral therapy

INTRODUCTION

During the last two decades, before the introduction of the new antiretroviral therapies, approximately one-third of the adults and one-half of the children with acquired
immunodeficiency syndrome (AIDS) eventually showed neurologic symptoms directly
due to HIV-1 infection of the central nervous system (CNS).[1] The CNS is exposed to
HIV-1 early in the natural history of infection, and evidence exists that direct infection
is the base for various neurologic dysfunctions at different stages of disease. However,
the most relevant determinant of pathogenetic susceptibility for CNS involvement by
HIV-1 remains the degree of immunosuppression resulting from chronic infection and
progressive depletion of cellular immunity. HIV-encephalopathy—alternatively known
as AIDS dementia complex or HIV-dementia (HIVD)—was in past years the main
and most typical CNS disorder in patients with AIDS.[2] Histologic abnormalities in
demented patients, such as astrocytosis, myelin pallor, infiltration by infected macrophages, resident microglia, and multinucleated giant cells, occur despite the absence of
direct infection of neurons. Mononuclear phagocytes in the brain are the main target of

Address for correspondence: Andrea Antinori, M.D., Instituto Nazionale per le Malattie
Infettive Diseases, "Lazzaro Spallanzani"—IRCCS, Via Portuense, 292, 00149 Rome, Italy.
Voice: +39-06-55170477-300; fax: +39-06-55170477.
antinori@inmi.it

HIV-1 infection and the site of productive viral replication.[3] The abnormal response of infected macrophages to viral stimulation leads to the release of large amounts of neurotoxic substances, which are the cause of neurologic damage.

Subclinical cardiac abnormalities are common in HIV+ patients.[4] Several studies have focused on the role of cytokines and other inflammatory products as mediators of cardiac abnormalities in HIV+ patients. The common pathway for neurologic and cardiac manifestations supports the relationship between advanced neurologic disease and cardiac dysfunction in HIV infection. Clinical observations suggest that cardiomyopathy may be associated with encephalopathy and that it may affect survival.[5]

Highly active antiretroviral therapy (HAART) is highly effective in suppressing plasma HIV-1 viral load, thereby preserving or restoring immune function and consequently reducing neurologic complications of disease. The global impact of HAART on the natural history of neurologic disorders is still largely unknown. Complex effects of antiretroviral therapy on the pathogenetic network that contributes to neurologic damage may be translated to cardiac manifestations of HIV disease.

CARDIAC INVOLVEMENT IN HIV-1 INFECTION

Pathogenetic Implications

Little is known about the etiology and pathogenetic mechanisms of dilated cardiomyopathy in the general population, even though genetic mutations, viral myocarditis, and autoimmune disease have been implicated. Nitric oxide (NO) is a biological mediator with multiple actions. Two NO-synthases invariably present in neuronal and endothelial cells were found, and a third form is inducible in many cells by cytokines such as interferon-γ, interleukin-1 and tumor necrosis factor alpha (TNF-α). High levels of TNF-α and increased production of NO have been associated with dilated cardiomyopathy (DCM). In particular, has been demonstrated that induced NO production has a negative inotropic effect on cardiac myocytes and that high levels of NO produced by inducible NO synthase (iNOS) are cytotoxic.[6] Moreover, iNOS gene expression has been associated with heart failure, and iNOS protein has been detected in ventricular myocytes from patients with end-stage heart failure diseases.[7] A relationship between TNF-α and iNOS is also suggested by the correlation between plasma concentration of acid-labile nitroso compound, end-products of NO methabolism, and TNF-α.[8]

Giving these findings, a pathway has been hypothesized with local NO production stimulated by TNF-α in the cardiac tissue leading to dilated cardiomyopathy via a chronic negative inotropic effect. Moreover, TNF-α has been found locally expressed predominantly in blood vessels but also in the cardiac myocytes of patients with DCM but not in patients with ischemic heart disease.[6] The increased levels of iNOS in DCM could depend on local availability of TNF-α resulting from an inflammatory response to causal agents, even though a role of other cytokines may be hypothesized. Moreover, it has been suggested that TNF-α production by cardiac myocytes *in vivo* may play a relevant pathophysiologic role not only in the pathogenesis of DCM but also in its progression in terms of progressive left ventricular dysfunction and enlargement of ventricular volume.[9]

In AIDS patients, prevalence of myocardial diseases is influenced by definition and diagnostic approach. Microscopic signs of focal myocarditis range from 15% to 50% in serial autopsies. Clinical cardiomyopathy defined as myocardial disease causing signs and symptoms of heart failure is relatively unusual (1–3% of AIDS patients). In prospective observations with serial echocardiography among HIV⁺ patients a prevalence of 4–8% with an annual incidence rate of 11–15.9 cases per 1000 patients was documented.[4,10] If only AIDS patients were included, the incidence would be more than 3% per year.

The pathogenesis of these disorders has not yet been definitively explained, even though current hypotheses include direct infection of myocardiocytes with HIV-1, coinfection with other viruses, postviral cardiac autoimmunity, cardiotoxicity related to psychotropic substances and pharmacologic agents (zidovudine, foscarnet, pentamidine, cytotoxic agents, etc.). HIV nucleic acid sequences were detected in a variable proportion of cardiac tissue sections (15–76%). In most patients histologic and immunohistologic examination found myocarditis. The extent of immunodeficiency, as assessed by a CD4 cell count less than 400 cells per cubic millimeter in HIV⁺ asymptomatic patients, has been demonstrated to be correlated with a higher incidence of DCM in adults. Furthermore, the role of myocarditis in the development of DCM has not been conclusively ascertained, and lymphocytic myocarditis has been found in 46–83% of patients with AIDS. The advanced stage of immunodeficiency may enhance the pathogenic role of HIV-1 and several other viruses such as coxsackievirus group B, cytomegalovirus, and Epstein-Barr virus, and the increased expression of MHC class I molecules suggests an active immune process in the myocardium.[4,11]

Studies investigating the characteristics and pathogenesis of HIV-associated cardiomyopathy in infected children identified progressive left ventricular dilatation with compensatory hypertrophy as the main cause of decreasing ventricular performance. Moreover, the abnormalities of left ventricular size occurred independently of zidovudine use.[12] Subclinical cardiac abnormalities are common and progressive in HIV⁺ children and correlated with immunodeficiency at baseline, even though CD4 count could not be a useful surrogate marker of progression of cardiac diseases.[5]

HIV-ENCEPHALOPATHY

Pathogenetic Implications

Neurologic disorders during natural history of HIV infection may occur either in presence of opportunistic infections or cancers, or may be directly attributable to infection of the brain by the HIV-1 itself. From a pathologic point of view, the characteristics of HIV-1 infection of the brain (HIV-encephalopathy) consist of reactive astrocytosis, infiltration by circulating macrophages, resident microglia and multinucleated giant cells, and myelin pallor. At the clinical level, these abnormalities determine the onset of the syndrome characterized by cognitive and motor deficits defined as AIDS dementia.[2] Nevertheless, the clinical progression of HIV-dementia seems to be due not to the direct infection of neurons by HIV-1 or to an autoimmune process induced by the virus, but there is a good evidence that the infection of the brain follows two steps mediated by macrophages. First, the viral coat glycoprotein gp120 binds a receptor on the macrophage surface such as CD4 and the virus is internalized by the macrophage. This process can stimulate macrophages to release low levels of neurotoxins, and similarly gp120, tat and nef could stimulate uninfected cells to release neurotoxins as well.[13,14] In the second step, the HIV-1 genome is integrated into the macrophage genome and active replication of the virus occurs. During this step the macrophage is induced to release a large amount of neurotoxic substances—eicosanoids and free radicals—which can contribute to neuronal damage by increasing the release of glutamate or decreasing its re-uptake.[15] TNF-α and IL-1β stimulate astrocytosis,[16] whereas platelet-activating factor from macrophages may cause neuronal death *in vitro* by increasing calcium ions and the release of glutamate.[17]

One of the substances released from macrophages in response to replication of HIV-1 is arachidonic acid and its metabolites. Arachidonic acid acts synergistically with endogenous glutamate to activate neuronal N-methyl-D-aspartate (NMDA) receptors, which mediate excitatory neurotransmission in the brain acting on channels permeable to calcium ions. Calcium ions may enter neurons that contain the constitutive form of nitric oxide synthase stimulating the formation of nitric oxide, which contributes to the cascade of neurotoxic events. In particular, NO is generated following activation of NO synthase (NOS), of which there are three isoforms, neuronal NOS (nNOS), endothelial NOS (eNOS), and inducible NOS (iNOS). nNOS regulates neuronal signals by overt glutamate excitoxicity. In this way, NO reacts with superoxid anion to form peroxynitrite that damages DNA, RNA, proteins, and lipids with mitochondrial impairment, loss of energy and cell death. The neuronal death following iNOS activation occurs slowly over time with the morphologic features of apoptosis.[18]

A role for iNOS in HIV dementia comes from both human post mortem studies and experimental models. A correlation between gp41 levels, iNOS expression and severity, and rate of progression of HIV dementia has been demonstrated, and the expression of gp41 and iNOS is predominantly localized to macrophage/microglia of the frontal lobe and basal ganglia.[19] Moreover, perivascular macrophage/microglia are the predominant source of iNOS in the HIV+ brain and its expression correlates with productive infection. This correlation, combined with the observation that iNOS is not induced in all stages of macrophage activation, suggests that immune activation may be not a sufficient condition for NO production in HIV+ brain, and this is also in agreement with *in vitro* observations that HIV+ monocytes, lipopolysaccharide- and TNF-α activated, produce more NO than either activated or infected monocytes alone.[20] Tat has also been demonstrated to induce iNOS causing neurotoxicity in culture, an effect that may be mediated by TNF-α.[21] Using these observations one may assume that the interaction between HIV proteins and various host signals forms a complex network that underlies the development of cerebral injury in response to HIV infection. Moreover, it has been recently demonstrated that there is a similar distribution of staining within the basal ganglia for TNF-α and activated NF-κB-α, a host transcriptional factor that upregulates the expression of HIV-1 and host proinflammatory factors, including cytokines, and which itself can be activated by TNF-α.[19] Putative NF-κB binding sites have been identified within the promoter region of the iNOS gene, suggesting a potential mechanism linking iNOS regulation to TNF-α expression in the HIV$^+$ brain. The complex network of activated cytokines is completed by the lack of IL-4 downregulation leading to uncontrolled activation of macrophages and production of neurotoxic mediators[22] (see FIGURE 1).

Moreover, it has been observed that cell death by apoptosis can occur in some oligodendrocytes in the presence of TNF-α, and this could imply a role of TNF-α in demyelinating processes. In particular, myelin-forming cells may be exposed chronically to TNF-α bound to or derived from activated microglia *in vivo*. This could result in the striking demyelination that can be observed in HIV-1 vacuolar myelopathy.[23]

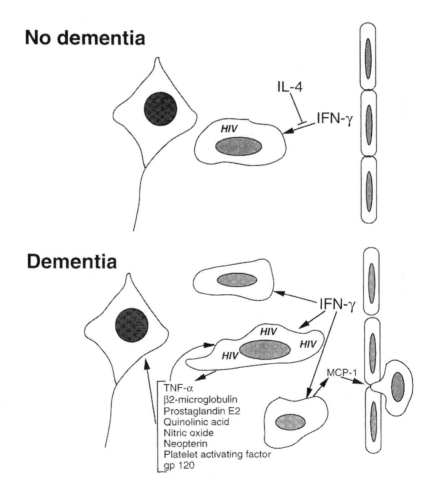

FIGURE 1. Uncontrolled macrophage activation and dementia pathogenesis during HIV infection. (From Griffin, D.E. 1997. J. Clin. Invest.[22])

CARDIOMYOPATHY AND ENCEPHALOPATHY IN
HIV-INFECTED PATIENTS

Several observations among children and adults with HIV infection suggested a strong clinical relationship between cardiomyopathy and encephalopathy. In HIV+ children, the development of encephalopathy was associated with a deterioration of left ventricular function, and this association has been confirmed in subsequent studies on HIV+ children and adults.[5] In particular, children who presented encephalopathy had depressed initial fractional shortening and this continued to decline during the follow-up period influencing survival. This defect, as well as the associated encephalopathy, did not correlate with CD4 count.

In another study, a diagnosis of cardiomyopathy was significantly more frequent in HIV+ children with encephalopathy (30% prevalence) than in those without encephalopathy (2%). No markers associated with time of onset of encephalopathy and cardiomyopathy were identified, even though high HIV-1 viral load in the first year of life may be associated with diagnosis of encephalopathy.[24] In HIV+ adults with dilated cardiomyopathy, those who also had encephalopathy had more abnormal echocardiographic functional parameters independent of the duration of documented cardiomyopathy, and these parameters tended to worsen progressively for patients with concomitant encephalopathy, who had a higher mortality rate (73%) for congestive heart failure.[25] These parameters were inversely correlated with HIV-1 RNA and CD4 cell count. There may be several causes for this strong association between cardiomyipathy and encephalopathy. Neuronal loss may occur as a result of highly productive infection with strong macrophage activation; moreover, mediators of the inflammation and HIV-1 viral proteins may act as neurotoxins, causing apoptosis of the neuronal cells. Furthermore, the involvement of the nervous system during HIV infection is associated with an alteration of the cardiac parasympathetic nervous system, which may cause a release of catecholamine, increased consumption of oxygen by myocardial tissue, downregulation of the myocardial β-adrenoceptors and subsequent progressive reduction of the contractile function of the myocytes. The HIV-1 virus itself could be responsible for some manifestations of cardiomyopathy and encephalopathy, as suggested by the positive signals for HIV-1 nucleic acid sequences found within the multinucleated giant cells of the cerebral cortex at autopsy in 79% of patients with encephalopathy who died of dilated cardiomyopathy. Moreover, in the same case series, a significantly higher proportion of patients with encephalopathy were positive for nucleic sequences of HIV-1 within myocardial cells than patients without encephalopathy.[25]

Other manifestations could however be due to immunological factors and cytokines: in particular the interaction between dendritic cells, responsible for the primary immunological response to HIV-1 and for the presentation of the antigen to T lymphocytes, and CD8 cells could induce a release of cytokines such as TNF-α, interleukin-1, interleukin-6, interleukin-10, producing neurocardiotoxic activities. A strong immunoreactivity for TNF-α and iNOS within cardiomyocytes was found in HIV+ patients with cardiomyopathy. The intensity of immunostaining was increased by the coexistence of HIV-encephalopathy and inversely related to absolute CD4 cell count. Moreover, a marked immunoreactivity for TNF-α and iNOS was found within glial cells and astrocytes of patients with encephalopathy who died of congestive heart failure. This specific pathway may be responsible for inducing apoptotic signaling in both myocardial and neuronal cells, especially in the presence of marked immunodeficiency.[25]

IMPACT OF HAART AND PERSPECTIVES

The introduction of potent combined antiretroviral therapy has strongly modified the clinical course and survival time of HIV[+] persons. The probabilty of survival after 24 months in HIV[+] patients with opportunistic infections increased from 49% of those diagnosed in 1993 to 80% in those diagnosed in 1997.[26] HAART has also had an impact on the main HIV-related neurologic diseases. Incidence rates of HIV dementia, cryptococcal meningitis, and CNS lymphoma have dramatically decreased since the introduction of HAART.[27,28] However, estimates on temporal trends and changes in the natural history of HIV-associated neurologic diseases such as HIV-dementia should be completely defined. Reduction trends were observed mostly in homosexual men with high treatment adherence and good virological response, but no definitive data were observed from other groups such as IV drug users or in patients with increasing resistance and virological failure. Studies on survival of HAART-treated neurologic cases documented a benefit of therapy also independent from virological effect, but in nonresponder populations a relevant role may be played by HIV-dementia and emerging disorders as PML or leukoencephalopathy of unknown origin[29] (see FIGURE 2). Cerebrospinal fluid (CSF) and plasma HIV-1 dynamics become increasingly independent in advanced HIV disease, and the

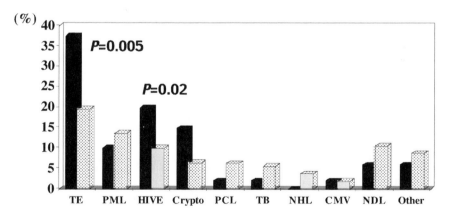

FIGURE 2. Specific neurologic diseases as proportion of CNS disorders by HAART exposure. Data from Italian Register Investigative Neuro AIDS (IRINA) Study. TE, toxoplasma encephalitis; PML, progressive multifocal leukoencephalopathy; Crypto, cryptococcal meningitis; PCL, primary cerebral lymphoma; TB, tubercular meningitis; NHL, nonHodgkin's lymphoma with secondary CNS involvement; CMV, cytomegalovirus encephalitis; NDL, not determined leukoencephalopathy; Other, other CNS disorders.

compartmental discrepancy was largest in HIVD.[30,31] Divergent evolution of HIV-1 in the two different compartments has been observed with different mutations conferring resistance.[32] Pharmacokinetic studies of antiretrovirals showed variable profiles of drugs in CSF, and in some cases the efficacy of therapy may be different between compartments. A divergent, independent replicative process in CNS could determine a unforeseeable scenario in neurologic expression of HIV disease in coming years. How these conditions may affect the parallel occurrence of cardiac dysfunction related to common pathways remains to be established.

ACKNOWLEDGMENTS

This work was supported by the Ricerca Finalizzata e Corrente degli IRCCS, Ministero della Sanità and by the Programma Nazionale di Ricerca sull'AIDS, Istituto Superiore di Sanità, Italy.

REFERENCES

1. BACELLAR, H. *et al.* 1994. Temporal trends in the incidents of HIV-1 related neurologic diseases. Neurology **44:** 1892–1900.

2. PRICE, R.W. *et al.* 1988. The brain and AIDS: central nervous system HIV-1 infection and AIDS dementia complex. Science **239:** 586–592.

3. KOENIG, S. *et al.* 1986. Detection of AIDS virus in macrophages in brain tissue from AIDS patients with encephalopathy. Science **233:** 1089–1093.

4. BARBARO, G. *et al.* 1998. Incidence of dilated cardiomyopathy and detection of HIV in myocardial cells of HIV-positive patients. N. Engl. J. Med. **339:** 1093–1099.

5. LIPSHULTZ, S.E. *et al.* 1998. Left ventricular structure and function in children infected with human immunodeficiency virus. Circulation **97:** 1246–1256.

6. HABIB, F.M. *et al.* 1996. Tumor necrosis factor and inducible nitric oxide synthase in dilated cardiomyopathy. Lancet **347:** 1151–1155.

7. HAYWOOD, G.A. *et al.* 1996. Expression of inducible nitric oxide synthase in human heart failure. Circulation **93:** 1087–1094.

8. TORRE-AMIONE, G. *et al.* 1995. Expression and functional significance of tumor necrosis factor receptors in human myocardium. Circulation **92:** 1487–1493.

9. SATOH, M. *et al.* 1999. Tumor necrosis factor-α-converting enzyme and tumor necrosis factor-α in human dilated cardiomyopathy. Circulation **99:** 3260–3265.

10. CURRIE, P.F. *et al.* 1994. Heart muscle disease related to HIV infection: prognostic implications. Br. Med. J. **309:** 1605–1607.

11. HERSKOWITZ, A. *et al.* 1994. Myocarditis and cardiotropic viral infection associated with severe left ventricular dysfunction in late-stage infection with human immunodeficiency virus. J. Am. Coll. Cardiol. **24:** 1025–1032.

12. LIPSHULTZ, S.E. *et al.* 1992. cardiac structure and function in children with human immunodeficiency virus infection treated with zidovudine. N. Engl. J. Med. **327:** 1260–1265.

13. WAHL, L.M. *et al.* 1989. Human immunodeficiency virus glycoprotein (gp120) induction of monocyte arachidonic acid metabolites and interleukin-11. Proc. Natl. Acad. Sci. USA **86:** 621–625.

14. HAYMAN, M. *et al.* 1993. Neurotoxicity of peptide analogues of the transactivating protein tat from Maedi-Visna virus and human immunodeficiency virus. Neuroscience **53:** 1–6.

15. GENIS, P. *et al.* 1992. Cytokines and arachidonic acid metabolites produced during human immunodeficiency virus (HIV)–infected macrophages-astroglia interactions: implications for the neuropathogenesis of HIV disease. J. Exp. Med. **176:** 1703–1718.
16. SELMAJ, K.W. *et al.* 1990. Proliferations of astrocytes in vitro in response to cytokines: a primary role for tumor necrosis factor. J. Immunol. **144:** 129–135.
17. LIPTON, S.A. 1994. HIV displays its coat of arms. Nature **367:** 113–114.
18. DAWSON, V.L. *et al.* 1994. Expression of inducible nitric oxide synthase causes delayed neurotoxicity in primary mixed neuronal-glial cortical cultures. Neuropharmacology **33:** 1425–1430.
19. ROSTASY, K. *et al.* 1999. Human immunodeficiency virus infection, inducible nitric oxide synthase expression, and microglial activation: pathogenetic relationship to the acquired immunodeficiency syndrome dementia complex. Ann. Neurol. **46:** 207–216.
20. BUKRINSKY, M.I. *et al.* 1995. Regulation of nitric oxide synthase in human immunodeficiency virus type 1-infected monocytes: implications for HIV-associated neurological diseases. J. Exp. Med. **181:** 735–745.
21. SHI, B. *et al.* 1998. Neuronal apoptosis induced by HIV-1 tat protein and TNF-α: potentiation of neurotoxicity by oxidative stress and implications for HIV-1 dementia. J. Neurovirol. **4:** 281–290.
22. GRIFFIN, D.E. 1997. Cytokines in the brain during viral infection: clues to HIV-associated dementia. J. Clin. Invest. **100:** 2948–2951.
23. WILT, S.G. *et al.* 1995. In vitro evidence for a dual role of tumor necrosis factor-α in human immunodeficiency virus type-1 encephalopathy. Ann. Neurol. **37:** 381–394.
24. COOPER, E.R. *et al.* 1998. Encephalopathy and progression of human immunodeficiency virus disease in a cohort of children with perinatally acquired human immunodeficiency virus infection. J. Pediatr. **132:** 808–812.
25. BARBARO, G. *et al.* 2000. Clinical course of cardiomyopathy in HIV-infected patients with or without encephalopathy related to the myocardial expression of tumor necrosis factor-α and nitric oxide synthase. AIDS **14:** 427–428.
26. LEE, L.M. *et al.* 2001. Survival after AIDS diagnosis in adolescents and adults during the treatment era, United States, 1984-1997. JAMA **285:** 1308–1315.
27. AMMASSARI, A. *et al.* 2000. AIDS-related focal brain lesions in the era of highly active antiretroviral therapy. Neurology **55:** 1194–1200.
28. SACKTOR, N. *et al.* 2001. HIV-associated neurologic disease incidence changes: Multicenter AIDS Cohort Study, 1990-1998. Neurology **56:** 257–260.
29. ANTINORI, A. *et al.* Shift of prevalence and selected characteristic in HIV-1-related neurologic disorders in HAART era: data from Italian Register Investigative Neuro AIDS (IRINA). Abstract of the 8th Conference on retrovirus and opportunistic infection (Chicago, IL): no. 8. Foundation for Retrovirology and Human Health.
30. STAPRANS, S. *et al.* 1999. Time course of cerebrospinal fluid responses to antiretroviral therapy: evidence for variable compartmentalization of infection. AIDS **13:** 1051–1061.
31. ELLIS, R.J. *et al.* 2000. Cerebrospinal fluid HIV-RNA originates from both local CNS and systemic sources. Neurology **54:** 927–936.
32. STINGELE, K. *et al.* 2001. Independent HIV replication in paired CSF and blood viral isolates during antiretroviral therapy. Neurology **56:** 355–361.

Cardiology and AIDS —
HAART and the Consequences

CHRISTIAN HOFFMANN AND HANS JAEGER

KIS–Curatorium for Immunedeficiency, Munich,Germany

ABSTRACT: Since the introduction of highly active antiretroviral therapy (HAART), AIDS has become a treatable disease. A steep decline in morbidity and mortality has been observed in most western countries. The HIV epidemic is now moving into middle-aged populations which are already at increased risk for cardiovascular disease. Since the cardiovascular system is frequently affected in HIV infection, reflections on traditional cardiovascular risk factors is a pressing issue. Moreover, during the last few years, complex lipodystrophic body changes in association with metabolic abnormalities such as dyslipidemia and insulin resistance have become a common feature in HIV$^+$ patients on HAART. Although the precise mechanisms are not fully understood, early reports on myocardial infarctions and vascular changes have raised concern about the possibility of an epidemic of cardiovascular events among HAART patients within the next decade. Not only more data on lipid-lowering drugs in the context of HAART, on switching strategies, and treatment interruptions, but also from intervention studies on traditional risk factors such as smoking, are urgently needed. In this review the key issues concerning cardiovascular aspects of HIV infection in the era of HAART and possible preventive strategies are discussed.

KEYWORDS: cardiovascular diseases; risk factors; HIV/AIDS; antiretroviral therapy; treatment strategies

INTRODUCTION

Since 1996 AIDS has become a treatable and chronic disease. With the introduction of highly active antiretroviral therapy (HAART), a steep decline in mortality and morbidity has been observed in most western countries. In the EuroSIDA study, a prospective multicenter study of more than 7,300 patients, the incidence of AIDS-defining events in 1998 had declined to less than a tenth that in 1994.[1] However, the most cited study reporting increased survival, conducted by Palella and colleagues,[2] could also be used to argument that impressive clinical benefit is achieved only in severely immunosuppressed patients. Furthermore, the sobering results of studies demonstrating, even in patients with prolonged viral suppression,[3–5] the persistence of HIV-1 transcription in latently infected cells underscores that eradication of HIV is currently an unrealistic goal.

More physicians are thus becoming aware that the "hit hard and early" practice, which focuses on the early suppression of viremia, may not be in the best interests

Address for correspondence: Dr. med. Christian Hoffmann, KIS, Mozartstraße 3, 80336 Munich, Germany. Voice: 0049 89 55 870 30; fax: 0049 89 550 39 41.
christian.hoffmann@mucresearch.de

of the patient. Since the major goal of HIV therapy is to maintain long-term health, factors other than viral suppression such as long-term toxicities should be considered. In this setting, diverse aspects including the increased age of the HIV population, reports of HAART-related metabolic abnormalities, and the evidence that the heart is a frequently affected organ in HIV infection have led to the growing importance of cardiology in HIV medicine. Moreover, recent reports of myocardial infarctions in young HIV$^+$ patients receiving HAART have raised concerns of premature cardiovascular disease. In this review discussion centers on the key issues of cardiovascular aspects of HIV infection in the era of highly active antiretroviral therapy.

CARDIOVASCULAR INVOLVEMENT IN HIV PER SE: THE EARLY YEARS

The heart is a frequently affected organ in HIV patients. Cardiac disease can be caused by HIV per se, cardiotropic viruses and other opportunistic infections, malignancies, or medical treatment, and can involve the pericardium, myocardium, endocardium, and blood vessels. In the pre-HAART era, the estimated prevalence of cardiac morbidity was 6–7%, although there was high variability, owing probably to different patient populations.[6] In intravenous drug abusers and in HIV$^+$ patients with more advanced disease, the prevalence of cardiac abnormalities seemed to be higher.[7,8]

The most common cardiac manifestations seen in AIDS patients in the pre-HAART era were pericardial effusion, myocarditis, and dilated cardiomyopathy. Autopsy studies revealed evidence of pericarditis and myocarditis in 20–50% of patients.[6,9,10] In a prospective echocardiographic study, evidence of pericardial effusion was found in 39 of 102 patients.[11] The most common and life-threatening cardiovascular complication of HIV infection is dilated cardiomyopathy, the development of primary heart muscle disease associated with severe global left ventricular dysfunction. One large trial, in which 952 asymptomatic HIV$^+$ patients underwent clinical and echocardiographic follow ups, identified 76 patients (8%) with dilated cardiomyopathy.[12] In 83% of these patients a histologic diagnosis of myocarditis was made; most of them had a positive hybridization signal for HIV, leading the authors to hypothesize that HIV has a direct effect on inducing myocarditis, and that there is a pathogenetic relation between myocarditis and dilated cardiomyopathy. Notably, the extent of immunodeficiency influenced the incidence of cardiomyopathy. Thus, in HIV patients with more advanced disease, the incidence of dilated cardiomyopathy may be higher.[12]

Pericarditis, myocarditis and dilated cardiomyopathy are not the only cardiac manifestations in HIV$^+$ individuals. Nonbacterial endocarditis, pulmonary hypertension, and malignant neoplasms have also been seen in AIDS patients.[13–15] Furthermore, a recent study emphasized the involvement of cardiovascular autonomic tone in advanced HIV infection; spectral analysis of heart rate variability revealed severe global autonomic dysfunction, which was not secondary to heart failure.[16]

Pathological studies have also provided evidence for a pathogenetically relevant vasculopathy in HIV infection by demonstrating that the endothelial cell pattern is clearly disturbed.[17–19] In comparison with an HIV-negative group, the aortic endothelium of 32 HIV$^+$ patients was characterized by chronic injury, activation, and increased leukocyte adhesion.[17] Autopsy examination of coronary arteries of young HIV+ patients with no associated risk factors demonstrated severe distal and proximal vascular lesions.[18] Another study analyzing the coronary arteries of 15 young HIV+ patients showed thickening of the intima in the proximal network to at least that of the media, caused by a proliferation of secreting cells phenotypically identified as smooth muscle cells.[19] In four cases arteriosclerosis had an unusual appearance in the form of mamillated vegetations with endoluminal protrusions. The authors concluded that lesions observed in HIV+ patients showed distinct features that were intermediate between lesions observed in common coronary atherosclerosis and in atherosclerosis associated with chronic rejection of cardiac transplants.[19]

The pathogenesis of HIV-related vasculopathy is not fully understood and would appear to be multifactorial. Elevated endothelial cell products may contribute to a procoagulant environment.[17,20] Chronic infection and inflammation may also play a role.[21] Since traditional risk factors cannot completely explain the incidence and trends in cardiovascular disease, recent interest has focused on the role of chronic infections by agents such as *Chlamydia pneumoniae*. In HIV+ patients it seems reasonable to assume that opportunistic and cardiotropic agents such as herpes viruses may directly induce endothelial damage.[18,22] There is also strong evidence that HIV+ per se, which has been shown to be able to infect endothelial cells *in vitro*,[23] may have cytotoxic effects on endothelial cell function via extracellular, circulating HIV-1 proteins.[24] Moreover, hypertriglyceridemia which was well described in HIV+ patients in the pre-ART era and which seems to be an independent risk in coronary disease, may contribute to vascular damage.[25,26]

Until now, however, cardiovascular abnormalities related to HIV have remained less well characterized than lesions of other organs–mainly because during the early years of the epidemic their clinical significance was questionable.

CONSIDER TRADITIONAL RISK FACTORS—EVEN IN HIV-INFECTED PATIENTS

Only with the introduction of potent antivirals, did consideration of cardiovascular risk factors in HIV+ patients become a more pressing issue. The threat of opportunistic infections and malignancies and the perception that death from AIDS was the inevitable outcome of the HIV diagnosis, led both patients and physicians to believe that concerns about lipids or blood pressure were irrelevant. Now, at least in western countries, the HIV epidemic is moving into middle-aged populations who are already at increased risk of cardiovascular disease. Patients who acquired HIV in the 1980s are currently in the 40- to 60-year age group.

The absolute risk of coronary heart disease in any individual is determined by a complex interplay of several risk factors, which include smoking, hypertension, older age, positive family history, elevated blood lipids, diabetes and other determinants. In addition to concern about the adverse effects of antiretroviral therapy, it is now high time to consider and evaluate these risk factors in HIV+ patients. For example, there is no intervention study of the value of smoking-cessation in the HIV population, despite the high prevalence of smoking in HIV+ patients.[27] Moreover, no clinical guidelines exist which specifically address smoking-cessation strategies in this population. Recent reports showed that up to 70% of HIV$^+$ patients smoke and that 80% of them had not considered and were not considering quitting smoking in the near future.[28] In our own cohort of more than 1,000 HIV$^+$ individuals, which matches the infection risk patterns in Germany, about two-thirds of the patients smoke (unpublished data). Smoking's well known impact on cardiovascular disease, and furthermore its association with increased incidences of opportunistic infections such as oral candidiasis, oral hairy leukoplakia, and other oral lesions, stress the importance of intervention studies concerning smoking cessation in HIV$^+$ individuals.

Hypertension may be another important issue. There are no recommendations for the treatment of hypertension in HIV$^+$ patients. Although one large study of outpatient HIV$^+$ individuals showed that hypertension is not frequent and that HIV$^+$ patients as a group do not exhibit a typical age-related increase in systolic blood pressure,[29] there exist several HIV-related pathomechanisms such as renal dysfunction which are able to induce a sustained elevation in blood presssure. With regard to hypertension, HIV patients should therefore not only be routinely evaluated for renal disease but also for hypothyroidism, hypogonadism and hepatic disease.

Physical inactivity, a sedentary lifestyle, and alcohol consumption may also have potentially adverse affects on the cardiovascular system, and attention to these factors is advisable.

Furthermore, many of the medications used to treat HIV and HIV-related diseases have the potential to cause cardiovascular events. The most frequently used medications with a known impact on cardiac function include erythropoetin, doxorubicin, zidovudine, and interferon alpha. Torsades de pointes may occasionally be triggered by anti-infectious agents such as pentacarinate or trimethoprime-sulfamethoxazole, and may also be seen in association with ketoconazole and terfenadine or cisapride.[30] Physicians should also consider that active drug abuse, in particular cocaine consumption, is often involved in cardiac disease. One recent study suggests that angiotensin-converting enzyme-inhibitor therapy may have potential for aiding in reduction of cocaine abuse and its complications.[31] These preliminary findings lead to the speculation that ACE-inhibitor therapy may offer a new pharmacological approach to the treatment of cocaine-abuse.

In conclusion, given that HIV$^+$ individuals can now enjoy the prospect of living longer, healthier and more productive lives, there is a clear need to create care models and intervention studies to improve their health risk profiles.

HAART AND THE CARDIOVASCULAR SYSTEM

Cardiac involvement is frequently observed in HIV$^+$ patients, especially in those in advanced stages of the disease. Since the extent of immunodeficiency influences the incidence of cardiac disease, the introduction of HAART and an immune recovery per se may be beneficial. One retrospective study showed that HAART significantly decreased the incidence of cardiac involvement, especially of pericarditis, arrhythmias, and dilated cardiomyopathy.[32] One could argue, however, that the decrease in HIV-related cardiac complications achieved by immune reconstitution and viral suppression will be overtaken by the consequences of HAART-induced metabolic syndromes.

ARE MYOCARDIAL INFARCTIONS (MI) MORE FREQUENT?

Since 1998 there have been many anecdotal reports of a close association between the initiation of protease inhibitors and the occurrence of severe vascular events.[33–36] A recent study reported a definite deterioration in 11 of 14 patients with confirmed coronary disease while on HAART. Although all patients had other risk factors such as smoking and hyperlipidemia, and a causal relationship between treatment and deterioration cannot be established by case observations, this remains an intriguing observation.[37] Some cohort studies have reported an increased incidence of myocardial infarction following the introduction of HAART.[38–39] In one cohort of nearly 5,000 patients, the incidence of MI per 1,000 patient-years increased from 0.59 (1991–94) to 3.41 (1995–98).[38] Reporting bias, reduced HIV-specific mortality, and changing risk factor profiles may have had an impact on these results. Thus, these studies do not prove whether HAART itself has an impact on the pathogenesis and clinical presentation of MI in HIV infected patients. An analysis of four Phase III clinical trials suggested that the risk of MI is not increased by protease inhibitors (PIs) as compared to non-PI-regimens;[40] however, the follow up was only 12 months, and longer periods of observation may yield a different result.

WHAT ABOUT THE VESSELS?

An increased thickness of the carotid artery has been shown to be predictive of an increased risk of myocardial infarction. Therefore, over the last two years this surrogate for cardiovascular disease has been assessed intensely in HIV+ patients.[41–45] Although different methods were employed, most studies demonstrated that the carotid intima media thickness (IMT) is frequently increased in HIV+ patients, especially in those individuals treated with protease inhibitors. In 10/29 (35%) patients undergoing ultrasonographic imaging, an increased IMT was observed; age and LDL cholesterol, but not duration of PI therapy, were significant risk factors.[41] In another study, the IMT was higher in 37 HIV+ patients, most of whom were on PIs, compared to matched healthy volunteers. A multivariate significant association of IMT was demonstrated for age and elevated cholesterol and decreased high density lipoprotein (HDL).[42] Other groups studied endothelial dysfunction in the brachial artery and showed that the flow-mediated diameter of the brachial artery is reduced in patients receiving PI therapy as compared to those on PI-sparing regimens.[43] The largest such study included 102 patients who were evaluated for premature atherosclerotic lesions of epiaortic vessels using both ultrasonographic and ultrasound color-power doppler techniques.[44] Of the PI-treated patients, 53% presented lesions of the vascular wall, whereas similiar lesions were found only in 15% of the PI naive group. In a control group of 104 healthy individuals, only 7% demonstrated such lesions. Cigarette smoking, hypertriglyceridemia, and CDC stage of HIV infection were significantly associated with an increased risk of vascular lesions. A slight correlation was found between carotid lesions and age, male sex and hypercholesterolemia. From a statistical viewpoint, the use of PIs exerted the greatest influence on development of carotid vessel lesions.[44] These results contrast with the findings of another large study in which age and smoking but not PI therapy were identified as independent factors associated with increased IMT.[45] Of note, a high prevalence of plaques (55%) was found in this cohort of 131 HIV[+] individuals.

However, most available data indicate that early carotid wall thickening is present in PI-exposed patients and is associated with age, smoking, and some but not all metabolic disturbances. Whether PIs, independent of their metabolic effects, contribute directly to endothelial dysfunction remains unclear. Furthermore, these findings have to be differentiated from the large vessel vasculopathy observed in HIV[+] patients, which may be of infective or immune complex origins.[22]

LIPODYSTROPHY—COMPLEX BUT FREQUENT

Antiretroviral therapy may be associated with a syndrome of peripheral fat loss (face, limbs, and buttocks) and central fat accumulation in abdomen, breasts and over the dorsocervical spine. The prevalence rates of this syndrome differ considerably from study to study, ranging from 30–80%, probably owing to the heterogenity of patient populations and the lack of an objective and validated case definition.[46] However, there is no HIV physician, who has not been made aware of characteristic body changes in a large proportion of HIV[+] patients. A large study which carefully evaluated physical abnormalities by questionnaires, physical examination and dual-energy X-ray absorptiometry, showed an 83% prevalence of lipodystrophy after only 21 months of therapy.[47]

Whereas the cause of this syndrome is still unknown, several hypotheses exist, indicating multifactorial causation and complex individual susceptibilities. One hypothesis is that protease inhibitors can inhibit lipid and adipocyte regulatory proteins that have partial homology to the catalytic site of HIV-1 protease.[48] Another hypothesis focuses on mitochondrial toxicity, which implicates the NRTIs, a class of drugs that block DNA polymerase gamma. As this enzyme is required for mitochondrial DNA replication, its inhibition and consequent mitochondrial dysfunction may also explain the well known side effects of NRTIs such as neuropathy, myopathy, pancreatitis, and lactate acidosis.[49] This hypothesis is supported by recent observations on subcutaneous fat biopsies, which revealed that individuals on ART exhibit a depletion of mitochondrial DNA that is greater in patients with lipoatrophy. Results among antiretroviral naive and uninfected control subjects showed no statistical difference.[50] Recent basic science investigations presented at the 2nd International Workshop on Adverse Drug Reactions and Lipodystrophy suggested that PIs (and to an extent also NRTIs) may act through modulation of adipocyte differentiation and/or reduction in the intracellular degradation of cellular proteins.[51–55] These studies demonstrate unambigously that antiretrovirals have direct metabolic effects and indicate that the problem may be not only toxicity as such, but rather dysregulation.

Several studies had identified risk factors for lipodystrophy such as cumulative time on stavudine, white race, a CD4 nadir below 200 cells/μL, age, PI use, and non-use of non-nucleoside reverse transcriptase inhibitors (NNRTIs).[56,57] The findings suggest a multifactorial etiology for lipodystrophy. Our group identified major risk factors as prolonged treatment with d4T and low CD4 cell count.[56] However, whether a definite causative hierarchy exists among antiviral drugs is unclear.

Although lipodystrophy can be observed without biological alterations, an association between fat distribution and metabolic changes (i.e., insulin resistance) is often experienced. It has not been clearly established whether all of these phenomena are interrelated. In one carefully matched study HIV[+] patients with lipodystrophy as compared with controls were shown to be more likely to have impaired glucose tolerance, diabetes, hypertriglyceridemia, reduced levels of HDL cholesterol levels, and diastolic hypertension. Most of these risk factors for cardiovascular disease were markedly attenuated in HIV patients without lipodystrophy.[58] One recent study demonstrated lack of a relationship between fat intake and body changes, suggesting that dietary fat reduction may be of little use in the management of lipodystrophy.[59]

INSULIN RESISTANCE

Insulin resistance is a well known risk factor for atherosclerosis being associated with endothelial dysfunction and diminished vasodilatation.[60] Impaired glucose tolerance accompanying peripheral insulin resistance resulting from HAART has been described frequently since 1998.[48,61,62] The prevalence of impaired glucose tolerance differed between 16 and 46%, and of diabetes mellitus between 7 and 13%. During the last months considerable progress has been made in clarification of HAART-induced insulin resistance.

With *in vitro* studies using a variety of cell lines PIs have been shown not only to increase basal glucose transport but also to increase the insulin-stimulated glucose transport that defines insulin resistance. The effect of the PIs was additive.[63] Since healthy controls show a decreased insulin sensitivity after four weeks on indinavir therapy, insulin sensitivity would appear to be a mechanism independent of effects due to HIV or immune function.[64] Other, however, have found a distinct relationship between the degree of insulin resistance and the levels of soluble type 2 tumor necrosis factor-α (TNF-α) receptor, which is used as an indicator of immune activation. This relationship suggests that an inflammatory stimulus is contributing to the development of HIV-associated lipodystrophy.[65] In one study, fasting concentrations and secretion response of insulin, proinsulin, and C-peptide to glucose ingestion were significantly increased in the PI-treated group, indicating a β cell dysfunction in addition to peripheral insulin resistance.[62]

Hyperinsulinemia was shown to be associated with increased levels of tissue plasminogen activation (tPA) and plasminogen activator inhibitor-1 (PAI-1). Both these latter proteins are new surrogate markers for atherosclerosis and markers of poor outcome.[66]

Recently, a randomized, double-blind, placebo-controlled pilot study of HIV[+] patients with fat redistribution and abnormal glucose tolerance tests has shown that a low dosage of metformin (500 mg BID) reduces insulin resistance, weight and diastolic blood pressure. No increases in lactate or liver transaminase levels were observed.[67] Although these results are encouraging, more studies are needed to estimate the risk of lactacidosis, which is a well known adverse effect associated with the use of both metformin and antiretrovirals. In patients with renal or hepatic dysfunction metformin should not be used.

DYSLIPIDEMIA AND MEDICAL INTERVENTION:
STATINS OR FIBRIC ACIDS?

Several cross-sectional and prospective studies of HIV patients receiving HAART have reported various combinations of lipid abnormalities.[47,62,68-70] Most of these showed a rapid and significant elevation of serum triglycerides in 50–70% of patients on PIs and to a lesser extent an increase in serum cholesterol, whereas plasma HDL-cholesterol levels remained unchanged. Lipoprotein A levels, an atherogenic lipoprotein, may also be elevated.[62,70] Lipid changes were generally evident within the first three months. Several studies have indicated that increases in cholesterol and triglycerides occur more frequently with regimens containing ritonavir and ritonavir/saquinavir as compared to those with indinavir, nelfinavir, and saquinavir alone.[47,68,71] However, it must also be borne in mind that HDL decreases and elevated triglycerides were well described in HIV infection prior to the introduction of effective antiretroviral treatment.[26,72]

Although the type and magnitude of lipid alterations suggest that an increased cardiovascular morbidity in ART-treated patients are to be expected, only preliminary recommendations for the evaluation and management of dyslipidemia in this population are available.[73] These propose that HIV$^+$ patients should be evaluated and treated on the basis of existing guidelines for dyslipidemia, preferably the Guidelines of the National Cholesterol Education Panel, which stratify treatment decisions and treatment goals based on low density lipoprotein levels and risk factors for cardiovascular disease.[74] However, the authors themselves point out that realizing recommendations may be difficult, in fact almost impossible, owing to the increasing evidence of severe interactions with ART.[73]

There are two main drug groups for treating hyperlipidemia. HMG-coenzyme A reductase inhibitors (statins) such as fluvastatin and pravastatin work predominantly by lowering cholesterol and have only slight impact on moderate to severe hypertriglyceridemia. The other medication group consists of fibric acid analogs such as gemfibrozil or fenofibrate. Gemofibrozil can effectively decrease serum triglycerides by inhibiting triglyceride synthesis and increasing lipoprotein lipase activity. Fenofibrate seems to have less interaction potential and is also effective.[75] In large trials in the general population both groups of drugs have been shown to be very effective in primary and secondary prevention of coronary artery disease.[76,77]

Only a few studies exist concerning HIV$^+$ patients with elevated lipids on PIs. However, the data on gemfibrozil, fenobrate, and various statins suggest that both classes of drugs can moderate lipid abnormalities.[75,78,79] Only one study has evaluated the combination of statins and fibric acids in HIV$^+$ patients on HAART. In a small group of patients with high lipid levels, in whom atorvastatin was added to gemfibrozil, the mean cholesterol and triglycerides concentration fell by 30% and 60%, respectively, over six months.[71] Many physicians have major reservations about this approach owing to problems associated with polypharmacy such as compliance, toxicity (rhabdomyolysis!), and drug interactions. For example, the side effects of HMG-CoAs include muscle weakness, muscle pain, and elevated liver enzymes, all of which may interfere with antiretroviral therapy. In a small study of 13 patients, two individuals receiving lovastatin, one with marked CK elevations, experienced myalgias.

In this context, a recent study on healthy volunteers has emphasized the interactions between PIs and statins which are metabolized by the p450 enzyme CYP3A4. In the presence of ritonavir and saquinavir, the median AUC for simvastatin and atorvastatin levels increased 31.6- and 4.5-fold, respectively.[81] In contrast, pravastatin concentrations declined. Although no significant adverse events occurred, this study has raised concern about strong and dangerous interactions between statins and PIs. Therefore, atorvastatin and simvastatin should be avoided in patients taking PIs. Another consideration is that to date it remains unclear whether the well-known association among the HIV⁻ population between metabolic changes and cardiovascular diseases can be extrapolated to HIV⁺ patients.[60]

WHAT ELSE CAN BE DONE?

There are several options for patients who experience metabolic changes while on HAART. Although so far there have been no studies comparing switching strategies versus addition of lipid-lowering drugs to a successful HAART, switching from PIs to PI-sparing regimens may be a reasonable option. Data indicate that this approach appears to be virologically and immunologically safe. However, the current prospective randomized studies on improvement of metabolic changes have produced inconclusive results. In the CNA30017 trial 105 patients were randomized to abacavir while 106 continued their PI regimen. Nucleoside reverse transcriptor inhibitors (NRTIs) were also continued. In the abacavir group there was evidence of a reduction in triglyceride and cholesterol levels and also of reversal of insulin resistance.[82] In another study, 80 patients on PI therapy with lipodystrophy syndrome were randomized to continue current ART or to continue NRTIs and substitute the PI(s) with abacavir, nevirapine, adefovir, and hydroxyurea. After 24 weeks, triglyceride, and total and LDL cholesterol levels were significantly decreased in the switch group. However, C-peptide, insulin, insulin resistance, and HDL cholesterol remained unchanged. Central fat declined more in the switch group as did total muscle mass.[83] In contrast, two other comparative studies showed that switching to nevirapine appeared to be associated with significant decreases in triglyceride levels, modest improvements in total cholesterol levels, and also with improvements in insulin resistance.[84,85] Our own experience concerning switching from a single-PI-containing to a PI-sparing regimen containing efavirenz appears to influence cholesterol but not triglycerides to a significant level.[86] In conclusion, there may be benefits to switching from a PI-based regimen to a PI-sparing regimen. However, resolution of the clinical abnormalities that may arise during PI therapy is incomplete, and metabolic improvement may be more prominent with nevirapine and abacavir than with efavirenz.

So-called drug holidays, or structured treatment interruptions, may be another option. Our own data from a prospective study on more than 110 patients taking drug holidays compared to 140 frequency-matched controls indicate that such structured treatment interruptions are clinically safe and lead to a significant decrease in blood lipids within a few weeks.[87]

In general, a detailed review of the case history of each individual patient is warranted. Many patients began their ART 1996–97, during the euphoric phase post-Vancouver.

In retrospect, there may be patients in whom treatment was started too early. In these cases, especially in those lipodystrophic patients with resistance and/or compliance problems or in patients where pretreatment viral load was low or unavailable, an interruption of therapy should be considered. A carefully monitored interruption of therapy may lead to prolonged periods of treatment-free time in patients with only modest rebound of viral load and slight decreases in CD4 counts.

In dyslipemic patients in whom a change of antiretroviral therapy appears inadvisable, one should consider lipid-lowering agents since diet and exercise often fail to control cholesterol or triglycerides. Although patient's adherence to lifestyle changes is often poor, more exercise, cessation of smoking and a more aggressive control of hypertension will contribute to a better risk profile in HIV$^+$ patients. One will also have to rethink that weight reduction is essential in obese patients—a difficult approach in a setting where, for many years, gaining or not losing weight were major goals for most patients. In diabetic patients, regular exercise and diet modifications are also strongly recommended. Sulfonylureas and metformin are reasonable choices. Acarbose should be avoided owing to diarrheal side effects.

CALCULATING THE RISKS AND BENEFITS OF HAART

The most important issue, however, may be to define the balance between the potential benefits of therapy in delaying clinical events and the potential morbidities associated with long-term side effects, that is, to identify those patients who need to be treated to avoid opportunistic infections and those who will be harmed by cardiovascular complications due to therapy. The hitherto most sophisticated model to address this issue was presented at the 40th ICAAC conference.[88] This elegant analysis by Matthias Egger included data from the Multicenter AIDS Cohort (MACS) Study on the risk of disease progression in the pre-HAART era[89] and data from the Swiss Cohort on the rate of progression in HAART-treated individuals.[90] A comparison between these large studies demonstrated that while HAART was associated with an 86% reduction in progression to AIDS among patients with CD4 cell counts of less than 200 cells/µl and a high viral load, only a 2% reduction was observed among patients with high CD4 cell counts of 200–350 cells/µl and a low viral load. Egger estimated that in the cohort with more advanced disease, the number of individuals who would need to be treated for one additional person to benefit was only 1–2, while for those who were less severely ill, this number was 50. Taking data from Carr et al. on HIV$^+$ patients with lipodystrophy[47] and from the Caerphilly Cohort in Southern Wales, which comprised more than 2,500 men aged 45–59 years with 5-year collections of data regarding risk factors for cardiovascular disease, Egger also estimated that the more severe forms of lipodystrophy that develop as a result of HAART can increase the risk of coronary artery disease by a factor of 3 to 4. He then focused on the number of individuals who would need to be treated for one additional person to be harmed. Calculation of the number needed to treat to produce harm resulted in values ranging from 10 to 200 subjects, based on different premorbid metabolic characteristics and factors such as gender, smoking status, and age.

Although these models may not be suitable for every individual and the overall analysis remains tilted in favor of treatment, they clarify that, at least for some subjects, there are circumstances in which the risk:benefit ratio of antiretroviral treatment is not beneficial. More studies addressing this issue are needed to define more clearly when antiretroviral treatment should be initiated.

CONCLUSIONS

There is evidence that cardiovascular problems are common in HIV+ patients and will increase with widespread use of HAART. This presents complex considerations for the physician. Although the current data do not warrant drastic changes in current antiretroviral therapy, more experience on switching strategies, treatment interruptions and delayed initiation of therapy is important. New guidelines on antiretroviral treatment should consider individual risk factor profile. Intervention studies on traditional risk factors such as smoking and hypertension, and more data on lipid-lowering drugs in the setting of HAART, are urgently needed in order to prevent an epidemic of cardiovascular events in HIV+ patients. Within the next decade, close collaboration between AIDS specialists and cardiologists presents an essential challenge.

ACKNOWLEDGMENTS

The authors would like to thank Dianne Lydtin and Elke Gersbacher for help in preparing the manuscript.

REFERENCES

1. MOCROFT, A., C. KATLAMA, A.M. JOHNSON, et al. 2000. AIDS across Europe, 1994–98: the EuroSIDA study. Lancet 356: 291–296.
2. PALELLA, F.J., K.M. DELANEY, A.C. MOORMAN, et al. 1998. Declining morbidity and mortality among patients with advanced human immunodeficiency virus infection. N. Engl. J. Med. 338: 853–860.
3. FINZI, D., J. BLANKSON, J.D. SILICIANO, et al. 1999. Latent infection of CD4+ T cells provides a mechanism for lifelong persistence of HIV-1, even in patients on effective combination therapy. Nat. Med. 5: 512–517.
4. FURTADO, M.R., D.S. CALLAWAY, J.P. PHAIR, et al. 1999. Persistence of HIV-1 transcription in peripheral-blood mononuclear cells in patients receiving potent antiretroviral therapy. N. Engl. J. Med. 340: 1614–1622.
5. ZHANG, L., B. RAMRATNAM, K. TENNER-RACZ, et al. 1999. Quantifying residual HIV-1 replication in patients receiving combination antiretroviral therapy. N. Engl. J. Med. 340: 1605–1613.
6. YUNIS, N.A. & V.E. STONE. 1998. Cardiac manifestations of HIV/AIDS: a review of disease spectrum and clinical management. J. Acquir. Immune Defic. Syndr. Hum. Retrovirol. 18: 145–154.
7. FRANCIS, C.K. 1990. Cardiac involvement in AIDS. Curr. Probl. Cardiol. 15: 574–639.
8. HERSKOWITZ, A., D. VLAHOV, S. WILLOUGHBY, et al. 1993. Prevalence and incidence of left ventricular dysfunction in patients with human immunodeficiency virus infection. Am. J. Cardiol. 71: 955–958.
9. KAUL, S., M.C. FISHBEIN & R.J SIEGEL. 1991. Cardiac manifestations of acquired immunodeficiency syndrome: a 1991 update. Am. Heart J. 122: 535–544.

10. BARBARO, G., G. DI LORENZO, B. GRISORIO, *et al.* 1998. Cardiac involvement in the acquired immunodeficiency syndrome: a multicenter clinical-pathological study. AIDS Res. Hum. Retroviruses **14:** 1071–1077.
11. CORALLO, S., M.R. MUTINELLI, M. MORONI, *et al.* 1988. Echocardiography detects myocardial damage in AIDS: prospective study in 102 patients. Eur. Heart J. **9:** 887–892.
12. BARBARO, G., G. DI LORENZO, B. GRISORIO, *et al.* 1998. Incidence of dilated cardiomyopathy and detection of HIV in myocardial cells of HIV-positive patients. N. Engl. J. Med. **339:** 1093–1099.
13. RERKPATTANAPIPAT, P., N. WONGPRAPARU, L.E. JACOBS, *et al.* 2000. Cardiac manifestations of acquired immunodeficiency syndrome. Arch. Intern. Med. **160:** 602–608.
14. MILEI J., D. GRANA, G.F. ALONSO, *et al.* 1998. Cardiac involvement in the acquired immunodeficiency syndrome—a review to push action. Clin. Cardiol. **21:** 465–472.
15. COTTON, P. 1990. AIDS giving rise to cardiac problems. JAMA **263:** 2149.
16. NEILD, P.J., A. AMADI, P. PONIKOWSKI, *et al.* 2000. Cardiac autonomic dysfunction in AIDS is not secondary to heart failure. Int. J. Cardiol. **74:** 133–137.
17. ZIETZ, C., B. HOTZ, M. STURZL, *et al.* 1996. Aortic endothelium in HIV-1 infection: chronic injury, activation, and increased leukocyte adherence. Am. J. Pathol. **149:** 1887–1898.
18. PATON, P., A. TABIB, R. LOIRE, *et al.* 1993. Coronary artery lesions and human immunodeficiency virus infection. Res. Virol. **144:** 225–231.
19. TABIB, A., C. LEROUX, J.F. MORNEX, *et al.* 2000. Accelerated coronary atherosclerosis and arteriosclerosis in young human-immunodeficiency-virus-positive patients. Coron. Artery Dis. **11:** 41–46.
20. LAFEUILLADE, A., M.C. ALESSI, J.A. GASTAUT, *et al.* 1992. Endothelial cell dysfunction in HIV infection. J. Acquir. Immune Defic. Syndr. **5:** 127–131.
21. MENDALL, M.A. 1998. Inflammatory responses and coronary heart disease. Br. Med. J. **316:** 953–954.
22. CHETTY, R., S. BATITANG & R. NAIR. 2000. Large artery vasculopathy in HIV-positive patients: another vasculitic enigma. Hum. Pathol. **31:** 374–379.
23. CONALDI, P.G., C. SERRA, A. TONIOLO, *et al.* 1995. Productive HIV-infection of human vascular endothelial cell requires cell proliferation and is stimulated by combined treatment with interleukin-1β plus tumor necrosis factor-α. J. Med. Virol. **47:** 355–363.
24. HUANG, M.B., M. HUNTER & V.C. BOND. 1999. Effect of extracellular human immunodeficiency virus type 1 glycoprotein 120 on primary human vascular endothelial cell cultures. AIDS Res. Hum. Retroviruses **15:** 1265–1277.
25. ASSMANN, G., H. SCHULTE, H. FUNKE, *et al.* 1998. The emergence of triglycerides as a significant independent risk in coronary artery disease. Eur. Heart J. **Suppl. M:** M8–M14.
26. GRUNWALD, C., D.P. KOTLER, R. HAMADEH, *et al.* 1989. Hypertriglyceridemia in the acquired immunodeficiency syndrome. Am. J. Med. **86:** 27–31.
27. NIAURA, R., W.G. SHADEL, K. MORROW, *et al.* 2000. Human immunodeficiency virus infection, AIDS, and smoking cessation: the time is now. Clin. Infect. Dis. **31:** 808–812
28. NIAURA, R., W.G. SHADEL, K. MORROW, *et al.* 1999. Smoking among HIV-positive persons. Ann. Behav. Med. **21**(Suppl.): 116.
29. MATTANA, J., F.P. SIEGAL, R.T. SANKARAN, *et al.* 1999. Absence of age-related increase in systolic blood pressure in ambulatory patients with HIV infection. Am. J. Med. Sci. **317:** 232–237.
30. MONSUEZ J..J., B. GALLET, L. ESCAUT, *et al.* 2000. Cardiac side effects of anti-HIV agents. Arch. Mal. Coeur Vaiss. **93:** 835–840.
31. MARGOLIN, A., S.K. AVANTS, J.F. SETARO, *et al.* 2000. Cocaine, HIV, and their cardiovascular effects: is there a role for ACE-inhibitor therapy? Drug Alcohol Depend. **61:** 35–45.
32. PUGLIESE, A., D. ISNARDI, A. SAINI, *et al.* 2000. Impact of highly active antiretroviral therapy in HIV-positive patients with cardiac involvement. J. Infect. **40:** 282–284.

33. HENRY, K., H. MELROE, J. HUEBSCH, *et al.* 1998. Severe premature coronary artery disease with protease inhibitors. Lancet **351:** 1328.
34. BEHRENS, G., H. SCHMIDT, D. MEYER, *et al.* 1998. Vascular complications associated with use of protease inhibitors. Lancet **351:** 1958.
35. FLYNN, T.E. & L.A. BRICKER. 1999. Myocardial infarction in HIV-infected men receiving protease inhibitors. Ann. Intern. Med. **131:** 548.
36. KARMOCHKINE, M. & G. RAGUIN. 1998. Severe coronary artery disease in a young HIV-infected man with no cardiovascular risk factor who was treated with indinavir. AIDS **12:** 2499.
37. FRIEDL, A.C., C.H. JOST, C. SCHALCHER, *et al.* 2000. Acceleration of confirmed coronary artery disease among HIV-infected patients on potent antiretroviral therapy. AIDS **14:** 2790–2792.
38. RICKERTS, V., H.R. BRODT, S. STASZEWSKI, *et al.* 2000. Incidence of myocardial infarctions in HIV-infected patients between 1983 and 1998: The Frankfurt HIV-Cohort Study. Eur. J. Med. Res. **5:** 329–333.
39. JUETTE, A., B. SALZBERGER, C. FRANZEN, *et al.* 1999. Increased morbidity from severe coronary heart disease in HIV-patients receiving protease inhibitors. Presented at the 6th Conference on Retroviruses and Opportunistic Infections, Chicago, IL, USA. Abstract 656.
40. COPLAN, P., A. NIKAS, A. SAAH, *et al.* 1999. No association observed between indinavir therapy for HIV/AIDS and myocardial infarction in 4 clinical trials with 2,825 subjects. Presented at the 6th Conference on Retroviruses and Opportunistic Infections, Chicago, IL, USA. Abstract 658.
41. LENORMAND-WELCKENAER, C., M. CAZAUBON, V. JOLY, *et al.* 2000. Carotid intima media thickness in protease inhibitor-treated HIV-1 infected patients with hyperlipemia. Presented at the 40th Interscience Conference on Antimicrobial Agents and Chemotherapy, Toronto, Ont., Canada. Abstract 1298.
42. CHEMINOT, N., J. GARIEPY, G. CHIRONI, *et al.* 2000. Diagnosis and determinants of subclinical arterial disease in HIV1-infected patients on HAART. Presented at the 7th Conference on Retroviruses and Opportunistic Infections, San Francisco, CA, USA. Abstract 31.
43. SOSMAN, J., M. KLEIN, J. BELLEHUMEUR, *et al.* 2000. Use of HIV protease inhibitors is associated with endothelial dysfunction. Antiviral Ther. **5**(Suppl. 5): 16.
44. MAGGI, P., G. SERIO, G. EPIFANI, *et al.* 2000. Premature lesions of the carotid vessels in HIV-1-infected patients treated with protease inhibitors. AIDS **14:** 123–128.
45. DEPAIRON M., S. CHESSEX, A. TELENTI, *et al.* 2000. Noninvasive morphological analysis of carotid and femoral arteries in protease-inhibitor-treated HIV-infected individuals. Presented at the 7th Conference on Retroviruses and Opportunistic Infections, San Francisco, CA, USA. Abstract 30.
46. CARR, A. & D.A. COOPER. 2000. Adverse effects of antiretroviral therapy. Lancet **356:** 1423–1430.
47. CARR, A., K. SAMARAS, A. THORISDOTTIR, *et al.* 1999. Diagnosis, prediction, and natural course of HIV-1 protease-inhibitor-associated lipodystrophy, hyperlipidaemia, and diabetes mellitus: a cohort study. Lancet **353:** 2093–2099.
48. CARR, A., K. SAMARAS, D.J, CHISHOLM, *et al.* 1998. Pathogenesis of HIV-1-protease inhibitor-associated peripheral lipodystrophy, hyperlipidaemia, and insulin resistance. Lancet **351:** 1881–1883.
49. BRINKMAN, K., J.A. SMEITINK, J.A ROMIJN, *et al.* 1999. Mitochondrial toxicity induced by nucleoside-analogue reverse-transcriptase inhibitors is a key factor in the pathogenesis of antiretroviral-therapy-related lipodystrophy. Lancet **354:** 1112–1115.
50. WALKER, U.A., M. BICKEL, S. VOLKSBECK, *et al.* 2000. Decrease of mitochondrial DNA content in adipose tissue of HIV-1-infected patients treated with NRTIs. Antiviral Ther. **5**(Suppl. 5): 5.
51. CARON, M., M. AUCLAIR, C. VIGOUROUX, *et al.* 2000. The HIV-protease inhibitor indinavir impairs adipocyte differentiation and induces insulin resistance by probably altering ADD 1/SREBP-1 maturation. Antiviral Ther. **5**(Suppl. 5): 4.

52. PARKER, R.A., D.S. MEYERS, B.A. ANDREWS, et al. 2000. Effects of nucleoside reverse transcriptase inhibitors and HIV protease inhibitors on adipogenesis and adipocyte metabolism. Antiviral Ther. 5(Suppl. 5): 4.
53. LIANG, J., O. DISTLER, D. COOPER, et al. 2000. HIV protease inhibitors increase secretion of apolipoproteins from hepatoma cells by preventing proteasomal degradation. Antiviral Ther. 5(Suppl. 5): 12.
54. DISTLER, O., J. LIANG, D. COOPER, et al. 2000. Direct effects of protease inhibitors on lipid metabolism in cultured mammalian cells. Antiviral Ther. 5(Suppl. 5): 13.
55. NGUYEN, A.T., A.M. GAGNON, J.B. ANGEL, et al. 2000. Ritonavir increases the level of active ADD-1/SREBP-1 protein during adipogenesis. AIDS 14: 2467–2473.
56. MAUSS, S., E. WOLF, M. CORZILLIUS, et al. 2000. Prevalence and risk factors for the HIV-associated lipodystrophy syndrome (HALS) in patients being 3 years on ART. Presented at the 40th Interscience Conference on Antimicrobial Agents and Chemotherapy, Toronto, Ont., Canada. Abstract 1287.
57. MALLAL, S.A., M. JOHN, C.B. MOORE, et al. 2000. Contribution of nucleoside analogue reverse transcriptase inhibitors to subcutaneous fat wasting in patients with HIV infection. AIDS 14: 1309–1316.
58. HADIGAN, C., J.B. MEIGS, C. CORCORAN, et al. 2001. Metabolic abnormalities and cardiovascular disease risk factors in adults with human immunodeficiency virus infection and lipodystrophy. Clin. Infect. Dis. 32: 130–139.
59. BATTERHAM, M.J., R. GARSIA & P.A. GREENOP. 2000. Dietary intake, serum lipids, insulin resistance and body composition in the era of highly active antiretroviral therapy 'Diet FRS Study.' AIDS 14: 1839–1843.
60. PASSALARIS, J.D., K.A. SEPKOWITZ & M.J. GLESBY. 2000. Coronary artery disease and human immunodeficiency virus infection. Clin. Infect. Dis. 31: 787–797.
61. WALLI, R., F.D. GOEBEL & T. DEMANT. 1998. Impaired glucose tolerance and protease inhibitors. Ann. Intern. Med. 129: 837–838.
62. BEHRENS, G., A. DEJAM, H. SCHMIDT, et al. 1999. Impaired glucose tolerance, beta cell function and lipid metabolism in HIV patients under treatment with protease inhibitors. AIDS 13: F63–70.
63. GERMINARIO, R.J., S.P. COLBY-GERMINARIO, C. CAMMALLERI, et al. 2000. The effects of a variety of protease inhibitors on insulin binding insulin-mediated sugar transport and cell toxicity in insulin target and non-target cell cultures. Antiviral Ther. 5 (Suppl. 5): 7.
64. NOOR, M., J. LO, K. MULLIGAN, et al. 2000. Metabolic effects of indinavir in healthy HIV-seronegative subjects. Antiviral Ther. 5(Suppl. 5): 8.
65. MYNARCIK, D.C., M.A. MCNURLAN, R.T. STEIGBIGEL, et al. 2000. Association of severe insulin resistance with both loss of limb fat and elevated serum tumor necrosis factor receptor levels in HIV lipodystrophy. J. Acquir. Immune Defic. Syndr. 25: 312–321.
66. HADIGAN, C., J. MEIGS, J. RABE, et al. 2000. Increased tPA antigen levels in the HIV lipodystrophy syndrome are reduced to response to metformin. Antiviral Ther. 5 (Suppl. 5): 15.
67. HADIGAN, C., C. CORCORAN, N. BASGOZ, et al. 2000. Metformin in the treatment of HIV lipodystrophy syndrome: a randomized controlled trial. JAMA 284: 472–477.
68. PERIARD, D., A. TELENTI, P. SUDRE, et al. 1999. Atherogenic dyslipidemia in HIV-infected individuals treated with protease inhibitors. The Swiss HIV Cohort Study. Circulation 100: 700–705.
69. SEGERER, S., J.R. BOGNER, R. WALLI, et al. 1999. Hyperlipidemia under treatment with proteinase inhibitors. Infection 27: 77–81.
70. KOPPEL, K., G. BRATT, M. ERIKSSON, et al. 2000. Serum lipid levels associated with increased risk for cardiovascular disease is associated with highly active antiretroviral therapy (HAART) in HIV-1 infection. Int. J. STD AIDS 11: 451–455.
71. HENRY, K., H. MELROE, J. HUEBESCH, et al. 1998. Atorvastatin and gemfibrozil for protease-inhibitor-related lipid abnormalities. Lancet 352: 1031–1032.
72. CONSTANS, J., J.L. PELLEGRIN, E. PEUCHANT, et al. 1994. Plasma lipids in HIV-infected patients: a prospective study in 95 patients. Eur. J. Clin. Invest. 24: 416–420.

73. DUBE, M.P., D. SPRECHER, W.K. HENRY, *et al.* 2000. Preliminary guidelines for the evaluation and management of dyslipidemia in adults infected with human immunodeficiency virus and receiving antiretroviral therapy: recommendations of the Adult AIDS Clinical Trial Group Cardiovascular Disease Focus Group. Clin. Infect. Dis. **31:** 1216–1224.

74. NATIONAL CHOLESTEROL EDUCATION PANEL. 1994. Detection, evaluation, and treatment of high blood cholesterol in adults (adult treatment panel II). Circulation **89:** 1333–1445.

75. THOMAS, J.C., M.F. LOPES-VIRELLA & V.E. DEL BENE. 2000. Use of fenofibrate in the management of protease inhibitor-associated lipid abnormalities. Pharmacotherapy **20:** 727–734.

76. SCANDINAVIAN SIMAVASTATIN SURVIVAL STUDY (4 S). 1994. Randomised trial of cholesterol lowering in 4444 patients with coronary heart disease. Lancet **344:** 1383–1389.

77. WEST OF SCOTLAND CORONARY PREVENTION STUDY. 1996. Identification of high-risk groups and comparison with other cardiovascular trials. Lancet **348:** 1339–1344.

78. HEWITT, R.G., M.J. SHELTON & L.D. ESCH. 1999. Gemfibrozil effectively lowers protease inhibitor-related hypertriglyceridemia in HIV-1-positive patients. AIDS **13:** 868–869.

79. MURILLAS, J., T. MARTIN, A. RAMOS, *et al.* 1999. Atorvastatin for protease inhibitor-related hyperlipidemia. AIDS **13:** 1424–1425.

80. PENZAK, S.R., S.K. CHUCK & G.V. STAJICH. 2000. Safety and efficacy of HMG-CoA reductase inhibitors for treatment of hyperlipidemia in patients with HIV infection. Pharmacotherapy **20:** 1066–1071.

81. FICHTENBAUM, C., J. GERBER & S. ROSENKRANZ. 2000. Pharmacokinetic interactions between protease inhibitors and selected HMG-CoA reductase inhibitors. Presented at the 7th Conference on Retroviruses and Opportunistic Infections, San Francisco, CA, USA. Abstract LB6.

82. GOEBEL, F. & R.K. WALLI for the CNA30017 STUDY TEAM. 2000. A novel use of abacavir to simplify therapy in PI experienced patients successfully treated with HAART: CNA30017. Presented at the 7th Conference on Retroviruses and Opportunistic Infections, San Francisco, CA, USA. Abstract 51.

83. CARR, A. & D.A. COOPER. 2000. A randomized, multicenter study of protease inhibitor substitution in aviremic patients with antiretroviral lipodystrophy syndrome. Presented at the 7th Conference on Retroviruses and Opportunistic Infections, San Francisco, CA, USA. Abstract 205.

84. BARREIRO, P., V. SORIANO, F. BLANCO, *et al.* 2000. Risks and benefits of replacing protease inhibitors by nevirapine in patients under long-term successful triple combination therapy. AIDS **14:** 807–812.

85. RUIZ, L., E. NEGREDO, P. DOMINGO, *et al.* 2000. Clinical, virological, and immunological benefit of switching the protease inhibitor by nevirapine in HAART experienced patients suffering lipodystrophy (LD): 36-week follow-up. Presented at the 7th Conference on Retroviruses and Opportunistic Infections, San Francisco, CA, USA. Abstract 206.

86. HOFFMANN C., E. JAEGEL-GUEDES, E. WOLF, *et al.* 2000. PI to Efavirenz (EFV) switch effect on lipids in HIV-positive patients. Presented at the XIIIth International AIDS Conference, Durban, South Africa Abstract WePeB4185.

87. HOFFMANN C., E. WOLF, S. MUELLER, *et al.* 2000. Drug holidays in HIV[+] patients—clinical issues. Presented at the Fifth International Congress on Drug Therapy in HIV Infection, Glasgow, Scotland. Abstract 68.

88. EGGER, M. 2000. Cardiovascular epidemiology in the context of HIV disease. Presented at the 40th Interscience Conference on Antimicrobial Agents and Chemotherapy, Toronto, Ont., Canada. Abstract 1374.

89. MELLORS, J.W., A. MUNOZ, J.V. GIORGI, *et al.* 1997. Plasma viral load and CD4[+] lymphocytes as prognostic markers of HIV-1 infection. Ann. Intern. Med. **126:** 946–954.

90. LEDERGERBER, B., M. EGGER, V. ERARD, *et al.* 1999. AIDS-related opportunistic illnesses occurring after initiation of potent antiretroviral therapy: the Swiss HIV Cohort Study. JAMA **282:** 2220–2226.

HIV Inhibitors: Problems and Reality

JÓZSEF TÖZSÉR

Department of Biochemistry and Molecular Biology, Faculty of Medicine, Debrecen University, H-4012 Debrecen, Hungary

ABSTRACT: The human immunodeficiency virus encodes three replication enzymes, which are required for a productive life-cycle. Currently, several anti-retroviral drugs are available for clinical use, and they are inhibitors of either the reverse transcriptase or the viral protease. The introduction of combination anti-retroviral therapy (HAART) changed the prognosis of HIV infection. However, current therapy is not able to eradicate the virus, only suppress it; therefore, long-term use of the drugs is required to keep the viral load under control. Most of the problems associated with the HIV therapy are the consequence of the necessarily long-term use of the drugs. The long-term effectiveness of current inhibitors as therapeutic agents is limited by the rapid development of drug-resistant variants. Furthermore, various side effects have been reported. These side effects include hypersensitivity, mitochondrial toxicity, lypodystrophy syndrome, insulin resistance and cardiovascular disorders. Further drug development is necessary to design new compounds that have efficacy similar to the currently used drugs in the management of HIV infection and that are potent against the resistant viruses but do not exhibit unwanted metabolic side effects.

KEYWORDS: HIV-1; replication enzymes; inhibitors; resistance; side effects

The human immunodeficiency virus (HIV) encodes three replication enzymes, a protease (PR), a reverse transcriptase (RT) which also contains a ribonuclease H (RNase H) activity, and an integrase (IN) that are assembled into the viral particle. The PR is required for proteolyic "maturation" of the viral particle, RT reverse transcribes the viral RNA into double stranded DNA, while IN carries out the integration of the viral DNA into the host-cell chromosome[1,2] (see FIGURE 1). Currently 15 anti-retroviral drugs are available for clinical use, and they are either RT or PR inhibitors. The introduction of combination anti-retroviral therapy (highly active anti-retroviral therapy; HAART) in 1995–1996 changed the prognosis of HIV infection. HIV-related morbidity and mortality rates in patients with advanced HIV infection have significantly declined. However, there are severe limits of HAART. Current anti-retroviral therapies do not allow viral eradication, therefore long-term use of the drugs is required. As a consequence, resistance develops in a significant portion of patients. Furthermore, several adverse metabolic side effects have been observed associated with the therapy.

Address for correspondence: Dr. József Tözsér, Department of Biochemistry and Molecular Biology, Faculty of Medicine, Debrecen University, H-4012 Debrecen, Hungary.
tozser@indi.biochem.dote.hu

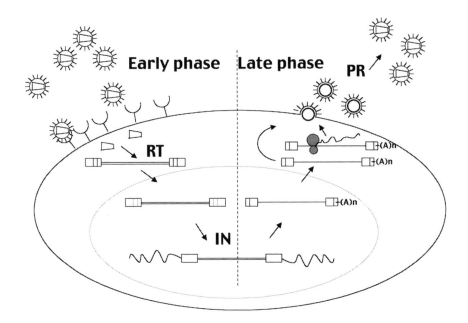

FIGURE 1. Replication cycle of HIV-1. The cycle starts by the receptor-envelope protein interaction on the surface of a susceptible cell, leading to fusion and entry of the cone-shaped core. Reverse transcription then generates a double-stranded DNA copy of the RNA genome (mediated by RT). The provirus is transported into the nucleus and integrated into chromosomal DNA (mediated by IN). In the late phase of the cycle, the viral DNA is transcribed by the cellular RNA polymerase II. The RNA is used as template for protein synthesis. Virion proteins and progeny RNA assemble at the plasma membrane, and progeny "immature" virus is released by a process of budding followed by PR-mediated "maturation" into infectious virus.

REPLICATION ENZYMES OF HIV-1: TARGETS OF CHEMOTHERAPY

Reverse Transcriptase

The RT possess three enzymatic activities: an RNA-dependent DNA polymerase, ribonuclease H, and a DNA-dependent DNA polymerase activities. By these activities the RT produces a double-stranded DNA copy from the plus-strand viral genomic RNA[1] in the early phase of viral replication cycle (FIG. 1). The HIV-1 RT is a heterodimer composed of a 66 kDa subunit (p66) and a 51 kDa subunit (p51) (see FIGURE 2). The p51 subunit is generated by PR-mediated processing of a p66 molecule (FIG. 2A). The X-ray crystal structures of HIV-1 RT revealed that the polymerase regions of p66 and p51 can be divided into four subdomains. Three of these subdomains are denoted "finger," "palm," and "thumb" owing to the anatomical resemblance of the structure to a right hand. The fourth subdomain lies between the polymerase and the RNase H domain, therefore it is called the "connection" subdomain. These subdomains are arranged differently in each subunit and thus the heterodimer is asymmetric (FIG. 2B). The polymerase active-site residues are located in the "palm" domain of p66. Kinetic studies with HIV-1 RT revealed an ordered reaction pathway similar to that of other polymerases, with binding of the template-primer as a first step, followed by the binding of the dNTP substrate. As a consequence of the absence of RT editing functions, retroviruses, like other RNA viruses, mutate at a much higher rate than cellular genes. In every replication cycle typically one nucleotide mutation occurs per genome. This yields a natural variation throughout the sequence unless selective pressure keeps the sequence (or at least part of it) conserved. Owing to the high replication rate and error-prone RT activity, HIV exists as a quasi-species within each infected individual.

The first drug used in HIV therapy was a nucleoside analog reverse transcriptase inhibitor (NRTI), 3'-azido-2',3'-dideoxythymidine (zidovudine, AZT). Later other NRTI drugs were also used in therapy (see FIGURE 3 A). These analogs are taken up by cells, become converted to the respective triphosphate forms, and presumably inhibit DNA synthesis as chain terminators. A group of non-nucleoside inhibitors (NNRTIs) have also been developed (FIG. 3 B). Unlike NRTIs, these drugs interact with the RT at an allosteric, non-substrate binding site. In spite of their structural diversity, NNRTIs bind to the same allosteric site of RT, close to the active site of the enzyme (FIG. 2 B).

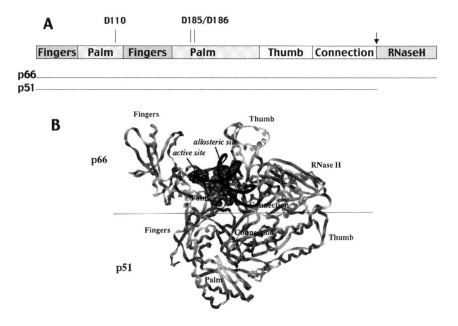

FIGURE 2. Linear map (**A**) and ribbon diagram (**B**) of the active p66/p51 heterodimer form of the reverse transcriptase. The active site residues of the polymerase domain are indicated above the linear map, while the *arrow* indicates the site of partial PR-mediated processing (RT/RH site as shown in FIG. 4). The four subdomains of the polymerase part of p66 and p51 have different relative orientations. The Asp residues of the active site of the polymerase domain as well as the residues of the allosteric NNRTI binding site are in space-filling representation. *Black ribbon* represents the RNA-DNA hybrid.

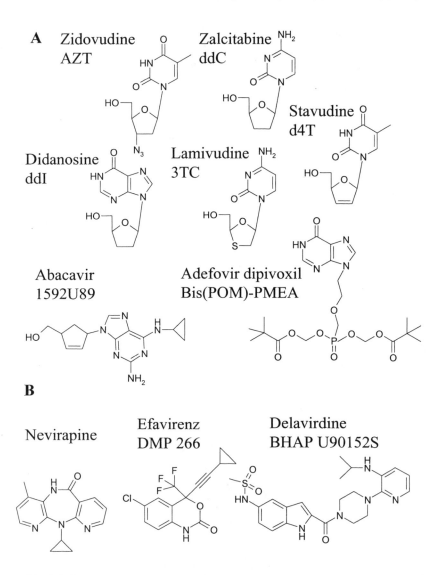

FIGURE 3. Name and structure of nucleoside type (**A**) and non-nucleoside type (**B**) reverse transcriptase inhibitors currently used in combination antiretroviral therapy.

Protease

In the late phase of viral replication, the Gag and Gag-Pro-Pol polyproteins are assembled together with the envelope proteins and the viral genomic RNA at the surface of the infected cell, and budding yields "immature" virions with a "doughnut-shaped" capsid structure (FIG. 1). The PR cleaves the viral polyproteins at a limited number of sites (see FIGURE 4 A), producing a condensed, "cone-shaped" core (FIG. 1).

Only the "mature" virion formed by these proteolytic events is infectious, therefore this function of the PR is critical for virus replication. As shown in Figure 4A, the PR is part of the Gag-Pro-Pol, and together with the Pol proteins it is synthesized by ribosomal frameshifting.[3] The relatively low frequency of frameshifting assures that the amount of replication enzymes in the virions is only about 5–10% of those of the structural proteins encoded at the *gag* gene. The cleavage sites where the polyproteins are processed are given in Figure 4B. It is a special feature of the PR that even though the enzyme is fairly specific it is not possible to give a consensus substrate sequence. There have been numerous studies on the specificity of the HIV-1 PR to resolve this apparent contradiction and provide data for inhibitor design. Early specificity studies revealed two types of cleavage sites, type 1 having aromatic residues and Pro, and type 2 having hydrophobic residues (excluding Pro) at the site of cleavage (Fig. 4B). These two types of cleavage sites seem to have different preferences for the surrounding positions.[4] The type 1 cleavage site is very important for several reasons. No other proteinase, except pepsin, is known to act at the imino side of a Pro residue. Indeed, the uniqueness of Pro in that position was recognized even before the discovery of the PR,[3] and it was suggested early that inhibitors based on the this type of cleavage site

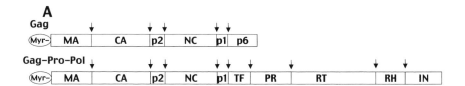

A

B	Site	Sequence	Type
	MA/CA	SQNY–↓–PIV	1
	CA/p2	ARVL–↓–AEA	2
	p2/NC	ATIM–↓–MQR	2
	NC/p1	RQAN–↓–FLG	–
	p1/p6	PQNF–↓–LQS	–
	TF/PR	SFNF–↓–PQI	1
	PR/RT	TLNF–↓–PIS	1
	RT/RH	AETF–↓–YVD	2
	RT/IN	RKIL–↓–FLD	2

FIGURE 4. Linear maps of the Gag and Gag-Pro-Pol polyproteins (**A**), and PR cleavage site sequences together with their classification (**B**). Both polyproteins are myristylated at their N-terminus. The polyproteins are processed into matrix (MA), capsid (CA), nucleocapsid (NC), three smaller fragments and proteins designated according to their molecular weight (e.g., p1, a kDa peptide), transframe protein (TF), protease (PR), reverse transcriptase (RT) which is active as p66/p51 having RNase H (RH) domain in the larger protein, and integrase (IN). Sites of cleavages are indicated by *arrows* above the maps. Classification of cleavage sites was done based on the sequence around the site of cleavage.[4]

should be specific against the retroviral PRs.[5] Detailed specificity studies as well as HIV-1 PR-inhibitor crystal structures appear to indicate that there is very strong sequence context-dependence of the specificity of PR.[4] In other terms, the interactions between the ligand side chains and respective binding pockets are not additive, they are complicated by various types of ligand side chain interactions. The strong sequence context-dependence should be taken into account in the design of proteinase inhibitors: a mutation in a substrate binding subsite of the PR indirectly could influence the specificity of the other binding sites.

The sequence of the HIV-1 PR is shown in FIGURE 5. Three characteristic conserved regions found also in other retroviral proteases are the active site triplet containing the catalytic aspartate, the so called flap region, and a third conserved region close to the C-terminal end. The natural variations of the sequence are also indicated in FIGURE 5; these residues were found in different HIV-1 clones in the absence of PR inhibitor treatment. The structure of the HIV-1 PR was discovered more than a decade ago, and it greatly facilitated rational inhibitor design. Currently it is the most represented structure in the structural databanks.[6] The HIV-1 PR is a

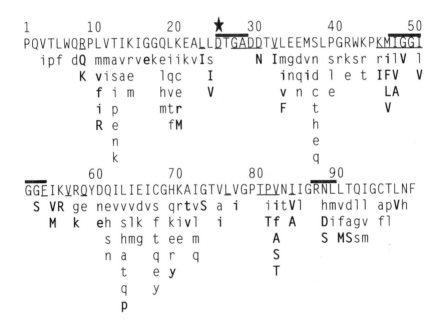

FIGURE 5. Sequence of the HIV-1 protease (HXB2 clone). Conserved regions characteristic of retroviral proteinases are indicated by *horizontal bars* above the sequence, while the active site aspartate is indicated by a *star*. Residues of the PR that are involved in ligand binding are underlined. Residues occurring as natural variations are indicated by lower case letters while those which have also been found as mutations occurring in drug resistance are in bold. Residues occurring only in drug-resistant mutants are indicated by capital bold letters. Sequences were taken from the HIV database (http://hiv-web.lanl.gov) and from Kozal *et al.*[38]

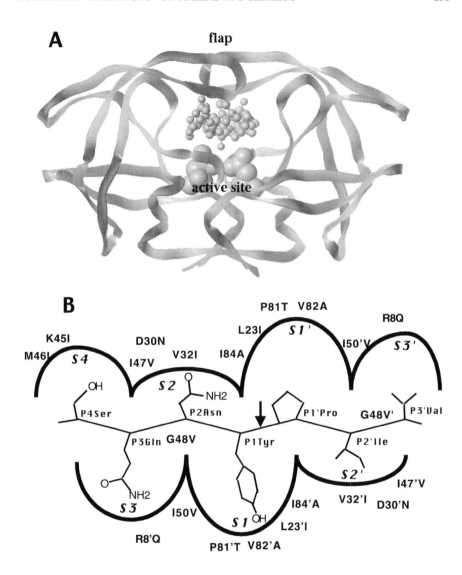

FIGURE 6. Ribbon diagram of the homodimeric active HIV-1 protease with a bound ligand (**A**) and a schematic representation of the substrate binding subsites of the enzyme (**B**). The active site aspartates and the ligand are shown in space filling and ball-and stick representations, respectively. The relative size of each subsite is indicated approximately by the area enclosed by the *curved line* around each substrate side chain. According to the nomenclature, residues of the ligand (substrate or inhibitor) interacting with the protease are designated as P1, P2, P3, etc. from the scissile bond towards the N-terminus of the substrate, and P1′, P2′, etc. towards the C-terminus. The respective substrate binding subsites are designated as S1, S2, and so forth. The relative location of residues forming the subsites (see FIG. 5) is also shown. Some of the mutations occurring in resistance are indicated as wild type residue/residue found in resistant viruses. Amino acid residues of the second subunit of the protease dimer are indicated by a prime.

Saquinavir
Invirase
Ro 31-8959

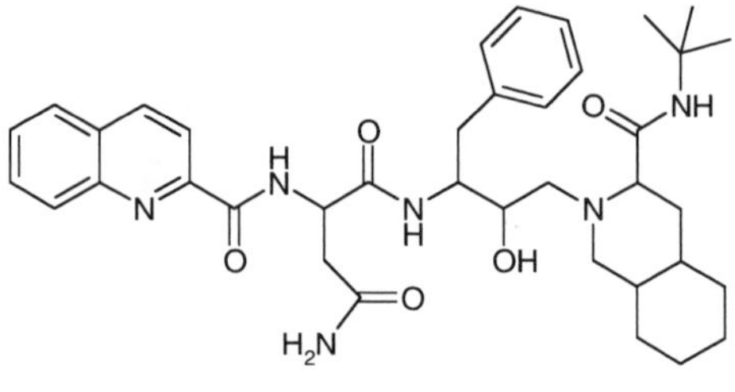

Indinavir
Crixivan
MK-639
L735,524

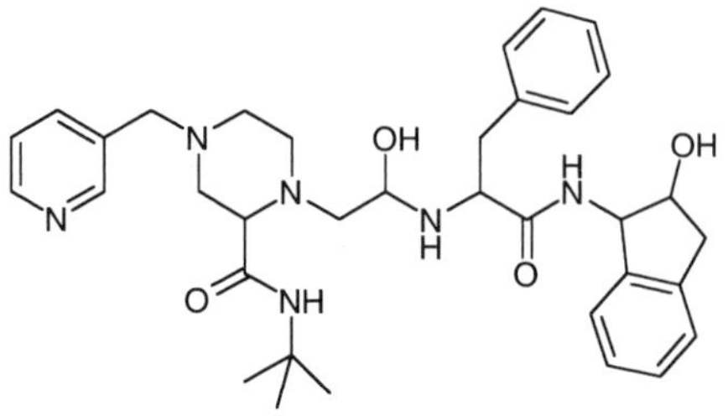

Ritonavir
Norvir
ABT-538

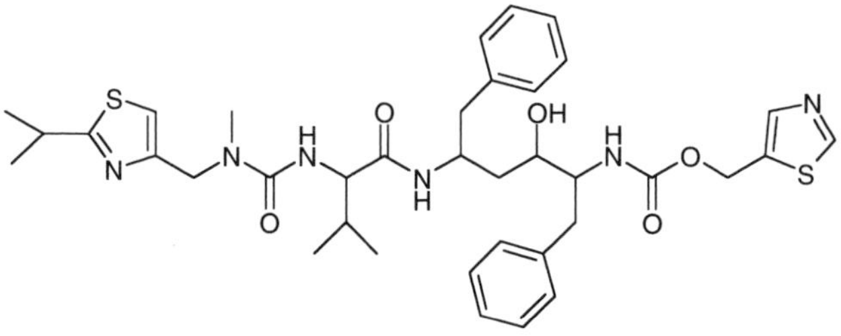

Nelfinavir
Viracept
Ag-1343

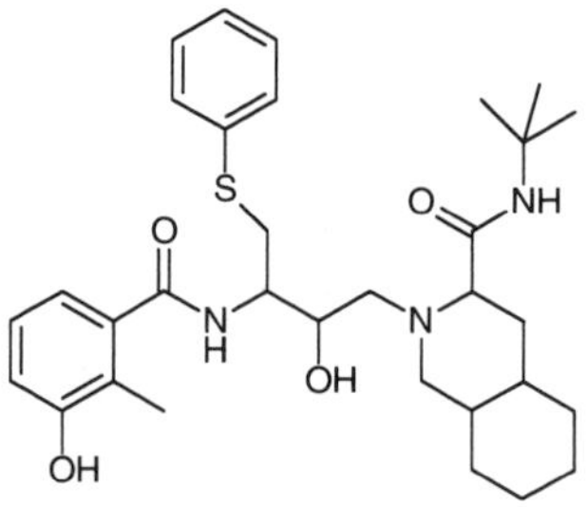

Amprenavir
Aguerase
VX-478

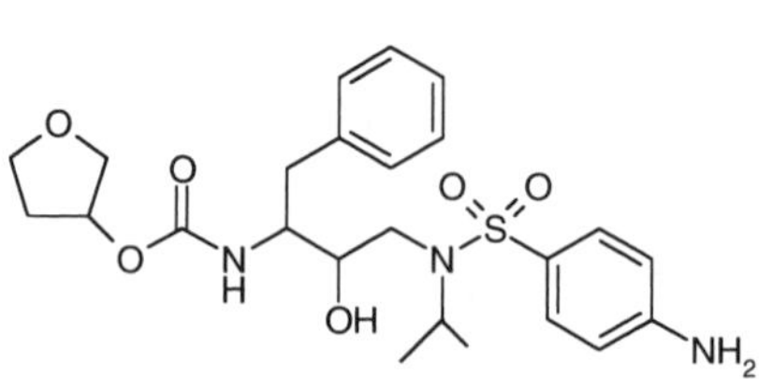

FIGURE 7. Name and structure of HIV-1 PR inhibitors used in antiretroviral therapy.

homodimeric aspartic protease of subunits 99 residues long. In the absence of ligand it is almost perfectly symmetrical.[6] It has two flap regions which are very flexible in the absence of ligand, but which are closed down on the bound inhibitors as well as substrates (see FIGURE 6A). A schematic diagram of the substrate binding site of HIV-1 PR with the modeled interaction of an oligopeptide representing the HIV-1 matrix/capsid cleavage site shows that the enzyme recognizes at least seven residues of a substrate, which are anchored in an extended beta sheet form (FIG. 6B). The side chains of the substrate fit into more or less well-defined substrate binding pockets (FIG. 6B). Inhibitors bind in a very similar way to the enzyme, so they mimic the enzyme-substrate interactions.

The names and structures of HIV PR inhibitors currently used in therapy are shown in FIGURE 7. A common feature of these compounds is that they are peptidomimetics, they mimic the substrates of the PR. The enzyme-inhibitor interactions, similar to the enzyme-substrate interactions, are primarily hydrophobic. Typically, these inhibitors contain a phenyl residue at the P1 position. Another common feature of these inhibitors is that they contain a nonhydrolyzable transition-state mimic, like a hydoxyethylamine group, at the site corresponding to the cleavable bond in the substrates. Saquinavir was the first approved HIV-1 PR drug. It is based on a type 1 cleavage site, in which the Pro was replaced by a saturated isoquinoline ring. Indinavir and nelfinavir also mimic the type 1 cleavage site; ritonavir was developed from a symmetric molecule, while amprenavir is a sulfonamide compound.

PROBLEMS ASSOCIATED WITH HIV THERAPY

Current anti-retroviral therapy is not able to eradicate the virus from the body of the infected individual, only suppress it, therefore long-term use of the antiretroviral drugs is required to keep the viral load under control. The existence of organ sanctuaries (e.g., brain, testis) and long-lived infected cells carrying proviral DNA contribute to the limits to eradication of virus.[7] Most of the problems associated with HIV therapy are the consequence of the necessarily long-term use of the drugs.

Development of Resistance

The first report on HIV drug resistance to zidovudine[8] was followed with a large number of reports documenting genotypic correlates of reduced drug susceptibility *in vitro*, and virological failure, *in vivo*. Viruses requiring only one mutation to generate high level resistance will very likely be represented within the prevailing HIV-1 quasi-species. When more than one mutation is required, there is a reduced chance of preexistence of these mutations as well as of their generation. The acquisition of high level zidovudine resistance requires several changes in the RT,[9] including at amino acid positions 41, 67, 70, 215, and 219. The emergence of resistance to ddI and ddC occurs more slowly than for zidovudine, and the mutations (at positions 65, 69, 74 and 184) lead to only modest loss of potency.[10] A high level of resistance is generated by the M184V mutation within RT, which occurs within weeks of monotherapy. Resistance against abacavir is associated with mutations at RT positions 65, 74, 115 and 184.[10] There is a variable cross-resistance between the approved drugs. In addition, combination therapies may select for novel mutations not observed in monotherapy studies.

Resistance against NNRTIs develop rapidly, resulting from mutations at the amino acid residues surrounding the NNRTI-binding site. Failure of NNRTIs is often caused by a single mutation, therefore it is likely that these variants pre-exist as natural sequence variations. Emergence of NNRTI-resistant HIV strains can be prevented if NNRTIs are combined with NRTIs and used from the beginning at sufficiently high concentrations.[11]

Resistance also develops against PR inhibitors. In most cases mutations occur in the PR gene. While most of the natural variations are outside the substrate binding sites, several of the mutations conferring resistance involve residues of the substrate binding subsites and therefore alter the specificity and catalytic power of the enzyme (FIG. 5). Recent studies showed, that in patients receiving HIV PR inhibitors, not only is the PR mutated, but mutations were also observed at the nucleocapsid/p1 and p1/p6 Gag cleavage sites. These mutations were first described in *in vitro* studies, but later they were also found in patients undergoing indinavir therapy.[12,13] These mutations occurred together with mutations in the PR gene, at positions 46, 54, 71, 82, 89 and 90.[13]

Metabolic Side Effects

Hypersensitivity

Drug hypersensitivity in HIV-1 infected patients is about 100 times more common than in the general population.[14] It manifests as a maculopapular rash, often with fever. All licensed NNRTIs, the NRTI abacavir, and the PR inhibitor amprenavir has been reported to cause hypersensitivity, which is rare with the other licensed antiretroviral drugs.[15] The pathogenesis of hypersensitivity is unknown.

Mitochondrial Toxicity

The NRTIs are phosphorylated intracellularly to active triphosphate forms, and are then incorporated into the newly synthesized DNA strands. The lack of 3′ hydroxyl in this type of inhibitors results in chain termination. The major toxicities of these inhibitors are thought to be due to inhibition of mitochondrial DNA polymerase γ, resulting in impaired synthesis of mitochondrial enzymes that generate ATP by oxidative phosphorylation. As a consequence, myopathy, neuropathy, hepatic steatosis, and lactic acidosis may develop.[15] The prevalence and severity of symptoms usually increase with the length of therapy. The relatively tissue-specific nature of these toxicities may be due to tissue-specific drug penetration and metabolism, to the level of natural nucleotides in the target tissues, and to the dependency of the target tissue upon mitochondria for function.[16] NNRTIs are usually less toxic than the NRTIs, likely as a consequence of the absence of similar allosteric site in cellular DNA polymerases.

Lipodystrophy Syndrome

The main clinical features of this symptom are peripheral fat loss and central fat accumulation (within the abdomen, breasts, and over the dorsocervical spine). The overall prevalence of at least on of this features is between 18% and 83% depending on the study and criteria used.[15] Metabolic features associated with the syndrome include hypertriglyceridemia, hypercholesterolemia, insulin resistance and type 2 diabetes mellitus. These metabolic abnormalities are more profound in those receiving protease inhibitors.[17] The prevalence of diabetes mellitus is about 8–10%, while a further 15% of patients have impaired glucose tolerance.[15]

The molecular mechanism of these symptoms is not known, although several proteins are suspected or verified to be able to interact with the antiretroviral drugs. The 3A isoform of cytochrome P450 (Cyp450A3) has been found to be inhibited by the PR inhibitors *in vitro*, at concentrations which correspond to the *in vivo* steady state concentration of these drugs during therapy.[18] Cyp450A3 is involved in the metabolism of several different drugs, including some NNRTIs, peptides and peptidomimetics.[19] As HIV patients are likely to be taking multiple prolonged drug regimens, this may lead to drug interactions as a result of enzyme induction or inhibition. This effect can also be utilized in AIDS therapy, since a fairly low concentration of ritonavir, the most potent inhibitor of Cyp450A3 among the PR inhibitors, can substantially increase the steady state concentration of other PR inhibitors used in combination. Other drugs like phenobarbital, rifampicin, which are inducers of Cyp450A3, may reduce the plasma concentrations of the PR inhibitors and reduce their antiviral efficacy.

Inhibition of Cyp450A3 has been associated with the development of lipodystrophy owing to its role of retinoid metabolism and signaling. It converts all *trans* retinoic acid to 9-*cis* retionic acid, which acts as a ligand of RXR receptor. RXR-peroxisome proliferator-activated receptor type gamma (PPARγ) heterodimers are involved in the adipocyte differentiation, so impaired activity of this heterodimer due to the decreased 9-*cis* retionic acid production may lead to increased adipocyte apoptosis.[20] In a recent study, PR inhibitors were found to augment or inhibit the differentiation of preadipocytes, but direct inhibition of PPARγ-mediated gene transciption was excluded.[21]

Other possible molecular targets are the LDL-receptor related protein (LRP) and cytoplasmic retinoic acid-binding protein type 1 (CRABP-1).[20] The sequence homology between the active site of HIV-1 PR (DTG) and parts of LRP and CRABP-1 are shown in FIGURE 8A. LRP is a hepatic receptor important for postprandial chylomicron clearance. In complex with lipoprotein lipase, it is also responsible for cleaving fatty acids from circulating triglycerides, permitting the entering of free fatty acids into adipocytes. CRABP-1 is a ubiquitous protein that bind virtually all cytosolic retinoic acid and presents it to cytochrome P450A3. However, there is no experimental verification of the inhibition of these molecules by protease inhibitors. Furthermore, the homology is also somewhat misleading. The N-terminal half of the homologous region (FIG. 8A) is mostly buried in the HIV-1 PR at the dimer interface and is not in contact with substrates or inhibitors. Although some of the residues at the C-terminal half of the homologous region could be involved in ligand binding, except in a few cases, the PR-ligand interaction is primarily hydrophobic; therefore, these residues, especially the aspartates are not involved in ligand recognition. As shown in FIGURE 8B, the region homologous to the substrate binding part of HIV-1 PR is in a loop region of CRABP-1, and is not involved in retinoic acid binding. If indeed LRP and CRABP-1 are able to bind the PR inhibitors, it could be due to the hydrophobic, lipid-like nature of these compounds and not to the sequence homology with HIV-1 PR. A recent study showed that HIV-1 PR inhibitors indeed affect retinoic acid metabolism, although the molecular mechanism has not been elucidated.[22]

The characteristic feature of lipodystrophy, peripheral fat wasting with central adiposity, may be the consequence of the different metabolism of these fat tissues. It has been hypothesized that peripherial adipocytes might synthesize lipids from glucose while abdominal adipocytes may obtain their lipid from circulating triglycerides.[23]

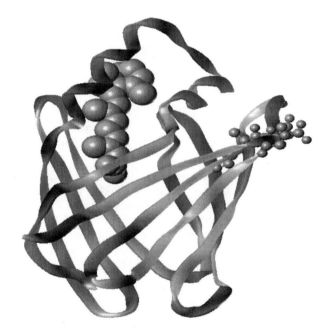

A-E-A-L-L-C-N-G-Q-D-D-C LRP (aa2919-2930)

K-E-A-L-L-D-T-G-A-D-D-T HIV PR (aa 19-30)

D-E-L-I-L-T-F-G-A-D-D-V CRABP-1 (aa 116-127)

FIGURE 8. Sequence around the active site of HIV-1 proteinase (A) together with the homologous regions of LDL-receptor-related protein (LRP) and cytoplasmic retinoid acid-binding protein type 1 (CRABP-1) based on Carr *et al.*,[20] and ribbon representation of the structure of CRABP-1 (B). The residues of HIV-1 protease that are involved in enzyme-ligand interactions (see FIG. 5) are underlined. The retinoic acid bound to CRABP-1 and residues with the highest homology with HIV-1 protease (bracketed in panel A) are given in space-filling and ball-and stick representations, respectively. (The accession number of the CRABP-1 structure in the Protein Data Bank: 1CBR.)

More recently, some features of the lipodystrophy syndrome have been suggested to represent mitochondrial toxicity of NRTIs, since lipoatrophy have been reported in patients who have received only such inhibitors, and similar symptoms occur in HIV[-] patients with mitochondrial defects.[24–26]

Mechanism of Insulin Resistance Caused by Protease Inhibitors

Shortly after the introduction of PR inhibitors into AIDS therapy, reports linking their use with the development of hyperglycemia and insulin resistance began to appear.[27–29] PR inhibitors were shown to inhibit insulin-stimulated glucose uptake of adipocytes *in vitro*, while the basal glucose transport was largely unaffected.[23] Insulin stimulates glucose uptake in muscle and fat cells mainly through GLUT4. Upon insulin binding, the intrinsic tyrosine kinase activity of the insulin receptor is activated, which in turn activates a signaling cascade.[30] Ultimately, there is a translocation of intracellularly sequestered glucose transporters, mainly the GLUT4 transporter isoform, to the plasma membrane.[31] PR inhibitors block the transport capability of GLUT4 and not its translocation to the plasma membrane.[23] GLUT4 is predominantly expressed in tissues responsible for the bulk of whole body glucose disposal (skeletal as well as cardiac muscle and fat)[32] and it is believed to be the principal transporter isoform mediating insulin-stimulated glucose uptake at these sites. Since glucose transport into muscle is the rate-limiting step for whole body glucose disposal,[33] the inhibition of GLUT4 by the PR inhibitors could be the cause of insulin resistance observed in HIV patients receiving this type of drugs. A knockout mouse lacking GLUT4 is insulin-resistant and almost devoid of fat tissue.[34] Thus, GLUT4 activity may be required for adipogenesis. Therefore, in addition to insulin resistance, the inhibition of GLUT4 by PR inhibitors may also contribute to the development of lipodystrophy.

PR Inhibitors and Cardiovasular Diseases

Cardiovasular diseases are becoming very important side effects of PR inhibitors. Dyslipidemia, as described before, at concentrations associated with increased cardiovascular disease occurs in about 70% of patients. Therefore, the metabolic changes caused by the PR inhibitors could indirectly lead to cardiovascular diseases. Several reports have described premature coronary-artery disease in patients with few or no risk factors who were receiving PR inhibitors.[35–37] However, some cases have occurred in patients who received very brief PR inhibitor therapy and may represent a prothrombotic effect of therapy rather than an arteriosclerotic effect.

In summary, since RT and PR inhibitors play a vital role in prolonging the lifespan of HIV patients and are often administered over an extended period of time, the metabolic side effects and their chronic consequences are likely to be more prevalent in the future. Further drug development is necessary to design new compounds that are equally potent against the resistant viruses as the drugs currently used in the management of HIV infection, but do not exhibit unwanted metabolic side effects.

ACKNOWLEDGMENTS

The research presented in this paper was funded in part by the following grants: OTKA T 22670, T 30092 (from the Hungarian Science and Research Fund), FKFP 1318/97 (from the Hungarian Ministry of Education).
I wish to thank Dr. Péter Bagossi for preparing figures and for valuable discussions.

REFERENCES

1. KATZ, R.A. & A.M. SKALKA. 1994. The retroviral enzymes. Ann. Rev. Biochem. **63:** 133–173.
2. VOGT, V.M. 1997. Retroviral virions and genomes. *In* Retroviruses. J.M. Coffin, S.H. Hughes & H.E. Varmus, Eds.: 27–69. Cold Spring Harbor Laboratory Press. Plainview, NY.
3. OROSZLAN, S. & R.B. LUFTIG. 1990. Retroviral proteinases. Curr. Topics Microbiol. Immunol. **157:** 153–185.
4. TŐZSÉR, J. 1997. Specificity of retroviral proteinases based on substrates containing tyrosine and proline at the site of cleavage. Pathol. Oncol. Res. **3:** 141–146.
5. COPELAND, T.D., E.M. WONDRAK, J. TŐZSÉR, *et al.* 1990. Substitution of proline with pipecolic acid at the scissile bond converts a peptide substrate of HIV proteinase into a selective inhibitor. Biochem. Biophys. Res. Commun. **169:** 310–314.
6. WLODAWER, A. & J. VONDRASEK. 1998. Inhibitors of HIV-1 protease: a major success of structure-assisted drug design. Annu. Rev. Biophys. Biomol. Struct. **27:** 249–284.
7. TELENTY, A. & G.P. RIZZARDI. 2000. Limits to potent antiretroviral therapy. Rev. Med. Virol. **10:** 385–393.
8. LARDER, B.A., G. DARBY & D.D. RICHMAN. 1989 HIV with reduced sensitivity to zidovudine (AZT) isolated during prolonged therapy. Science **243:** 1731–1734.
9. LARDER, B.A. 1994. Interactions between drug resistance mutations in human immunodeficiency virus type 1 reverse transcriptase. J. Gen. Virol. **75:** 951–957.
10. PILLAY, D., S. TAYLOR & D.D. RICHMAN. 2000. Incidence and impact of resistance against approved antiretroviral drugs. Rev. Med. Virol. **10:** 231–253.
11. DE CLERCQ, E. 1998. The role of non-nucleoside reverse transcriptase inhibitors (NNRTIs) in the therapy of HIV-1 infection. Antiviral Res. **38:** 153–179.
12. CROTEAU, G., L. DOYON, D. THIBEAULT, *et al.* 1997. Impaired fitness of human immunodeficiency virus type 1 variants with high-level resistance to protease inhibitors. J. Virol. **71:** 1089–1096.
13. ZHANG, Y.M., H. IMAMICHI, T. IMAMICHI, *et al.* 1997. Drug resistance during indinavir therapy is caused by mutations in the protease gene and in its Gag substrate cleavage sites. J. Virol. **71:** 6662–6670.
14. ROUJEAU, J.-C. & R.S. STERN. 1994. Severe adverse cutaneous reactions to drugs. N. Engl. J. Med. **331:** 1272–1285.
15. CARR, A. & D.A. COOPER. 2000. Adverse effects of antiretroviral therapy. Lancet **356:** 1423–1430.
16. LEWIS, W. & M.C. DALAKAS. 1995. Mitochondrial toxicity of antiviral drugs. Nat. Med. **1:** 417–421.
17. TSIODRAS, S., C. MANTZOROS, S. HAMMER & M. SAMORE. 2000. Effects of protease inhibitors on hyperglycemia, hyperlipidemia and lipodystrophy. Arch. Intern. Med. **160:** 2050–2056.
18. KOUDRIAKOVA, T., E. IATSIMIRSKAIA, I. UTKIN, *et al.* 1998. Metabolism of the human immunodeficiency virus protease inhibitors indinavir and ritonavir by human intestinal microsomes and expressed cytochrome P4503A4/3A5: mechanism-based inactivation of cytochrome P450A3 by ritonavir. Drug Metab. Dispos. **26:** 552–561.
19. WACHER, V.J., J.A. SILVERMAN, Y. ZHANG & L.Z. BENET. 1998. Role of P-glycoprotein and cytochrome P450 3A in limiting oral adsorption of peptides and peptidomimetics. J. Pharmacol. Sci. **87:** 1322–1330.

20. CARR, A., K. SAMARAS, D.J. CHRISHOLM & D.A. COOPER. 1998. Pathogenesis of HIV protease inhibitor-associated syndrome of peripheral lopodystrophy, hyperlipidaemia and insulin resistance. Lancet **351:** 1881–1883.
21. ZHANG, B., K. MACNAUL, D. SZALKOWSKI, et al. 1999. Inhibition of adipocyte differentiation by HIV protease inhibitors. J. Clin. Endocrinol. Metab. **84:** 4274–4277.
22. IKEZOE, T., E.S. DAAR, J. HISATAKE, et al. 2000. HIV-1 protease inhibitors decrease proliferation and induce differentiation of human myelocytic leukemia cells. Blood **96:** 3553–3559.
23. MURATA, H., P.W. HRUZ & M. MUECKLER. 2000. The mechanism of insulin resistance caused by HIV proteinase inhibitor therapy. J. Biol. Chem. **275:** 20251–20254.
24. CARR, A., J. MILLER, M. LAW & D.A. COOPER. 2000. A syndrome of lipoathrophy, lactic acidemia and liver dysfunction associated with HIV nucleoside analogue therapy: contribution to protease inhibitor-related lipodystrophy syndrome. AIDS **14:** F25–F32.
25. SAINT-MARC, T., M. PARTISANI, I. POIZOT-MARTIN, et al. 1999. A syndrome of peripheral fat wasting (lipodystrophy) in patients receiving long-term nucleoside analogue therapy. AIDS **13:** 1659–1667.
26. BRINKMAN, K., J.A. SMEITINK, J.A. ROMIJN & P. REISS. 1999. Mitochondrial toxicity induced by nucleoside-analogue reverse-transcriptase inhibitors is a key factor in the pathogenesis of antiretroviral-therapy-related lipodystrophy. Lancet **354:** 1112–1115.
27. DUBÉ, M.P., D.L. JOHNSON, J.S. CURRIER & J.M. LEEDOM. 1997. Protease inhibitor-associated hyperglycaemia. Lancet **350:** 713–714.
28. VISNEGARWALA, F., K.L. KRAUSE & D.M. MUSHER. 1997. Severe diabetes associated with protease inhibitor therapy. Ann. Intern. Med. **127:** 947.
29. EASTONE, J.A. & C.F. DECKER. 1997. New-onset diabetes mellitus associated with use of protease inhibitors. Ann. Intern. Med. **127:** 948.
30. CZECH, M.P. & S. CORVERA. 1999. Signaling mechanisms that regulate glucose transport. J. Biol. Chem. **274:** 1865–1868.
31. PESSIN, J.E., D.C. THURMOND, J.S. ELMENDORF, et al. 1999. Molecular basis of insulin-stimulated GLUT4 vesicle trafficking. Location! Location! Location! J. Biol. Chem. **274:** 2593–2596.
32. BIRNBAUM, M.J. 1989. Identification of a novel gene encoding an insulin-responsive glucose transporter protein. Cell **57:** 305–315.
33. CLINE, G.W., K.F. PETERSEN, M. KRSSAK, et al. 1999. Impaired glucose transport as a cause of decreased insulin-stimulated muscle glycogen synthesis in type 2 diabetes. N. Engl. J. Med. **341:** 240-246.
34. KATZ, E.B., A.E. STENBIT, K. HATTON, et al. 1995. Cardiac and adipose tissue abnormalities but not diabetes in mice deficient in GLUT4. Nature **377:** 151–155.
35. BEHRENS, G., H. SCHMIDT, D. MEYER, et al. 1998. Vascular complications associated with use of HIV protease inhibitors. Lancet **351:** 1598.
36. HENRY, K., H. MELROE, J. HUEBSCH, et al. 1998. Severe premature coronary artery disease with protease inhibitors. Lancet **351:** 1328.
37. FLYNN, T.E. & L.A. BRICKER. 1999. Myocardial infarction in HIV-infected men receiving protease inhibitors. Ann. Intern. Med. **131:** 548.
38. KOZAL. M.J., N. SHAH, N. SHEN, et al. 1996. Extensive polymorphism observed in HIV-1 clade B protease gene using high-density oligonucleotide arrays. Nat. Med. **2:** 753–759.

Apoptosis and the Heart

A Brief Review

L. DAVID TOMEI AND SAMUIL R. UMANSKY

Xenomics Inc., Richmond, California 94805, USA

ABSTRACT: Cardiomyopathies are observed with increasing frequency in association with AIDS and HIV infection. Although indirect evidence exists suggesting an association between apoptosis regulation and HIV infection, there is yet no direct evidence that HIV-associated cardiomyopathies involve increased level of apoptosis in the heart. However, since it is now known that apoptosis plays a significant role in heart injury associated with other conditions such as ischemia/reperfusion and heart failure, there is a possibility that dysregulation of apoptosis plays a similarly important role in HIV-associate cardiomyopathies. Here we will briefly review the evidence that apoptotic death of cardiomyocytes occurs and what novel therapeutic strategies may be suggested.

KEYWORDS: apoptosis; heart; cardiomyopathy

INTRODUCTION

In 1994, the Annals of the New York Academy of Sciences published a collection of papers focused on then current views of the biochemical and molecular bases of myocardial damage associated with ischemia and reperfusion injury.[1] At that time the prevailing hypotheses involved several views of the molecular nature of cellular damage expressed in terms of free radical–mediated processes, calcium ion overloading, and loss of sarcolemal phospholipids.[2] Since that time, a fundamentally new approach to understanding the nature of heart damage has emerged which followed the introduction of the concept of apoptosis[3,4] (see also review[5]). In this new view cellular damage is considered to be a signaling event producing a transduction cascade(s) leading to expression of factors that either suppress or promote nuclear, mitochondrial, and plasma membrane changes collectively known as apoptosis. During the last few years, much has been learned about the details of apoptotic signal transduction pathways and the role of specific gene expression regulating whether a cell dies or survives. From the viewpoint of modern molecular medicine, this is a significant step toward more effective therapeutic intervention in acute myocardial infarction and heart failure.

For many years it has been believed that necrosis is the predominant form of cardiomyocyte death following ischemia and subsequent reperfusion.[6–8] However, within the past few years many investigators have reported evidence that apoptosis

Address for correspondence: Dr. L.D. Tomei, Xenomics Inc., 6034 Monterey Ave., Richmond, CA 94805. Voice: 510-234-8045.

ldtomei@xenomics.net
sumansky@xenomics.net

plays a significant role in acute myocardial infarction and the pathogenesis of other forms of heart failure (see review[5] and refs. 9–11). The question of whether cardiomyocytes die by apoptosis or necrosis is not of purely theoretical significance because strategies for therapeutic intervention for the modification of necrotic versus apoptotic cell death are quite different. In order to inhibit necrotic death we can only endeavor to prevent the cell injury by early reperfusion and introduction of antioxidants, the key elements of such a therapeutic strategy. However, apoptosis can also be prevented by interfering with the signaling mechanisms and the apoptotic pathway(s) after cells have already been damaged by ischemia or other means.

Apoptosis has had a great deal of intuitive appeal to scientists especially recently. However, the concept has always been and continues to be controversial because it challenges our ability to apply the simple definitions of what constitutes a living versus a dead cell. In contrast to simple *in vitro* models, the physiologically complex dynamic nature of a living heart and the effects of sudden disruption of coronary blood flow have put the concept of apoptosis to the test. Future studies demand more rigorous methodologies for measurement of molecular processes related to signal transduction pathways, gene expression, structural and functional changes in nuclear DNA, and the fate of muscle cells. It appears that there is little tolerance of acute cell death in the coordinated electromechanical matrix uniquely subject to global failure. It is thus evident that apoptosis, programmed cell death, appears to be a challenging, often paradoxical concept.

CELL DEATH IN THE MYOCARDIUM

In *in vitro* models of simulated ischemia and reperfusion both necrotic and apoptotic myocytes were detected.[12–15] Apoptotic cells were identified by morphological analysis, flow cytometry, detection of internucleosomal DNA cleavage, and activation of apoptosis-related biochemical events, including caspase activation, cytochrome c release, and decrease in mitochondrial transmembrane potential. However, *in vivo* detection of apoptotic cells in general, and cardiomyocytes in particular, is not methodologically trivial.[16–19] Chromatin condensation and margination, considered "classical" characteristics of apoptotic morphology, are not typically observed in apoptotic cardiomyocytes and other contractile cells *in vivo*. Cardiomyocytes are not capable of phagocytosis of neighboring apoptotic cells as in other tissues and apoptotic cardiomyocytes remain within the microarchitecture that is mechanically, electrically, and metabolically very active. Activation of lysosomal enzymes in these early stage apoptotic myocytes is expected, which likely leads rapidly to secondary necrosis. Based on current knowledge of apoptotic pathways, it is unlikely that early stage apoptotic myocytes in a functioning heart would be capable of sustaining coordinated metabolic processes for orderly completion of DNA internucleosomal fragmentation and eventual physical breakup into apoptotic bodies.

Internucleosomal DNA fragmentation has been detected in the myocardium after ischemia and reperfusion.[20–22] This fragmented DNA is probably not only from myocytes, but can also originate from infiltrating cells during reperfusion. Among the most recent methods for identifying apoptotic cells in the heart during ischemia and reperfusion, the technique of detection of annexin V–binding cells looks very promising.[23,24] Other indications of apoptosis in myocardium have come from analysis of processes involved in apoptotic pathways, namely activation of caspases, release of cytochrome c, etc. An indirect, yet especially useful technique for demonstrating that apoptosis occurs in the heart is the fact that specific apoptosis inhibitors prevent DNA degradation when introduced after ischemia, during reperfusion.[25] In some cases infarct size can be reduced by post-ischemic application of compounds that do not affect the damage of cardiomyocytes but interfere with the apoptotic pathway.[18,19]

The general concept that apoptosis mediates a significant portion of ischemia/reperfusion injury has not changed since its introduction.[5,26] Cumulative cell damage during ischemia initiates apoptotic pathways which, however, cannot proceed in the absence of energy production. If ischemia goes on too long, massive and irreversible cell injury produces rapid irretrievable necrotic death. Restoration of blood flow to ischemic regions prevents additional cell damage but creates conditions for continuation of apoptotic processes induced during ischemia. Currently accumulated experimental results demonstrate that a significant portion of this apoptotic cell death during reperfusion can be prevented by interference with the apoptotic pathway. This can lead to beneficial clinical outcome in the form of reduction of infarction size.

APOPTOSIS AND THERAPEUTIC INTERVENTION

Historically, an early and key observation lead to the concept that cells that had been damaged would subsequently die but as a consequence of an independent pathway and not as a direct consequence of damage (see ref. 27). Moreover, this simple observation suggested that it was more important to understand the nature of this as-yet-undefined pathway rather than the nature of the molecular damage that initiated it. This insight was based upon the ability of phorbol esters to block cell death following gamma irradiation without any evidence that these agents either reduced radiation damage, or promoted repair of the damage. These studies demonstrated that apoptosis could be inhibited by therapeutic drug intervention after the initial cell damage and without the need for pretreatment. These data further suggested the existence of a previously unrecognized cause of cell death which was confirmed to be apoptosis. This is similar to the studies of reperfusion death in ischemic myocardium which had been believed to be an immediate consequence of lethal oxidative damage—thus the term reperfusion oxidative damage was widely used to account for subsequent infarction. In 1994, it was suggested that oxidative damage, although it may occur, was not the immediate cause of cell death since apoptosis inhibition before or after ischemia/reperfusion was capable of inhibiting the appearance of infarction.[12,20]

The potential for involvement of apoptotic cell death in the pathogenesis of heart injury is not limited to acute regional ischemia or subsequent reperfusion. Rather, a wide range of phenomena are associated with injury to the heart, including most notably age, the presence of infectious disease, and stress. Cytoprotective effects of ACE inhibitors have been examined and it has been reported that apoptosis associated with chronic heart failure in dogs is reduced.[28] Angiotensin II receptor activation as well as adrenergic stimulation play a significant role in heart failure. Yellon and Baxter[29] discuss the evidence that several peptide growth factors including TGF-β_1, insulin, IGF-1, and others act to suppress myocardial reperfusion injury perhaps through a common growth factor–signaling pathway involving p42/p44 MAP kinase. These data and that of many other groups imply that apoptosis suppression will reduce heart damage in acute regional ischemia and chronic heart failure. Naturally, the cardioprotective activity of a variety of drugs and treatments may not act on the apoptotic pathways directly. Depending upon the sequence of events, agents that inhibit a wide variety of cell damage can reasonably be expected to effectively reduce the downstream sequelae including apoptosis without providing any insight into the apoptotic process itself.

Recently, Elsasser et al.[16] reviewed the role of apoptosis in the pathogenesis of myocardial injury associated with coronary insufficiency, ischemia, and reperfusion. These authors examine the molecular and histological evidence that apoptotic internucleosomal DNA fragmentation occurs and whether various widely used methods yield consistent and reproducible results. What emerges from such studies is the general confirmation that a significant portion of myocardial ischemia-reperfusion damage is marked by initiation of apoptosis. The major questions posed by these authors focus on the unresolved molecular and temporal details which may be necessary to rationally design drugs specifically directed to modify the ability of cardiomyocytes to live or die. In addition, they feel that it is not clear that all dead cells are post-apoptotic and that some cells die as a direct consequence of the loss of plasma membrane integrity and ion control.

APOPTOSIS AND SIGNAL TRANSDUCTION IN THE MYOCARDIUM

The nature of signal(s) that initiates apoptosis in cardiomyocytes during ischemia and reperfusion is not finally understood. The possible involvement of ceramide, a secondary lipid messenger, in initiation of the apoptotic pathway in cardiomyocytes both in vitro and in vivo was investigated by several groups.[30–32] Synthetic, cell-permeable C2-ceramide induced apoptotic death of rat neonatal cardiomyocytes in vitro. Accumulation of ceramide in cardiomyocytes during ischemia and reperfusion was demonstrated both in vitro and in vivo. Inhibitors of caspases 3 and 8 but not of other caspases inhibit ceramide-induced death of cardiomyocytes. Thus, ceramide is a serious candidate for a signaling molecule in ischemia/reperfusion–induced apoptosis.

Involvement of TNF and Fas in myocardial apoptosis has been discussed in several publications.[33–35] However, the role of these signaling systems in acute myocardial infarction as well as in chronic heart failure is not clear because in both cases increase in soluble forms of Fas receptor, which should inhibit Fas response, has been observed.[20,36] There are also data that indicate a positive effect of TNF in acute myocardial infarction.[37,38]

Yaoita et al.[39] discuss the evidence that early apoptosis-signaling pathways converge leading to mitochondrial failure and cell death. They propose that therapeutic intervention must target events prior to mitochondrial damage in order to possibly reduce infarction. This suggests that the earliest irreversible steps toward cell death are mitochondrial rather than nuclear. This is in accord with substantial data from many groups indicating that DNA laddering and TUNEL assay results frequently do not correlate well with measurements of organ damage and failure. Similarly, caspase-3 has been found to be involved in mediation of apoptosis progression, yet inhibitors of caspases have been reported to have inconsistent effects on infarct size even in the presence of a reduction of TUNEL-positive myocytes.[40] In our laboratory using an ischemia reperfusion model, caspase-3 inhibition prevented DNA fragmentation but did not reduce the relative number of dead cells. It is likely that the temporal sequence of molecular events involving the caspase family of proteases are not well understood or controlled in current experimental designs. It is also possible that the TUNEL assay is not an accurate method of estimating the number of apoptotic cells in the risk area following acute regional ischemia.

PREVENTION OF APOPTOSIS IN MYOCARDIUM

Different approaches have been used to inhibit apoptotic death of cardiomyocytes following ischemia and reperfusion. Among the most convincing results is evidence of the ability of the anti-apoptotic Bcl-2 protein to prevent cardiomyocyte death obtained by Brocheriou et al.[41] and Chen et al.[42] These investigators generated a line of transgenic mice that carry a human Bcl-2 transgene under the control of a mouse α-myosin heavy chain promoter. The transgenic mice were subjected to ligation of the coronary artery followed by reperfusion. The infarct sizes, expressed as a percentage of the area at risk, were significantly smaller in the transgenic mice than in the nontransgenic mice.

In our laboratory, we found that expression of SARP family members was tissue specific encoding secreted proteins that possess a cysteine-rich domain (CRD) homologous to the CRD of frizzled proteins but lack putative membrane-spanning segments.[43] Expression of SARPs modifies the intracellular levels of β-catenin, suggesting that SARPs interfere with the Wnt-frizzled protein signaling pathway. Further, we analyzed the effect of overexpression of another anti-apoptotic protein, sFRP-2 (SARP1), on death of rat neonatal cardiomyocytes in vitro (Melkonyan et al., unpublished results). In these experiments, cells were infected with sFRP-2 (SARP1) gene–bearing adenovirus and their apoptotic death was initiated by serum/glucose deprivation or by adriamycin treatment. In both cases survival of cells overexpressing SARP1 was significantly higher than in control cells infected with β-Gal expressing adenovirus. Purified recombinant SARP1 also significantly reduced serum deprivation–induced death of cardiomyocytes.

Several groups tried to reduce apoptotic death of cardiomyocytes with caspase inhibitors both in vivo and in vitro.[40,44,45] In all cases caspase inhibitors prevented internucleosomal DNA degradation. However, data on the ability of caspase inhibitors to prevent cardiomyocyte death or to reduce the infarct size appear to be contradictory. In some publications evidence of reduction of infarct size is presented. However, in many others report that neither cell death nor the infarct were affected. It should be noted that data on the anti-apoptotic effects of caspase inhibitors in other model systems are also contradictory. Caspase inhibitors block apoptosis induced through Fas or TNF receptor in hepatocytes and lymphocytes, an observation that can be explained by the inhibition of caspases involved in the death signal transduction in these systems.[46,47] At the same time they prevent DNA degradation but usually have no effect on cell death induced by other pro-apoptotic agents, such as staurosporine, VP-16, actinomycin D, perforin, and granzyme B, as well as by Fas signaling in many other cell types.[48–52] Recent studies performed with caspase gene "knock-out" mice have also revealed differential effects of caspase ablation on apoptosis induced by a variety of stimuli. Seven lines of caspase-deficient mice have been generated (caspase 1,2,3,9, and 11), all of which exhibit abnormalities in cell death. However, no global suppression of apoptosis has been observed; rather it was tissue- and cell-type–specific and stimulus-specific apoptosis that was affected.[53] This phenomenon can be explained by the existence of several known independent and parallel apoptotic pathways that can be initiated by the same factors. Alternatively, it may be more likely that downstream branch points exist in the apoptotic pathway, as suggested by the observation that some apoptosis suppressors prevent both DNA degradation and death of cardiomyocytes and lead to reduction in infarct size.

Alternatively, suppression of both apoptosis and reduction of myocardial infarct size has been observed using post-ischemia treatment with lysophosphatidic acid (LPA) and several of its analogs.[54] In these experiments using primary cultures of rat neonatal cardiomyocytes, LPA prevented all steps in apoptotic cell death including caspase-3 activation, internucleosomal DNA degradation, cell permeabilization, and final detachment as dead cells. Caspase-3 activity increased approximately twofold by the end of ischemia and a further twofold during the first 12 h of reperfusion. However, the caspase inhibitor z-VAD prevented DNA degradation, as reported by others,[46] yet had no effect on cell death. LPA was equally effective at inhibiting cardiomyocyte death when added either prior to or immediately following *in vitro* simulated ischemia followed by simulated reperfusion. It is also noteworthy that LPA prevents cardiomyocyte death induced by serum deprivation, ischemia and reperfusion, and ceramide but has no effect on cell death induced by cycloheximide, puromycin, adriamycin, staurosporine, *cis*-platinum, or menadione. This is an indirect indication that LPA interferes with some but not all signaling pathways. Several LPA receptors and some details of LPA signaling mechanisms have been recently described.[55,56] However, it is unclear now which of these receptor(s) mediates anti-apoptotic activity of LPA.

CONCLUDING REMARKS

It remains to be determined whether insights into the molecular processes of apoptosis associated with myocardial injury will extend to HIV-associated cardiomyopathies. However, there is some indirect evidence that there is a close linkage between HIV infection and dysregulation of apoptosis (see review[57]). Some evidence has been published indicating that viral sequences are to be found in the myocardium of HIV[+] children and may be associated with the progression of heart disease in these patients.[58] However, it is not known whether HIV-associated cardiomyopathies involve increased levels of apoptotic myocytes. Furthermore, no evidence has been published to date suggesting that factors known to suppress myocardial apoptosis may provide benefit to HIV[+] patients who experience such cardiomyopathies. None the less, as we learn more about the role of apoptosis in the myocardium, we gain more insight into new means of therapeutic intervention. This is not only applicable to treatment of ischemia/reperfusion injury, but also drug-related injury and cardiomyopathies secondary to HIV infection.

REFERENCES

1. DAS, D.K., Ed. 1994. Cellular, Biochemical, and Molecular Aspects of Reperfusion Injury. Ann. N.Y. Acad. Sci. **723**.
2. DAS, D.K. 1994. Introduction. Ann. N.Y. Acad. Sci. **723**: xii–xvi.
3. LEWIS, W. 2000. Cardiomyopathy in AIDS: a pathophysiological perspective. Prog. Cardiovasc. Dis. **43**: 151–170.
4. KAN, H. *et al.* 2000. HIV gp120 enhances NO production by cardiac myocytes through p38 MAP kinase-mediated NF-kappa B activation. Am. J. Physiol. Heart Circ. Physiol. **27**: H3138–H3143.
5. UMANSKY, S.R. & L.D. TOMEI. 1997. Apoptosis in the heart. *In* Advances in Pharmacology. Scott H. Kaufmann, Ed. **41**: 383–407. Academic Press. San Diego, CA.
6. ALPERT, J.S. 1989. The pathophysiology of acute myocardial infarction. Cardiology **76**: 85–95.
7. WALLER, B.F. 1988. The pathology of acute myocardial infarction: definition, location, pathogenesis, effects of reperfusion, complications, and sequelae. Cardiol Clin. **6**: 1-28.
8. REIMER, K.A. *et al.* 1993. Reperfusion in acute myocardial infarction: effect of timing and modulating factors in experimental models. Am. J. Cardiol. **72**: 13G–21G
9. HONG, F. *et al.* 2001. Insulin-like growth factor-1 protects H9c2 cardiac myoblasts from oxidative stress-induced apoptosis via phosphatidylinositol 3-kinase and extracellular signal-regulated kinase pathways. Life Sci. **68**: 1095-1105.
10. OSKARSSON, H.J. *et al.* 2000. Antioxidants attenuate myocytes apoptosis in the remote non-infarcted myocardium following large myocardial infarction. Cardiovasc. Res. **45**: 679–687.
11. GOTTLIEB, R.A. & R.L. ENGLER. 1999. Apoptosis in myocardial ischemia-reperfusion. Ann. N.Y. Acad. Sci. **874**: 412–426.
12. UMANSKY, S. *et al.* 1995. Post-ischemic apoptotic death of rat neonatal cardiomyocytes. Cell Death & Differ. **2**: 235–241.
13. WANG, G.W. *et al.* 2001. Inhibition of hypoxia/reoxygenation-induced apoptosis in metallothionein-overexpressing cardiomyocytes. Am. J. Physiol. Heart Circ. Physiol. **280**: H2292-H2299.
14. HALESTRAP, A.P. *et al.* 2000. Mitochondria and cell death. Biochem. Soc. Trans. **28**: 170–177.
15. BIALIK, S. *et al.* 1999. The mitochondrial apoptotic pathway is activated by serum and glucose deprivation in cardiac myocytes. Circ. Res. **85**: 403–414.
16. ELSASSER, A. *et al.* 2000. Unresolved issues regarding the role of apoptosis in the pathogenesis of ischemic injury and heart failure. J. Mol. Cell Cardiol. **32**: 711–724.
17. TAKASHI, E. & M. ASHRAF. 2000. Pathologic assessment of myocardial cell necrosis and apoptosis after ischemia and reperfusion with molecular and morphological markers. J. Mol. Cell Cardiol. **32**: 209–224.
18. OHNO, M. *et al.* 1998. "Apoptotic" myocytes in infarct area in rabbit hearts may be oncotic myocytes with DNA fragmentation: analysis by immunogold electron microscopy combined with in situ nick end-labeling. Circulation **98**: 1422–1430.
19. SARASTE, A. & K. PULKKI. 2000. Morphologic and biochemical hallmarks of apoptosis. Cardiovasc. Res. **45**: 528–537.
20. GOTTLIEB, R.A. *et al.* 1994. Reperfusion injury induces apoptosis in rabbit cardiomyocytes. J. Clin. Invest. **94**: 1621–1628.
21. UMANSKY, S.U. *et al.* 1996. Dog cardiomyocyte death induced in vivo by ischemia and reperfusion. Basic & Applied Myol. **6**: 227–235.
22. ITOH, G. *et al.* 1995. DNA fragmentation of human infarcted myocardial cells demonstrated by the nick end labeling method and DNA agarose gel electrophoresis. Am. J. Pathol. **146**: 1325–1331.

23. DUMONT, E.A. *et al.* 2000. Cardiomyocyte death induced by myocardial ischemia and reperfusion: measurement with recombinant human annexin-V in a mouse model. Circulation **102:** 1564–1568.
24. HOFSTRA, L. *et al.* 2000. Visualisation of cell death in vivo in patients with acute myocardial infarction. Lancet **356:** 209–212.
25. OKAMURA, T. *et al.* 2000. Effect of caspase inhibitors on myocardial infarct size and myocyte DNA fragmentation in the ischemia-reperfused rat heart. Cardiovasc. Res. **45:** 642-650.
26. FREUDE, B. 2000. Apoptosis is initiated by myocardial ischemia and executed during reperfusion. J. Mol. Cell Cardiol. **32:** 197-208.
27. COPE, F.O. & L.D. TOMEI. 1994. Preface. *In* Apoptosis II: The Molecular Basis of Apoptosis in Disease. L.D. Tomei & F.O. Cope, Eds. Curr. Commun. Cell & Mol. Biol. **3:** 1–4. Cold Spring Harbor Laboratory Press. Plainview, NY.
28. GOUSSEV, A. *et al.* 1998. Effects of ACE inhibition on cardiomyocyte apoptosis in dogs with heart failure. Am. J. Physiol. **275:** H626–H631.
29. YELLON, D.M. & G.F. BAXTER. 1999. Reperfusion injury revisited: is there a role for growth factor signaling in limiting lethal reperfusion injury? Trends Cardiovasc. Med. **9:** 245–249.
30. BIELAWSKA, A.E. *et al.* 1997. Ceramide is involved in triggering of cardiomyocyte apoptosis induced by ischemia and reperfusion. Am. J. Pathol. **151:** 1257–1263.
31. CORDIS, G.A. *et al.* 1998. HPTLC analysis of sphingomylein, ceramide and sphingosine in ischemic/reperfused rat heart. J. Pharm. Biomed. Anal. **16:** 1189–1193.
32. WANG, J. *et al.* 2000. Involvement of caspase 3- and 8-like proteases in ceramide-induced apoptosis of cardiomyocytes. J. Card. Failure **6:** 243–249.
33. JEREMIAS, I. *et al.* 2000. Involvement of CD95/Apo1/Fas in cell death after myocardial ischemia. Circulation **102:** 915–920.
34. FERRARI, R. 1999. The role of TNF in cardiovascular disease. Pharmacol. Res. **40:** 97–105.
35. KROWN, K.A. *et al.* 1996. Tumor necrosis factor alpha-induced apoptosis in cardiac myocytes. Involvement of the sphingolipid signaling cascade in cardiac cell death. J. Clin. Invest. **98:** 2854–2865.
36. FIORINA, P. *et al.* 2000. Soluble antiapoptotic molecules and immune activation in chronic heart failure and unstable angina pectoris. J. Clin. Immunol. **20:** 101–106.
37. MICHAEL, L.H. *et al.* 2000. Endogenous tumor necrosis factor protects the adult cardiac myocyte against ischemic-induced apoptosis in a murine model of acute myocardial infarction. Proc. Natl. Acad. Sci. USA **97:** 5456–5461.
38. KURRELMEYER, K.M. *et al.* 2000. Soluble antiapoptotic molecules and immune activation in chronic heart failure and unstable angina pectoris. J. Clin. Immunol. **20:** 101–106.
39. YAOITA, H. *et al.* 2000. Apoptosis in relevant clinical situations: contribution of apoptosis in myocardial infarction. Cardiovasc. Res. **45:** 630–641.
40. OKAMURA, T. *et al.* 2000. Effect of caspase inhibitors on myocardial infarct size and myocyte DNA fragmentation in the ischemia-reperfused rat heart. Cardiovasc. Res. **45:** 642-650.
41. BROCHERIOU, V. *et al.* 2000. Cardiac functional improvement by a human Bcl-2 transgene in a mouse model of ischemia/reperfusion injury. J. Gene Med. **2:** 326–333.
42. CHEN, Z. *et al.* 2001. Overexpression of Bcl-2 attenuates apoptosis and protects against myocardial I/R injury in transgenic mice. Am. J. Physiol. Heart Circ. Physiol. **280:** H2313–H2320.
43. MELKONYAN, H.S. *et al.* 1997. SARPs: a family of secreted apoptosis-related proteins. Proc. Natl. Acad. Sci. USA **94:** 13636–13641.
44. MOCANU, M. *et al.* 2000. Caspase inhibition and limitation of myocardial infarct size: protection against lethal reperfusion injury. Br. J. Pharmacol. **130:** 197–200.
45. HOLLY, T.A. *et al.* 1999. Caspase inhibition reduces myocyte cell death induced by myocardial ischemia and reperfusion in vivo. J. Mol. Cell. Cardiol. **31:** 1709–1715.
46. KRAMMER, P.H. 1999. CD95(APO-1/Fas)-mediated apoptosis: live and let die. Adv. Immunol. **71:** 163–210.

47. ZHENG, T.S. *et al.* 1998. Caspase-3 controls both cytoplasmic and nuclear events associated with Fas-mediated apoptosis in vivo. Proc. Natl. Acad. Sci. USA **95:** 13618–13623.
48. AMARANTE-MENDES, G.P. *et al.* 1998. Anti-apoptotic oncogens prevent caspase-dependent and independent commitment for cell death. Cell Death Differ. **5:** 298–306.
49. JANICKE, R.U. *et al.* 1998. Caspase-3 is required for DNA fragmentation and morphological changes associated with apoptosis. J. Biol. Chem. **273:** 9357–9360.
50. KUROKAWA, H. *et al.* 1999. Alteration of caspase-3 (CPP32/Yama/apopain) in wild-type MCF-7, breast cancer cells. Oncol. Rep. **6:** 33–37.
51. LEMAIRE, C. *et al.* 1998. Inhibition of caspase activity induces a switch from apoptosis to necrosis. FEBS Lett. **425:** 266–270.
52. WEIL, M. *et al.* 1998. Are caspases involved in the death of cells with a transcriptionally inactive nucleus? Sperm and chicken erythrocytes. J. Cell Sci. **111:** 2707–2715.
53. GREEN, D. 1998. Apoptotic pathways: the roads to ruin. Cell **94:** 695–698.
54. UMANSKY, S.R. *et al.* 1997. Prevention of rat neonatal cardiomyocyte apoptosis induced by simulated in vitro ischemia and reperfusion. Cell Death Differ. **4:** 608–616.
55. SWARTHOUT, J.T. & H.W. WALLING. 2000. Lysophosphatidic acid: receptors, signaling and survival. Cell Mol. Life Sci. **57:** 1978–1985.
56. FUKUSHIMA, N. & J. CHUN. 2001. The LPA receptors. Prostaglandins **64:** 21–32.
57. REED, J.C. 2000. Mechanisms of apoptosis. Am. J. Pathol. **157:** 1415–1430.
58. BOWLES, N.E. *et al.* 1999. The detection of viral genomes by polymerase chain reaction in the myocardium of pediatric patients with advanced HIV disease. J. Am. Coll. Cardiol. **34:** 857–865.

Cardiac Manifestations of HIV Infection in Infants and Children

MARCIE J. KEESLER,[a] STACY D. FISHER,[b] AND STEVEN E. LIPSHULTZ [c]

[a]*Division of Pediatric Cardiology, University of Rochester Medical Center and Strong Children's Hospital, Rochester, New York 14642, USA*

[b]*Department of Medicine, University of Rochester School of Medicine and Dentistry and Department of Cardiology, University of Rochester Medical Center and Strong Children's Hospital, Rochester, New York 14642, USA*

[c]*Department of Pediatrics and Oncology, University of Rochester School of Medicine, Department of Pediatric Cardiology, University of Rochester Medical Center and Strong Children's Hospital, Rochester, New York 14642, USA*

ABSTRACT: Cardiac manifestations of HIV infection in children are common, but etiologies, contributing factors, and the natural history are largely unexplored. The Pediatric Pulmonary and Cardiovascular Complications of Vertically Transmitted Human Immunodeficiency Virus Infection Study (P^2C^2 HIV Study) was initiated in 1989 by the National Heart, Lung and Blood Institute, USA. A primary objective of this study is to examine the epidemiology of cardiovascular problems associated with HIV infection in a cohort of children vertically infected. Findings of the study thus far show that cardiovascular problems associated with HIV infection including left ventricular dysfunction and increased left ventricular mass are common and clinically important indicators of survival for children infected with HIV.

KEYWORDS: HIV; AIDS; cardiovascular; pediatric cardiomyopathy; congestive heart failure

INTRODUCTION

Worldwide, over one million children under the age of 15 are currently living with HIV/AIDS. [1] In an era of advanced therapy and associated increased longevity, cardiac complications are emerging as an important clinical problem in children infected with HIV. The Pediatric Pulmonary and Cardiac Complications of Vertically Transmitted HIV Infection Study group (P^2C^2 HIV Study) was created in 1989 by the National Heart, Lung and Blood Institute in response to a need to understand related illness in a growing HIV/AIDS epidemic. There are five participating United States clinical centers: Baylor College of Medicine/Texas Children's Hospital, Children's Hospital/Harvard Medical School, Mount Sinai School of Medicine, Presbyterian Hospital/Columbia University College of Physicians and Surgeons, and

Address for correspondence: Steven E. Lipshultz, M.D., Division of Pediatric Cardiology, University of Rochester School of Medicine, 601 Elmwood Avenue, Box 631, Rochester, NY 14642. Voice: 716-275-6096; fax: 716-275-7436.
steve_lipshultz@urmc.rochester.edu

UCLA School of Medicine. The clinical coordinating center for the study was established at the Cleveland Clinic. A primary objective of the P^2C^2 HIV Study was to study the epidemiology of cardiovascular problems associated with HIV infection in a cohort of infants and children vertically infected. The cohort studied is made up of 205 infants and children enrolled after 28 days of age and 612 fetuses and infants of HIV^+ mothers enrolled prenatally or postnatally at age less than 28 days. The cohort was followed at set intervals with cardiac, pulmonary, immunologic, and infectious examination and studies to observe the natural history of these patients.[2] Current findings and background from other studies in children are discussed.

As the number of children living with HIV infection increases so will the number that suffer from cardiovascular complications.[3] Cardiac disease as an underlying cause of death increases in frequency with increasing age. FIGURE 1 illustrates that as HIV^+ children grow older they are more likely to succumb to chronic cardiac disease. It is not normally seen in infancy or in early childhood but increases to 25% of deaths in children over 10 years of age in a review of 93 infants and children who died of HIV-related conditions.[3] Older children are also more likely to die of wasting syndrome. Fifty-one percent of the children with HIV-related deaths had chronic cardiac disease diagnosed prior to death.[3] Serious cardiac events were found in 28% of patients after AIDS diagnosis.[4] Cardiac dysfunction was found in 35% of patients who died during the study. FIGURE 2 illustrates the length of time after AIDS diagnosis to the occurrence of a serious cardiac event in these children. A serious cardiac event includes: transient and chronic congestive heart failure, hypotension, severe

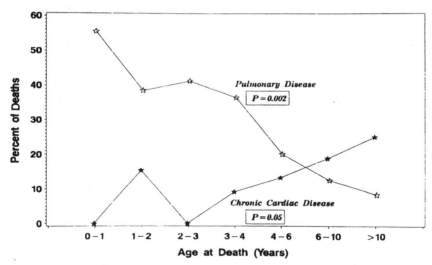

No. Cases: Cardiac Disease ($n=11$), Pulmonary Disease ($n=27$)

FIGURE 1. Linear age trends for the underlying cause of death in 93 HIV-related deaths. (From Langston, C., E.R. Cooper, J. Goldfarb, *et al.* 2001. HIV-related mortality in infants and children: data from the Pediatric Pulmonary and Cardiovascular Complications of Vertically Transmitted HIV Study. Pediatrics **107**(2): 328–336,[3] used with permission).

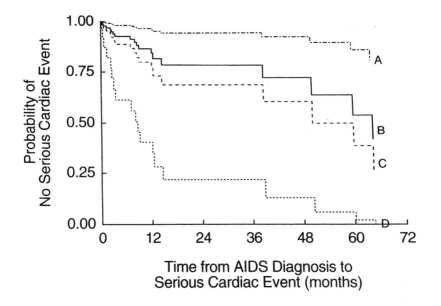

FIGURE 2. Time to occurrence of a serious cardiac event (transient and chronic congestive heart failure, hypotension, severe dysrhythmia, cardiac tamponade, cerebrovascular accident associated with hemodynamic instability, and cardiac arrest) in AIDS patients in 1992. Wasting and prior cardiac events at the time of AIDS diagnosis were significant predictors of subsequent serious cardiac events in multivariable analyses. Curve **A** represents AIDS patients with no wasting and no prior cardiac events. The curve marked **B** represents AIDS patients with no wasting but with a history of prior cardiac events. The curve marked **C** represents AIDS patients with wasting and no prior cardiac events. The curve marked **D** represents AIDS patients with wasting and a history of prior cardiac events. (From Al-Attar, I., E.J. Orav, V. Exil, *et al.* 1995. Predictors of cardiac morbidity and related mortality in children with the acquired immune deficiency syndrome. Pediatr. Res. **37:** 169A[4]).

dysrhythmia, cardiac tamponade, cerebrovascular accident associated with hemodynamic instability, or cardiac arrest.

RISK FACTORS FOR CARDIAC DISEASE

Encephalopathy, wasting, decreased CD4 count, and a prior history of a serious cardiac event are all predictors of cardiac complications associated with HIV infection in children.[4] Rapid progressors (those children who have an AIDS-defining condition other than lymphoid interstitial pneumonia/pulmonary hyperplasia or severe immunosupression in the first year of life) are also at an increased risk for cardiac complications. Rapid progressors have been found to have increased respiratory rate, increased heart rate, and decreased fractional shortening on serial echocardiographic measurements.[5] Cardiac abnormalities that are present in rapid progressors lead to poor outcomes including an increased mortality rate.

FETAL AND CONGENITAL CARDIOVASCULAR ASSOCIATIONS WITH HIV INFECTION

The vast majority of HIV$^+$ children under the age of 15 were born to HIV$^+$ mothers and acquired the virus before or during birth.[6] The rate of vertical transmission has substantially decreased in the past few years because of the administration of zidovudine (AZT) or other antiretroviral regimens to HIV$^+$ women during pregnancy and delivery. According to the Center for Disease Control between 1992 and 1998 perinatally acquired HIV infection cases declined 75% in the United States.[7]

As part of the P^{2}C^2 HIV study, fetal echocardiography was performed in 173 fetuses, and this revealed that fetuses of HIV$^+$ mothers may have abnormal cardiovascular structure and function irrespective of the HIV status of the infant.[8] Infants of HIV$^+$ mothers were also found to have increased right and left ventricular wall thickness.[8] A hostile maternal environment including maternal malnutrition or illness may affect both HIV$^+$ and HIV$^-$ infants born to HIV$^+$ women.

Congenital cardiovascular malformations have also been described in children with HIV infection. When comparing rates of congenital cardiovascular malformations in HIV-infected and -uninfected children no statistically significant difference was found in the prevalence rate between the two groups of children.[9] Rates from the P^{2}C^2 HIV study (12.3%) of congenital cardiovascular malformations were found to be five- to tenfold higher than traditionally reported in the population, but not higher than in normal populations similarly screened.[9] Malformations found in HIV$^+$ children in the P^{2}C^2 HIV study include atrial and ventricular septal defects, patent ductus arteriosus, tricuspid valve prolapse, valvar pulmonary stenosis, mitral valve prolapse, subaortic stenosis, and single coronary artery system.

The presence of cardiac abnormalities in fetuses of HIV$^+$ women is confounded by various maternal factors. These fetuses may also be exposed to smoking, illicit drug use, nutritional deficits, or co-infections that may affect the fetus regardless of HIV status.

LEFT VENTRICULAR DYSFUNCTION

Left Ventricular Systolic Function

Left ventricular dysfunction is a frequent manifestation of HIV infection in children. Although it is commonly found in HIV$^+$ children, the clinical significance is not fully understood. In a study of 193 children with vertically transmitted HIV, baseline echocardiograms were performed. Mortality was found to be higher in children who at baseline had decreased left ventricular fractional shortening and increased LV dimension, thickness, mass or wall stress.[10] FIGURE 3 illustrates these findings. Increased wall thickness and decreased fractional shortening were also found to be risk factors for mortality independent of CD4 count.[10,11]

The P^{2}C^2 HIV study also found that in 130 vertically infected children, 25% had a fractional shortening more than two standard deviations below normal and 42% of these patients also had depressed contractility.[12] FIGURE 4 shows the cumulative incidence of an episode of decreased left ventricular fractional shortening.

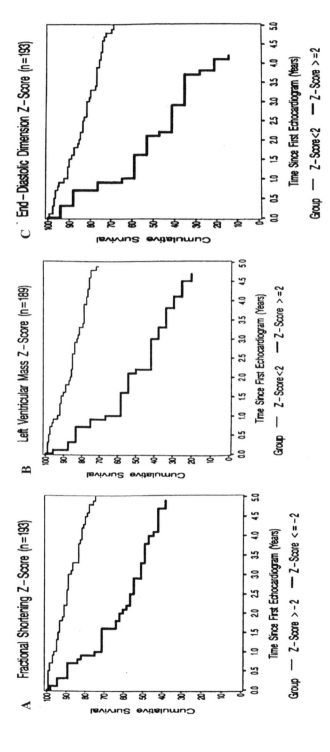

FIGURE 3. Kaplan Meier cumulative survival for 193 HIV⁺ children according to baseline clinical characteristics and baseline echocardiographic measurements. **A:** fractional shortening, **B:** left ventricular mass, and **C:** end-diastolic dimension. (From Lipshultz, S.E., K.A. Easley, E.J. Orav, *et al.* 2000. Cardiac dysfunction and mortality. The prospective P²C² HIV multicenter study. Circulation **102:** 1542–1548.[10] used with permission.)

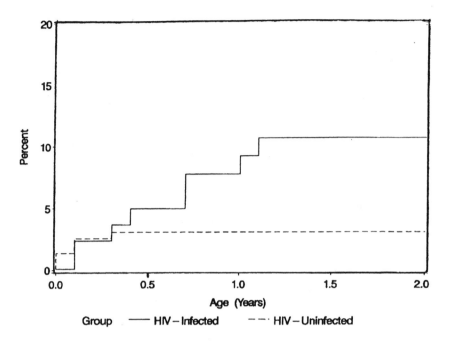

FIGURE 4. Kaplan Meier cumulative incidence of an initial episode of decreased left ventricular fractional shortening (not more than 25%) in HIV-infected and noninfected children over the first two years of life ($p = 0.01$; log-rank test). (From Starc, T.J., S.E. Lipshultz, S. Kaplan, *et al.* 1999. Cardiac complications in children with human immuno-deficiency virus infection. Pediatrics **104:** e14, used with permission).

The prevalence of decreased left ventricular function in HIV[+] children was 5.7% (FS $\leq$ 25%) with a two year cumulative incidence of 15.3%.[13] The incidence of decreased left ventricular fractional shortening among children infected with HIV in the neonatal period was 10.7% compared to 3.1% of children not infected. The cumulative incidence of left ventricular end diastolic diameter enlargement was 11.7% after two years in 205 HIV vertically infected infants. Twenty percent of HIV[+] children developed left ventricular dilation or depressed left ventricular function.[13] The incidence of congestive heart failure or the need for cardiac medications was 10% in this cohort. Left ventricular hypertrophy is also commonly seen in HIV[+] children. Hypertrophy in this population is the result of ventricular dilation over time resulting in an increase in left ventricular mass. HIV[+] children have been found to have a mean cardiac weight 184% higher than that of HIV[-] children.[14]

Increased mortality in children who at baseline had depressed left ventricular fractional shortening or contractility, increased left ventricular dimension, thickness, mass, or wall stress, or increased heart rate or blood pressure was found in 193 vertically infected children.[10] Also predicative of increased mortality rates were decreased left ventricular fractional shortening and increased left ventricular wall thickness independent of CD4 count.[10] These results suggest that measures of left ventricular function are clinically significant and may predict an increased risk of death in HIV$^+$ children.

HIV$^+$ children have increased mortality if malnutrition and wasting are also present clinically. There exists and inverse relationship between heart rate and nutritional status that suggests an increase in basal metabolic rate where malnutrition, altered cardiac muscle mass, and left ventricular dysfunction are interdependent.[15]

MYOCARDITIS

A common cause of left ventricular systolic dysfunction is myocarditis. The most common viruses found by PCR in affected tissues were adenovirus and CMV in HIV$^+$ children.[16] The presence of viral nucleic acids in the myocardium may also be associated with the development of myocarditis, dilated cardiomyopathy, or congestive heart failure in HIV$^+$ children.

Infections are not indicative of cardiomyopathy in all cases. EBV infection rate was similar between HIV$^+$ and HIV$^-$ children.[17] Similarly, CMV rates were equal for infected and uninfected children.[18] However, children who acquired CMV infection by 18 months of age had a higher rate of cardiomyopathy than those with HIV infection without CMV infection.

OTHER CARDIAC MANIFESTATIONS OF HIV INFECTION

Vascular disease has also been described in children infected with HIV. Arteriopathy, inflammatory lesions, and atherosclerotic lesions are frequently reported. Aortic root dilation that is either mildly progressive or stable over time was recently described in children with vertically transmitted HIV infection aged two to nine years. Aortic root dilation was found to be associated with increased viral load and lower CD4 count suggesting a direct pathogenic effect of the HIV virus.[19]

Electrocardiograph abnormalities are prominent in children infected with HIV. Abnormalities include tachycardia in 49–70% of HIV$^+$ children and ventricular hypertrophy in 20–30% of HIV$^+$ children.[14,20–22] Among the rhythm disturbances found in HIV$^+$ children are sinus arrhythmia, atrial ectopy, and ventricular arrhythmias.[22,23] Uncontrolled factors exist such as cocaine exposure and the prenatal environment which may also affect the electrocardiogram.

Pericardial disease, cardiovascular tumors and pulmonary hypertension have also been documented in children infected with HIV. Pericardial disease particularly pericardial effusion has a prevalence rate of 16 to 26% in HIV$^+$ children.[14,22,24–26] Pericardial effusions in children are generally small and asymptomatic. Cardiovascular tumors found in HIV$^+$ children include Kaposi's sarcoma and leiomyosarcoma. Left ventricular dysfunction, recurrent bronchopulmonary disease, and primary pulmonary hypertension are possible causes of pulmonary hypertension in HIV$^+$ children.[27,28]

CARDIAC COMPLICATIONS OF THERAPY

A risk of cardiac and skeletal muscle myopathies has been associated with the use of zidovudine (AZT) in animal models.[29,30] This has not been evident in clinical data in children. In a cohort of 24 children with symptomatic HIV infection that were treated with AZT, the cardiac structure and function by echocardiography were not altered by the administration of AZT when compared to those that were not exposed.[31] A group of infants that were exposed to zidovudine in the perinatal period were also followed from birth until five years of age and zidovudine was not associated with abnormalities of left ventricular structure or function.[32] These results suggest that neonatal and perinatal AZT use does not adversely affect cardiac development and function and careful thought must be given before withholding treatment with AZT.

SUMMARY

Cardiovascular effects of HIV infection in children are now being recognized with the help of prospective observational trials such as the P^2C^2 HIV study. Recent epidemiological studies have shown that cardiac disease in HIV^+ children is common and will continue to occur more and more frequently as children live longer with HIV. The P^2C^2 HIV study was created to help explore the fundamental effects of HIV, comorbid illness, and standard therapies on the cardiovascular system of children over their lifetime.

Left ventricular dysfunction and increased left ventricular mass have been shown to occur frequently and to be associated with mortality early in children with rapidly progressive disease and late in those with more latent infection. Understanding, monitoring and beginning early therapy of cardiovascular risk factors and disease associated with HIV infection will hopefully help to improve the quality and duration of life in children living with HIV infection in the future.

REFERENCES

1. UN AIDS. 2000. Report on the global HIV/AIDS epidemic [Web Page]. http://www.unaids.org.
2. THE P^2C^2 HIV STUDY GROUP. 1996. The pediatric pulmonary and cardiovascular complications of vertically transmitted human immunodeficiency virus infection study: design and methods. J. Clin. Epidemiol. **49**(11): 1285–1294.
3. LANGSTON, C., E. COOPER, J. GOLDFARB, et al. 2001. HIV-related mortality in infants and children: Data from the Pediatric Pulmonary and Cardiovascular Complications of Vertically Transmitted HIV Study. Pediatrics **107**(2): 328–336.
4. AL-ATTAR, I., E. ORAV, V. EXIL, et al. 1995. Predictors of cardiac morbidity and related mortality in children with acquired immune deficiency syndrome (abstract) Pediatr. Res. **37**: 169A.
5. SHEARER, W.T., S.E. LIPSHULTZ, K.A. EASLEY, et al. 2000. Alterations in cardiac and pulmonary function in pediatric rapid human immunodeficiency virus type 1 disease progressors. Pediatrics **105**(1): 1–8.
6. UNAIDS: JOINT UNITED NATIONS PROGRAMME ON HIV/AIDS. 1999 World AIDS Campaign Facts & Figures [Web Page]. http://www. unaids.org/wac/1999/statistics.html.

7. CENTERS FOR DISEASE CONTROL. HIV/AIDS Surveillance Report [Web Page]. http://www.cdc.gov/hiv/stats.
8. HORNBERGER, L., S.E. LIPSHULTZ, K.A. EASLEY, *et al.* 2000. Cardiac structure and function in fetuses of mothers infected with HIV: the prospective P^2C^2 HIV multicenter study. Am. Heart J. **140:** 575-84.
9. LAI, W.W., S.E. LIPSHULTZ, K.A. EASLEY, *et al.* 1998. Prevalence of congenital cardiovascular malformations in children of human immunodeficiency virus infected women. J. Am. Coll. Cardiol. **32**(6): 1749–1755.
10. LIPSHULTZ, S.E., K.A. EASLEY, E.J. ORAV, *et al.* 2000. Cardiac dysfunction and mortality. The Prospective P^2C^2 HIV Infection Study Group. Circulation **102:** 1542–1548.
11. LIPSHULTZ, S.E., K.A. EASLEY, E.J. ORAV, *et al.* 1998. Left ventricular structure and function in children infected with human immunodeficiency virus: the prospective P^2C^2 HIV multicenter study. Circulation **97**(13): 1246–1256.
12. LIPSHULTZ, S.E. 1993. Pediatric pulmonary and cardiovascular complications of vertically transmitted HIV infection study group. Progressive cardiac dysfunction in HIV-infected children (abstract). Proc. IXth International Conf. on AIDS **9**(1): 48.
13. STARC, T., S.E. LIPSHULTZ & S. KAPLAN. 1999. Cardiac complications in children with human immunodeficiency virus infection. Pediatrics **104**(2): 1–9.
14. LIPSHULTZ, S.E., S. CHANOCK, S.P. SANDER, *et al.* 1989. Cardiovascular manifestations of human immunodeficiency virus infection in infants and children. Am. J. Cardiol. **63**(20): 1489-97.
15. MILLER, T., E.J. ORAV, S. COLAN, *et al.* 1997. Nutritional status and cardiac mass and function in children infected with the human immunodeficiency virus. Am. J. Clin. Nutr. **66:** 660–664.
16. BOWLES, N.E., D.L. KEARNEY, J. NI, *et al.* 1999. The detection of viral genomes by polymerase chain reaction in the myocardium of pediatric patients with advanced HIV disease. J. Am. Coll. Cardiol. **34**(3): 857–865.
17. JENSON, H., K. MCINTOSH, J. PITT, *et al.* 1999. Natural history of primary Epstein-Barr virus infection in children of mothers infected with human immunodeficiency virus type 1. J. Infect. Dis. **179**(6): 1395–1404.
18. KOVACS, A., M. SCHLUCHTER, K. EASLEY, *et al.* 1999. Cytomegalovirus infection and HIV-1 disease progression in infants born to HIV-1-infected women. N. Engl. J. Med. **341**(2): 77–84.
19. LAI, W.W., S. COLAN, K.A. EASLEY, *et al.* Dilation of the aortic root in children infected with human immunodeficiency virus type 1. Am. Heart J. In press.
20. LOBATO, M.N., B. CALDWELL, P. NG & M.J. OXTOBY. 1995. Encephalopathy in children with perinatally acquired human immunodeficiency virus infection. J. Pediatr. **126**(5, Pt. 1): 710–715.
21. GRENIER, M.A., S.S. KARR, T.A. RAKUSAN & G.R. MARTIN. 1994. Cardiac disease in children with HIV: relationship of cardiac disease to HIV symptomatology. Pediatr. AIDS HIV Infect.: Fetus Adolesc. **5:** 174–178.
22. KAVANAUGH-MCHUGH, A.L., A.J. RUFF, S.A. ROWE, *et al.* 1991. Cardiac abnormalities in a multicenter interventional study of children with symptomatic HIV infection. Pediatr. Res. **29:** 176A.
23. LUGINBUHL, L.M., E.J. ORAV, K. MCINTOSH & S.E. LIPSHULTZ. 1993. Cardiac morbidity and related mortality in children with HIV infection. J. Am. Med. Assoc. **269**(22): 2869–2875.
24. ISSENBERG, H.J., M. CHARYTAN & A. RUBINSTEIN. 1985. Cardiac involvement in children with acquired immune deficiency (abstract). Am. Heart J. **110:** 710.
25. SHERRON, P., A.S. PICKOFF, P.L. FERRER, *et al.* 1985. Echocardiographic evaluation of myocardial function in pediatric AIDS patients (abstract). Am. Heart J. **110:** 710.
26. MAST, H.L., J.O. HALLER, M.S. SCHILLER & V.M. ANDERSON. 1992. Pericardial effusion and its relationship to cardiac disease in children with acquired immunodeficiency syndrome. Pediatr. Radiol. **22**(7): 548–551.
27. LIPSHULTZ, S.E. 1994. Cardiovascular manifestations of pediatric HIV infection. *In* Pediatric AIDS. The Challenge of HIV Infection in Infants, Children, and Adolescents, 2nd edit. P.A. Pizzo, Ed.: 483–511. Williams & Wilkins. Baltimore.

28. PETITPRETZ, P., F. BRENOT, R. AZARIAN, *et al.* 1994. Pulmonary hypertension in patients with human immunodeficiency virus infection. Comparison with primary pulmonary hypertension. Circulation **89**(6): 2722–2727.
29. CUPLER, E.J., M.C. DANON, C. JAY, *et al.* 1995. Early features of zidovudine-associated myopathy: histopathological findings and clinical correlations. Acta Neuropathol. **90**(1): 1–6.
30. LAMPERTH, L., M.C. DALAKAS, F. DAGANI, *et al.* 1991. Abnormal skeletal and cardiac muscle mitochondria induced by zidovudine (AZT) in human muscle in vitro and in an animal model. Lab. Invest. **65**(6): 742–751.
31. LIPSHULTZ, S.E., E.J. ORAV, S.P. SANDERS, *et al.* 1992. Cardiac structure and function in children with human immunodeficiency virus infection treated with zidovudine. N. Engl. J. Med. **327**(18): 1260–1265.
32. LIPSHULTZ, S.E., K.A. EASLEY, E.J. ORAV, *et al.* 2000. Absence of cardiac toxicity of zidovudine in infants. N. Engl. J. Med. **343**(11): 759–805.

Drugs and Cardiotoxicity in HIV and AIDS

M. FANTONI,[a] C. AUTORE,[b] AND C. DEL BORGO[a]

[a]Department of Infectious Diseases, Catholic University, Rome, Italy

[b]Department of Cardiovascular and Respiratory Sciences,
"La Sapienza" University, Rome, Italy

ABSTRACT: The advent of potent antiretroviral drugs in recent years has had an impressive impact on mortality and disease progression in HIV-infected patients, so that issues related to long-term effects of drugs are of growing importance. Hyperlipidemia, hyperglycemia, and lipodystrophy are increasingly described adverse effects of highly active antiretroviral therapy (HAART), in particular when protease inhibitors are used. Hyperlipidemia is strikingly associated with the use of most available protease inhibitors, with an estimated prevalence of up to 50%. Because of the short observation period and the small number of cardiovascular events, epidemiological evidence for an increased risk of coronary heart disease in HIV-infected patients treated with HAART is not adequate at present; however, it is likely that shortly more data will accumulate to quantify this risk. Before starting HAART and during treatment it is reasonable to evaluate all patients for traditional coronary risk factors, including lipid profile. Among the drugs that are currently used in HIV+ patients, antibacterials, antifungals, psychotropic drugs and anti-histamines have been associated with QT prolongation or torsade de pointe, a life-threatening ventricular arrhythmia. Among the risk factors that may precipitate an asymptomatic electrocardiographic abnormality into a dangerous arrhythmia is the concomitant use of drugs that share the CYP3A metabolic pathway. Since most protease inhibitors are potent inhibitors of CYP3A, clinicians should be aware of this potentially dangerous effect of HAART. Anthracyclines are potent cytotoxic antibiotics that have been widely used for the treatment of HIV-related neoplasms. Their cardiotoxicity is well known, ranging from benign and reversible arrhythmias to progressive severe cardiomyopathy. The increased survival and quality of life of HIV+ patients emphasize the importance of a high awareness of adverse drug-related cardiac effects.

KEYWORDS: cardiotoxicity; antiretrovirals; HAART; dyslipidemia; cardiomyopathy

Cardiac involvement in HIV disease is estimated to be approximately 6–7%.[1] A proportion of cardiac morbidity may be ascribed to the toxic effect of drugs used for the treatment of HIV+ patients. The pharmacological treatment of AIDS and HIV-related diseases includes the use of antiretroviral and other anti-infective or anti-neoplastic drugs. Moreover, patients with HIV infection are at higher risk for conditions such as psychiatric diseases or allergic diseases that require additional drug treatments. Until recently the prognosis for people with the acquired immunodeficiency

Address for correspondence: Massimo Fantoni, M.D., Dipartimento di Malattie Infettive, Università Cattolica S. Cuore, Laro F. Vito 1, 00168 Rome, Italy.
   crif@rm.unicatt.it

syndrome (AIDS) was so poor that concerns about long-term effects of drug treatment were relatively minor. The advent of potent antiretroviral drugs in recent years has had an impressive effect on mortality, disease progression, and incidence of HIV-related disorders.[2,3] Indeed, in an increasing proportion of patients HIV disease should be considered a chronic condition and issues related to long-term drug are of growing importance.[4] Some of the drugs that are presently prescribed have been used for years or decades and are well known, whereas some of the most frequently prescribed antiretrovirals are of recent origin and their long-term toxicities have not yet been assessed. Cardiotoxicity related to the use of anthracyclines, amphotericin B, zidovudine, macrolides, and interferon have been extensively described,[5–9] although the molecular mechanisms of all their effects have not been thoroughly assessed. A most important field of research is the possible increase of cardiovascular risk in patients treated with protease inhibitors. Some drugs commonly prescribed in HIV$^+$ patients have a direct effect on the myocyte, others cause electrophysiologic impairment, others are possibly involved in vascular alterations. The present review focuses on the cardiotoxicity of the drugs used for HIV disease.

ANTIRETROVIRAL THERAPY

The clinical management of HIV$^+$ patients is based on antiretroviral therapy, which has been demonstrated to provide clinical benefit in all patients with advanced disease and immunosuppression.[10] Although there is indeed a theoretical benefit in treating also asymptomatic individuals, the decision on when to start an aggressive treatment, with significant side effects and drug interactions, must take into account many factors, including patient adherence to treatment[11] and quality of life.[4] Until 1996, before the use of triple combination treatments, the effect of antiretroviral therapy on disease progression and overall survival was not very impressive. Nowadays, the improved survival, the availability of a number of antiretroviral agents, and the possibility of complex individualized combination regimens underscores the need for long-term treatment programs.

There are three classes of drugs that are presently used for people with HIV infection (see TABLE 1): the nucleoside reverse transcriptase inhibitors (NRTIs), including zidovudine (AZT), didanosine (DDI), zalcitabine (DDC), stavudine (D4T),

TABLE 1. Antiretroviral drugs

Nucleoside transcriptase inhibitors (NRTIs)	Non-nucleoside transcriptase inhibitors (NNRTIs)	Protease inhibitors (PIs)
Zidovudine (AZT)	Nevirapine	Saquinavir
Didanosine (DDI)	Delavirdine	Ritonavir
Zalcitabine (DDC)	Efavirenz	Indinavir
Stavudine (D4T)		Nelfinavir
Lamivudine (3TC)		Amprenavir
Abacavir		Lopinavir

lamivudine (3TC), and abacavir; the non-nucleoside reverse transcriptase inhibitors (NNRTI) including nevirapine and efavirenz; and the protease inhibitors (PIs), including ritonavir, saquinavir, indinavir, nelfinavir, amprenavir, and lopinavir. The standard of treatment is a PI or a NNRTI in combination with 2 NRTIs. Recent data indicate that the use of reduced doses of 2 PIs in combination with 2 NRTIs can achieve the same virological and immunological benefits of standard regimens with improved pharmacocynetic properties and possibly better patient adherence.[10]

Cardiomyopathy

Zidovudine (AZT) was the first antiretroviral drug to be widely used[12] and it is presently prescribed in combination regimens. AZT is also widely used in pregnant mothers and newborns after the demonstration of a dramatic decrease of perinatally transmitted HIV infection.[13] Soon after the widespread use of AZT, one report was published on the role of the drug in inducing dilated cardiomyopathy in a small number of adult patients. In this report the discontinuation of treatment resulted in an improved left ventricular function.[7] In a prospective study performed in Italy on an adult population, among patients receiving AZT the incidence of cardiomyopathy was greater in those with a higher degree of immunosuppression.[14,15] In a retrospective study, treatment of HIV+ children with zidovudine has been associated with a greater risk of developing cardiomyopathy.[16] More recently, in two large prospective studies, infants born to HIV+ mothers, exposed to AZT *in utero* and perinatally, were followed up from birth to as long as five years of age and no clinically relevant cardiotoxicity was observed.[17,18] Side-effects of NRTIs more frequently encountered than cardiotoxicity include myopathy, bone-marrow and hepatic toxicity, and neuropathy. The mechanism of all these adverse events is a toxic effect on mitochondria. The damage of cardiac mitochondrial ultrastructures and inhibition of mitochondrial DNA replication has been observed in animal models.[19] AZT acts as a competitive and non-competitive inhibitor of mitochondrial DNA polymerase.[19,20] The inhibitory action of NRTIs on DNA polymerase-γ, the only DNA polymerase involved in mitochondrial DNA replication, does interfere *in vitro* with mitochondrial replication and function.[21] Mitochondrial damage has been also indicated as a putative etiology for lipodystrophy, a debilitating adverse effect of potent combination antiretroviral therapy. Molecular mechanisms of cardiotoxicity other than mitochondrial damage have been hypothesized. In an animal model, the short term cardiotoxicity of DDC was not the direct consequence of mitochondrial DNA-related damage, but of reactive oxygen species (ROS)-mediated signaling through poly- and mono-ADP-ribosylation reactions and depression of heat shock protein (HSP)70 levels.[22]

The clinical relevance of combined regimens of NRTIs has not yet extensively been studied with regard to mitochondrial toxicity. Prospective clinical and *in vitro* studies are warranted, since the use of NRTIs combination regimens is likely to increase over time.

Dyslipidemia and Cardiovascular Risk

Hyperlipidemia, hyperglicemia, and lipodystrophy are increasingly described adverse effects of potent antiretroviral combination therapy, in particular when PIs are used.[23] According to Carr[24] the metabolic and somatic alterations in PI-treated subjects could be ascribed to the homology of the catalytic region of HIV protease, the molecular target of PIs, to regions of two human proteins that regulate lipid metabolism: cytoplasmic retinoic-acid binding protein 1 (CRABP-1) and low density lipoprotein-receptor-related protein (LRP). The hypothesis is that PIs inhibit CRABP-1-modified and CYP3A-mediated synthesis of *cis*-9-retinoic acid and peroxisome proliferator-activated receptor type-γ (PPAR-γ) heterodimer. This results in an increased apoptosis of adipocytes and in a reduced differentiation from pre-adipocytes to adipocytes, with the final effect of a reduced triglyceride storage and increased lipid release. PI binding to LRP would impair hepatic chylomicron uptake and endothelial triglyceride clearance, resulting in hyperlipidemia and insulin resistance.

Patients treated with NRTIs who have never used PIs can also experience hyperlipidemia and lipodystrophy, suggesting alternative or additional pathogenetic mechanisms,[20] related to the inhibition of mitochondrial DNA polymerase-γ. Indeed, it has been hypothesized that the mitochondrial toxicity of NRTIs is similar to the mitochondrial dysfunction observed in multiple symmetrical lipomatosis (MSL) or Madelung's disease.[25] Also NNRTIs can have adverse effects on lipid levels, although more limited data are presently available.[26]

Hyperlipidemia is strikingly associated with the use of most available PIs, with an estimated prevalence of up to 50%.[27–29] Data from large published series indicate that there is a wide variation in the degree of hyperlipidemia, with an average increase of total cholesterol and triglyceride levels of 28% and 96%, respectively, compared with pre-treatment levels.[23,29–32] The level of increase seems to be proportional to the duration of therapy[30] and to the type of drug.[31]

In a prospective study the administration of ritonavir, indinavir, nelfinavir or ritonavir/saquinavir, nelfinavir/saquinavir to HIV$^+$ subjects was associated with a significant compound-specific increase in plasma levels of both cholesterol and triglycerides. The mean duration of treatment was 470 ± 22 days; the proportion of subjects with total cholesterol level greater than 6.2 mmol/L (cardiovascular risk threshold according to National Cholesterol Education Program) rose from 7% to 44% in the ritonavir group, from 5% to 33% in the nelfinavir group and from 12% to 35% in the indinavir group. Moreover, a 48% increase in plasma levels of lipoprotein(a) was detected in treated subjects with pre-treatment values greater than 20 mg/dL.[31] In another study that involved 292 patients, hypercholesterolemia seemed to be reversible after PI discontinuation, whereas the levels of lipoprotein, insulin and plasminogen activator inhibitor 1 were constantly increased after 12 month follow-up.[33]

Although abnormalities of lipid metabolism in HIV$^+$ patients have been described in the pre-HAART era, recent reports of myocardial infarctions in young patients receiving PIs has focused interest in examining the associations between HIV infection, antiretroviral therapy, and coronary artery disease. Cardiovascular events closely associated with PI therapy were anecdotally described.[34–37] Now that the prolonged survival of HIV$^+$ patients is well established, the risk of premature cardiovascular events caused by coronary artery disease in HAART-treated patients is likely to become a key issue in the near future. In a study from the French Hospital Data Base on HIV it was found that patients treated with PIs had a 2.79-fold increased risk of myocardial infarction when compared with untreated patients.[38]

The study however was limited by the small number of events. An American retrospective case-control study examined 15 HIV$^+$ individuals with a recent cardiovascular event and compared them with matched controls. In this study HAART did not appear to be a risk factor in a multivariate analysis.[39] Also, the issue of surrogate markers of subclinical atherosclerosis has been addressed. A study was performed on a cohort of French HIV$^+$ patients to measure the intima-media thickness and assess indirectly the cardiovascular risk. In this population no independent link between intima-media thickness, lipodystrophy and HAART was observed.[40,41]

Many prospective trials are presently addressing this important aspect of HAART, but until now quantitative data on the risk of premature atherosclerosis and risk of coronary events in PI-treated subjects are lacking or uncertain. The rapid development of atherosclerosis has not yet been demonstrated in PI-treated individuals, owing to the relatively short observation period since the widespread use of HAART. This possibility is worrisome, since rapidly forming plaques can be unstable and more easily prone to rupture with consequent acute coronary event. More consistent data will be available by merging large cohorts and analyzing prospectively the cardiovascular risk related to drug-induced metabolic alterations. However, the observation that drug-induced changes in lipid levels has resulted in an increased cardiovascular risk in other diseases[42–44] is a reason for concern in HIV$^+$ patients, as clinical experience with HAART continues to grow. In some HIV$^+$ groups, such as i.v. drug users, heavy cigarette smoking is highly prevalent, adding a well-known risk factor for ischemic heart disease. Moreover, the role of non-traditional risk factors for coronary artery disease that may possibly be more prevalent in HIV$^+$ populations; for example the use of cocaine and anabolic steroids, must be taken into account.

Preliminary guidelines for the evaluation and management of dyslipidemia in HIV$^+$ patients receiving HAART have recently been published.[45] Key points of these recommendations are the routine screening of HIV$^+$ patients for coronary risk factors, a comprehensive analysis of the fasting lipid profile before starting antiretroviral therapy and the treatment of selected cases. In case of hypercholesterolemia, except for those patients with extreme elevations in cholesterol (greater than 400 mg/dL) a first attempt of treatment should include dietary interventions and reduction or abolishment of correctable risk factors for coronary disease, such as cigarette smoking, physical inactivity, diabetes mellitus, and hypertension. Eventually, the 3-hydroxy-3-methylglutaryil coenzyme A reductase inhibitors or statins can be prescribed. Since many of these compounds are cytochrome P 450 substrates, the concomitant use with PIs could retard their metabolism, with an increase of toxicity. The safest drugs in this respect have proved to be pravastatin[46] and atorvastatin.[27] Hypertriglyceridemia should also be treated initially with non-pharmacological therapies, such as diet, exercise, smoking cessation. Marked increases in triglyceride serum levels are a risk factor not only for coronary disease, but also for pancreatitis and should be treated with lipid-lowering agents. Fibrates are the most effective drugs used for the treatment of hypertriglyceridemia and have been proposed as possible first-line drugs for patients with both hypercholesterolemia and hypertriglyceridemia.[45] Genfibrozil has been used successfully in dyslipidemic HIV$^+$ patients receiving PIs.[27]

Another frequent side-effect of PI therapy is hyperinsulinemia, an independent risk factor for coronary artery disease.[47] Among PI-treated patients a prevalence of 25–62% of insulin resistance was reported.[23,29]

At present, the optimal time for initiation of HAART takes into account the clinical stage of disease, baseline viral load, and CD4+ counts. For asymptomatic persons with relatively high CD4+ counts and low or undetectable viral load it is important to balance the possible long-term adverse events, the decreasing adherence to treatment over time, and the emergence of viral resistance. There are patients with a high atherosclerotic co-morbidity or risk, a high CD4+ cell count, and a low plasma viral load; for such patients it is possible that the risk/benefit ratio of treating with HAART will be demonstrated to be not beneficial.[48]

DRUGS USED FOR HIV-RELATED DISORDERS

In the HAART era, the use of drugs for HIV-related opportunistic infections and neoplasms has significantly decreased, owing to the declining incidence of these conditions.[2] Nonetheless, there are circumstances in which HAART regimens fail, as a consequence of acquired drug resistance, poor patient adherence or treatment discontinuation for side-effects, especially in advanced stage patients. In such conditions, the incidence of HIV-related disorders may rise, leading to the use of drugs commonly administered in the pre-HAART era.

Drugs used for HIV-related diseases may have adverse cardiac effects including cardiomyopathy (as was extensively studied for anthracyclines), changes of the action potential of the myocardium leading to prolongation of the electrocardiographic QT-interval (as observed with many antimicrobials), and various other cardiac effects as described with the use of immunomodulators (see TABLE 2).

Cardiomyopathy is a disorder of cardiac muscle that produces systolic and less frequently diastolic dysfunction. The 1995 WHO/ISFC Report classifies cardiomyopathies as dilated, hypertrophic, restrictive and arrhythmogenic right ventricular cardiomyopathy.[49] The anthracyclines, anticancer drugs widely used for the treatment

TABLE 2. Drugs with potential cardiotoxicity used for HIV+ persons

Drugs	Use in HIV+ Persons	Potential Cardiotoxicity
NRTIs	HIV disease	Cardiomyopathy?
NNRTIs	HIV disease	Increased C.V. risk?
PIs	HIV disease	Increased C.V. risk?
Anti-infective drugs	Opportunistic infections	Prolonged QT interval
Psychotropic drugs	Psychotic disorders, depression	Prolonged QT interval
Antihistamines	Allergic reactions	Prolonged QT interval
Anthracyclines	HIV-related neoplasms	Cardiomyopathy
Interferon	KS, HIV/HCV coinfection	CHD, cardiomyopathy
Interleukin-2	HIV disease	CHD, cardiomyopathy

TABLE 3. Anti-infective drugs with QT-prolonging potential used for HIV^+ persons

Anti-infective Drugs	Use in HIV^+ Persons
Erythromycin	Bacillary angiomatosis
Clarithromycin	Mycobacterial diseases
TMP/SMX	PCP treatment and prophylaxis
Pentamidine	PCP treatment and prophylaxis
Fluoroquinolones	Mycobacterial diseases, other bacterial infections
Amphotericin B	Disseminated fungal infections
Azole antifungals	Mucosal and disseminated fungal infections

of HIV-related neoplasms, may be toxic to the myocardium and produce a specific cardiomyopathy characterized by mild dilation and impaired contraction of the left ventricle or, less commonly, of both ventricles. The pathologic features of anthracycline cardiomyopathy are unique, showing myocyte vacuolization progressing to cell drop out.

The prolongation of the electrocardiographic QT interval indicates an increased risk for the development of life-threatening arrhythmias, in particular of torsade de pointe, a polymorphous ventricular arrhythmia, that may cause syncope and degenerate into ventricular fibrillation.[50] Although the clinical relevance of asymptomatic QT interval prolongation is yet to be established, it should be considered a useful

TABLE 4. Other drugs with QT-prolonging potential used for HIV^+ persons

Antidepressants	
	Amitryptiline
	Doxepine
	Desipramine
	Imipramine
	Clomipramine
Antipsychotics	
	Thioridazine
	Chlorpromazine
	Pimozide
	Sertindole
	Haloperidol
Antihistamines	
	Astemizole
	Terfenadine

surrogate marker of cardiotoxicity of both cardiac and non-cardiac drugs. An important issue is the identification of co-factors that, together with the prescription of potentially cardiotoxic drugs, may precipitate a malignant arrhythmia. These factors are hepatic or renal impairment, electrolyte imbalance (especially hypokalemia and hypomagnesemia), and the concomitant use of diverse drugs with QT-prolonging potential. Among the drugs that are currently used in HIV$^+$ patients, antibacterials, antifungals, psychotropic drugs, and anti-histamines have been associated with QT prolongation or torsade de pointe (see TABLES 3 and 4). In most cases the effect is dose-dependent and/or associated with co-factors or concomitant treatment with CYP3A4 isoenzyme inhibitors.[51] The common mechanism with which so many chemically unrelated compounds prolong the QT interval is thought to be the blockade of myocardial ion channels, particularly the rapidly activating delayed repolarizing potassium current (I_{Kr}).[51,52] For most drugs QT prolongation and torsades de pointe should be considered a rare side-effect. In fact, most case-reports refer to concomitant use of drugs that share a QT-prolonging potential.

Anti-Infective Drugs

Macrolide antibiotics have a QT interval-prolonging potential. Erythromycin was the most extensively studied drug in this respect and its effects on electrocardiogram are well established, especially with i.v. administration.[51] As has been shown for antiarrhythmic drugs, a female predominance of erythromycin-associated arrhythmias was found.[53] Erythromycin has had wide applications in anti-infective therapy, but it has limited specific indications in HIV$^+$ patients. Clarithromycin, which is chemically closely related to erythromycin has wider applications in AIDS patients and it is currently recommended for the treatment of mycobacterial diseases. Its potential for electrocardiographic alterations and cardiac arrhythmias is not as high as erythromycin, but cases have been reported of QT prolongation and torsades de pointes.[54,55] Case reports of QT prolongation have been published both with clarithromycin used in combination and alone.[56,57]

Isolated cases of QT prolongation and torsades de pointes associated with the use of *trimethoprim/sulfametoxazole* in HIV-uninfected patients have been reported.[58,59] However, this must be considered an extremely rare event, since in the pre-HAART era trimethoprim/sulfamethoxazole has been extensively used at very high dosages in AIDS patients with *Pneumocystis carinii* pneumonia and among the frequent and severe side-effects, electrocardiographic abnormalities were not reported.

The use of *fluoroquinolones* has also been associated with QT prolongation, mostly with sparfloxacin.[60–63] Since the use of this class of antimicrobials is very extensive worldwide, the QT prolongation potential, especially when they are used in combination, should be carefully assessed.[64,65] Fluoroquinolones have wide indications in both HIV-related and unrelated infections. *Amphotericin B and azole antifungals*—ketoconazole, fluconazole, itraconazole—all have a QT prolongation potential.[66–69] The use of antifungal agents is most common in HIV$^+$ patients. *Candida* spp. infections range from mild oral thrush to life-threatening multi-organ involvement. Aspergillosis, as in non-HIV$^+$ patients, usually causes malignant lung or sinus abscesses. Amphotericin B, the most potent and most toxic of the commonly used antifungals, can also cause hypokalemia, precipitating the long-QT syndrome and arrhythmias.[70] Amphotericin B was also reported to cause bradycardia.[71] The more recent liposomal formulations of amphotericin B have improved the overall tolerability of the drug, but the potential for electrolyte unbalance and QT prolongation remains.[72,73] QT prolongations associated with the use of azole antifungals were believed to occur by inhibition of the hepatic metabolism of other QT-prolonging drugs;[70–77] however, a direct effect was also observed.[78]

Pentamidine is a second-line drug structurally similar to procainamide used for the treatment and prophylaxis of *Pneumocystis carinii* pneumonia. Pentamidine in several anecdotal reports and prospective studies was considered responsible for QT-prolongation and ventricular arrythmias.[79–83] The adverse cardiac electrophysiologic effects of pentamidine in fact occur in only a small proportion of patients and are enhanced by hypomagnesemia and hypokalemia.[84,85] When using other drugs with QT-prolongation potential it must be remembered that appreciable tissue levels of pentamidine may be present months after the discontinuation of the drug.[86]

Ganciclovir and foscarnet are first-line drugs for the treatment of cytomegalovirus (CMV) infections. In AIDS patients retinal or life-threatening disseminated CMV infections are common, although the prevalence has dropped with the advent of successful antiretroviral therapy. Anecdotal reports of cardiotoxicity with the use of ganciclovir and foscarnet were published. Two patients developed ventricular tachycardia during intravenous infusion of ganciclovir[87] and one patient developed reversible cardiomyopathy when treated with foscarnet.[88] The mechanism of cardiotoxicity of the drugs was not apparent. CMV can itself affect the myocardium, suggesting that in the cases described there was a possible concomitant effect of the drugs and the virus.

Antihistamines

Antihistamines may have potential indications in HIV$^+$ patients, since allergic reactions are much more frequent than in the general population.[89] Two non-sedating anti-histamines, astemizole and terfenadine, have a well known effect on QT interval, and torsades de pointe and sudden death have also been reported.[51,90–93] The newer non-sedating anti-histamines (ebastine, loratadine, cetirizine, acrivastatina, fexofenadine, and mizolastatine) seem to be safer,[93,94] but some of them do have an effect on I_{Kr} and their cardiotoxic potential needs to be assessed further. The cardiotoxicity of antihistamines is dose-dependent and usually influenced by the concomitant use of other drugs with a QT prolongation effect or inhibition of cytochrome P450.

Psychotropic Drugs

Psychotropic drugs have a potential cardiotoxicity related to their QT-prolonging effect. The tricyclic anti-depressants amitriptyline, doxepine, desipramine, imipramine and clomipramine have all been associated with QT prolongation, and sudden death was reported with desipramine, clomipramine and imipramine.[95,96] Antipsychotic agents in the butyrophenones and phenotiazine classes appear to be significantly cardiotoxic[97] both at therapeutic and supra-therapeutic doses. Case reports or treatment of healthy volunteers pointed out the cardiotoxicity of thioridazine,[98] chlorpromazine, haloperidol,[99–101] pimozide[102] and sertindole.[103] In numerous studies psychiatric morbidity in HIV^+ patients ranges widely according to definitions, study populations, and study design. There is however general agreement that psychiatric disorders, ranging from mild anxiety to major depression and psychosis, are far more prevalent than in the general population.[104–108] In a study that examined HIV^+ persons in a large outpatient clinic, 53% of the women and 70% of the men met Structural Clinical Interview for DSM-III-R criteria for psychiatric disorders.[109] The increased survival of HIV^+ patients with the need to cope with complex therapeutic regimens, adverse effects, and alterations of body image due to lipodystrophy could also potentially increase the long-term psychiatric morbidity. Since psychotropic drugs are routinely used in HIV^+ patients, there is the need for careful monitoring of potentially dangerous side-effects, including cardiac toxicity.

Drugs Used for HIV-related Neoplasms

The effects of anthracyclines on myocardial structure and function have been extensively studied.[110–113] Anthracyclines are potent cytotoxic antibiotics that have been widely used also in patients with AIDS-related neoplasms, but their use is limited by cardiotoxicity. A variety of cardiac effects have been described, ranging from benign and reversible arrhythmias to progressive severe cardiomyopathy. The most common cardiac toxicity is a cardiomyopathy that can lead to congestive heart failure. Endomyocardial biopsy is the most sensitive and specific test for the diagnosis of cardiomyopathy, but its routine use is limited by its invasiveness. Serial echocardiographic evaluation of left ventricular ejection fraction has also proved to be a valuable tool to guide therapy and promptly identify a cardiomyopathy. A 10% reduction of the ejection fraction from baseline or a value below 50% is an indication to discontinue therapy. A baseline ejection fraction less than 30% is generally considered a contraindication to starting a treatment with anthracyclines. A relevant issue is the progression of anthracycline-induced cardiomyopathy to chronic heart failure, after the cure of the tumor. A significant proportion (23–38%) of patients successfully treated with antracyclines have a persistent decrease of the ejection fraction. Of these, approximately 5% will eventually develop chronic heart failure. The overall increased survival of HIV^+ persons, including those with HIV-related malignancies will perhaps cause increased concern over this issue. Anthracycline toxicity is believed to be related to the generation of highly reactive oxygen species which cause direct damage to cardiac myocyte membranes.[114] The heart tissue is able to generate free radicals from anthracyclines at multiple cellular sites, including mitochondria, cytosol and sarcoplasmic reticulum.[115] Doxorubicin impairs glutathione peroxidase activity, a key mechanism of peroxidase removal, and cardiac tissue has low levels of catalase, the principal enzyme for the removal of hydrogen peroxide. In spite of this mechanism, free radical scavenger drugs have not proved effective in the prevention of anthracycline-related toxicity, suggesting an alternative mechanism. In fact, it was demonstrated that doxorubicin has a high binding activity to iron and that an iron-doxorubicin complex was the potent catalyzer of many free oxygen species. Consistent with these findings, iron chelators have proven effective in the prevention of anthracycline cardiac toxicity.[116] The myocardial degenerative process is dose-dependent and related to the high peak plasma level reached after the bolus dose of the drug and by the cumulative dose, with a significant increase of risk above the dose of 550 mg/m^2. However, there is significant individual variability in this dose-dependent toxic effect. Risk factors for increased toxicity include prior chest radiation, age over 70, pre-existing heart disease, and female gender. A less common cardiac effect of anthracyclines is an acute toxicity that is unrelated to cumulative dose and that can be observed hours or days after the administration of the drugs. This acute syndrome presents as supraventricular or ventricular arrhythmias, heart block, and acute congestive heart failure. Asymptomatic electro-cardiographic abnormalities including ST-T changes, decreased QRS voltage, pro-longation of QT-interval occur in up to 30% of cases. These changes usually regress within weeks and do not prompt the discontinuation of treatment. Patients that develop an early cardiotoxicity after anthracycline therapy are more likely to progress towards late congestive heart failure.[113] In recent years there have been efforts to prevent the cardiotoxicity of anthracyclines while preserving their anticancer effects by the administration of continuous infusions, lower doses at more frequent intervals,[117] the use of agents that selectively block the cardiotoxicity,[118] and the use of liposomial formulations.[119,120]

Anthracyclines are used for the treatment of a wide range of hematological and solid malignancies. In AIDS patients the risk of Kaposi's sarcoma (KS) and B-cell non-Hodgkin's lymphoma is greatly increased.[121] The clinical presentation of KS is highly variable, ranging from slow-growing and isolated cutaneous lesions to disseminated muco-cutaneous and visceral involvement. For less aggressive or localized KS, treatment options can be intralesional chemotherapy, radiation or systemic interferon. Many patients with immune reconstitution consequent to successful anti-retroviral therapy have experienced remission of KS lesions.[122] For disseminated or rapidly progressing KS, systemic chemotherapy is indicated and can be life-saving. At present two liposomal-formulated anthracyclines, liposomal daunorubicin and liposomal doxorubicin, have largely replaced the formerly used combination regimen ABV (i.e. adriamycin-bleomycin-vincristine) for the treatment of disseminated KS.[123] Liposomal anthracyclines appear to have an efficacy comparable to ABV, while being better tolerated.[124] In AIDS patients treated with pegylated liposomal doxorubicin compared with historical controls, a reduced cardiotoxicity was demonstrated by cardiac biopsy.[125]

In approximately 3% of AIDS patients a non-Hodgkin's lymphoma occurs. The treatment of AIDS-related lymphomas is generally based on cycles of combined chemotherapeutic agents. Among others, m-BACOD, CHOP, CDE, ACVB have been proposed, all containing anthracyclines. Mitoxantrone is a completely synthetic analog of the anthracyclines that has been proposed in combination regimens for the first-line or second-line treatment of AIDS-related lymphomas.[126,127] Mitoxantrone does cause cardiotoxicity, but less than the anthracyclines.[128] When treating AIDS patients with lymphoma, clinicians must be aware of the risk of cardiotoxicity related to anthracyclines, especially if the patients are receiving other cardiotoxic drugs or have underlying conditions that cause myocardial dysfunction.

Immunomodulators

Interferon

Interferons (IFNs) are human cytokines that have been used in therapy since the late 1950s. In the early years of the HIV epidemic treatment with α- and β-interferon was proposed for its antiviral effect. After disappointing results, this approach was abandoned. At present, recombinant human α-interferon is approved for the treatment of early stage Kaposi's sarcoma (KS) in patients with CD4 cell counts more than 200/mm³. In the HAART era KS still remains the most commonly diagnosed malignancy in HIV⁺ persons. α-Interferon is also approved for the treatment of chronic hepatitis C in HIV⁻ as well as in HIV⁺ patients. Common side effects of interferon include an early flu-like syndrome, fatigue, behavioral changes, autoimmune disorders, neutropenia.[129] While tachycardia and hypo- or hypertension have frequently been reported, there have also been occasional reports of other interferon-induced cardiovascular manifestations. Supraventricular arrhythmias are frequently reported after the first dose of IFN and may be related to the flu-like reaction. In a review of 44 cases of cancer patients from 15 reports in the literature the most common cardiac adverse events were arrhythmia, ischemic heart disease, and dilated cardiomyopathy.[130] In many of these patients there were underlying cardiovascular risks, including the use of anticancer drugs known to be cardiotoxic. The various manifestations of IFN cardiac toxicity suggest different mechanisms. The pathogenesis of interferon-related cardiomyopathy is not clear. In the 3 HIV⁺ patients of the review it was suggested that cardiomyopathy resulted from a combined effect of interferon and HIV.[131] The common flu-like syndrome itself, with fever, chills and increased oxygen consumption may precipitate acute cardiovascular events, including arrhythmias and acute coronary events. No relationship has been demonstrated between IFN toxicity and dose or duration of treatment. Taken together, the data on IFN cardiotoxicity seem to indicate that many cases of arrhythmia and coronary artery disease are related to drug-induced peripheral vasodilation and increased cardiac work load. Accordingly, IFN should not be administered in patients with unstable ischemic disorders.

Interleukin-2

Interleukin-2 (IL-2) is an immunoregulatory cytokine that induces production of other lymphokines, including interleukin-6 and γ-interferon. Moreover, IL-2 enhances the cytolitic activity of NK cells and induces the differentiation of T-cell precursors transforming them into LAK cells, which have an anti-neoplastic activity. One of the first immunologic defects described in HIV⁺ patients was impaired IL-2 production, with consequently reduced NK activity. Recombinant IL-2 has been used for the treatment of HIV⁺ patients in all stages of disease, with or without malignancies, although its widespread use has been limited by significant side-effects and high cost. Recently, a pooled analysis of controlled trials of IL-2 therapy in HIV disease showed significant immunological and virological benefits in treated patients.[132] Phase II/III trials are ongoing to evaluate the effects of combination treatment with IL-2 and HAART. IL-2 has a potential cardiotoxicity, that is believed to be dose dependent.[133] In 199 consecutive patients with metastatic melanoma or renal cell carcinoma, arrhythmias occurred in 6% of the courses, hypotension in 53%, and elevated creatine kinase levels with elevated MB isoenzymes in 2.5%.[134] Acute myocardial infarction, cardiomyopathy, and asymptomatic electrocardiographic changes were also reported.[133] The possible pathogenetic mechanism could be the production of secondary-message molecules such as nitric oxide and myocardial stunning.[135] Owing to the potential benefit of combination treatment with IL-2 and HAART, a variety of treatment schedules are being evaluated in HIV$^+$ patients to minimize IL-2 toxicity.[136]

ANTIRETROVIRAL THERAPY AND DRUG INTERACTIONS

Many antiretroviral agents share metabolic pathways with a great number of drugs commonly prescribed for HIV$^+$ persons. Some of the consequent drug interactions are clinically relevant and suggest the need for a close monitoring of potential side-effects. The most important drug interactions are between PIs and drugs that are substrates for the cytochrome P450 3A (CYP3A). The cytochrome P450 mixed function oxidases are a family of enzymes that account for most oxidative transformations of exogenous and endogenous biological compounds.[137] The isoforms of human CYP3A include 3A3, 3A4, 3A5, and 3A7. CYP3A4 is the predominant form of CYP3A in adult humans and it is one of the most important enzymes, since it biotransforms approximately 60% of oxidized drugs.[138] Cytochrome P450 activity is conditioned by age,[139] sex,[140] and liver disease.[141] In HIV$^+$ individuals, the variability in activity of CYP3A4 may be even greater than in uninfected persons.[142] The effect of these variables must be taken into account when prescribing drugs and combinations of drugs that are metabolized by the CYP3A4. Many drugs from a wide range of therapeutic groups are substrates for CYP3A4. A significant rise in plasma levels of various drugs, with consequent increase of dose-related toxicity, has been observed when they were co-administered with PIs, especially with ritonavir, the most potent CYP3A inhibitor of the class. Relevant interactions have been described between PIs and antimycobacterials, antifungals, macrolide and quinolone antibacterials, antihistamines, psychotropic drugs, anti-arrhythmics, cisapride (a gastrointestinal prokinetic), statins, anti-epileptics, and anti-neoplastic alkaloids. Some of these interactions can yield potentially cardiotoxic effects. As was previously noted, many medications that are CYP3A4 substrates may produce an electrocardiographic QT prolongation and torsades de pointe. An increased risk of arrythmias is present when all PIs are co-administered with bepridil, and this combination must be avoided. Potentially dangerous interactions that require close monitoring or dose adjustment can occur between PIs and amiodarone, disopyramide, flecainide, lignocaine, mexiletine, propafenone, and quinidine. Co-administration of PIs with astemizole, terfenadine or cisapride is contraindicated, owing to the risk of life-threatening arrhythmias. Many antipsychotic, antidepressant and anticonvulsant drugs interact with PIs. Some of these interactions are clinically relevant and contraindicate concomitant use or require dose adjustment. In everyday practice, clinicians should be aware of the potential severity of the cardiac side-effects caused by drug interactions between PIs and CYP3A substrates.

CONCLUSIONS

Drug-induced cardiotoxicity has been described in HIV$^+$ patients in the early years of the epidemic. Initially, however, this issue did not raise widespread concern, because the progression of HIV infection was much faster than drug-induced heart diseases. In addition, acute cardiotoxicity was relatively infrequent, when compared to other major drug toxicities. A new scenario was created by the advent of potent anti-retroviral therapies, with significant immune reconstitution, dramatically increased survival of patients, and the recognition of new adverse effects of HAART. In this new situation it is likely that an increase of drug-related cardiac adverse effects will be observed. Probably the major issue is the possibility of HAART-induced accelerated atherosclerosis with increased risk of coronary events. Dyslipidemia and insulin resistance caused by PIs is well established and large epidemiological studies are ongoing to quantify cardiovascular risk of patients treated with HAART. Other important information will derive from studies addressing the issues of abnormalities of endothelium and coagulation in HIV+ patients. It will be also necessary to understand if in HAART-treated patients there are additional co-factors, other than the traditional ones, that influence lipid and glucose metabolism. It is likely that all these data will have an impact on the development of future guidelines for the treatment of HIV+ persons, especially on the timing of treatment initiation. Until definitive data are available, it is reasonable to evaluate all HIV+ patients also for traditional coronary disease risk factors, including lipid metabolism. First line treatment of dyslipidemia should include dietary interventions and reduction or abolishment of correctable risk factors for coronary disease. Pharmacological treatment of dyslipidemia should be proposed only if significant drug interactions between lipid-lowering agents and antiretroviral drugs can be excluded.

Many drugs used in HIV disease have a QT interval prolonging potential. The identification and widespread knowledge of risk factors that may precipitate this asymptomatic electrocardiographic abnormality into a life-threatening arrhythmia is an important issue. Among these factors is the concomitant use of drugs that share the CYP3A metabolic pathway. Since most PIs are potent inhibitors of CYP3A, clinicians involved in the treatment of HIV patients should be particularly aware of these potentially dangerous effects of HAART.

The increased survival and quality of life of HIV patients emphasizes the importance of a high awareness of drug-related cardiac adverse effects, since the success of HAART may be frustrated by the risks related to unrecognized toxicity.

REFERENCES

1. YUNIS, N.A. & V.E. STONE. 1998. Cardiac manifestations of HIV/AIDS: a review of disease spectrum and clinical management. J. Acquir. Immune Defic. Syndr. Hum. Retrovirol. **18:** 145–154.
2. PALELLA, F.J. JR., K.M. DELANEY, A.C. MOORMAN, et al. 1998. Declining morbidity and mortality among patients with advanced human immunodeficiency virus infection. HIV Outpatient Study Investigators. N. Engl. J. Med. **338:** 853–860.
3. KAPLAN, J.E., D. HANSON, M.S. DWORKIN, et al. 2000. Epidemiology of human immunodeficiency virus-associated opportunistic infections in the United States in the era of highly active antiretroviral therapy. Clin. Infect. Dis. **30:** S5–S14.
4. WU, A.W. 2000. Quality of life assessment comes of age in the era of highly active antiretroviral therapy. AIDS **14:** 1449–1451.
5. GRENIER, M.A. & S.E. LIPSHULTZ. 1998. Epidemiology of anthracycline cardiotoxicity in children and adults. Semin. Oncol. **25:** 72–85.
6. ARSURA, E.L., Y. ISMAIL, S. FREEDMAN, et al. 1994. Amphotericin B-induced dilated cardiomyopathy. Am. J. Med. **97:** 560–562.

7. HERSKOWITZ, A., S.B. WILLOUGHBY, K.L. BAUGHMAN, *et al.* 1992. Cardiomyopathy associated with antiretroviral therapy in patients with HIV infection: a report of six cases. Ann. Intern. Med. **116:** 311–313.
8. MCCOMB, J.M., N.P. CAMPBELL, J. CLELAND, *et al.* 1984. Recurrent ventricular tachycardia associated with QT prolongation after mitral valve replacement and its association with intravenous administration of erythromycin. Am. J. Cardiol. **54:** 922–923.
9. SONNENBLICK, M. & A. ROSIN. 1991. Cardiotoxicity of interferon. A review of 44 cases. Chest **99:** 557–561.
10. CARPENTER, C.C., D.A. COOPER, M.A. FISCHL, *et al.* 2000. Antiretroviral therapy in adults: updated recommendations of the International AIDS Society-USA. JAMA **283:** 381–390.
11. MURRI, R., A. AMMASSARI, K. GALLICANO, *et al.* 2000. Patient-reported non-adherence to HAART is related to protease inhibitor levels. J. Acquir. Immune Defic. Syndr. **24:** 123–128.
12. VOLBERDING, P.A., S.W. LAGAKOS, M.A. KOCH, *et al.* 1990. Zidovudine in asymptomatic human immunodeficiency virus infection. A controlled trial in persons with fewer than 500 CD4-positive cells per cubic millimeter. The AIDS Clinical Trials Group of the National Institute of Allergy and Infectious Diseases. N. Engl. J. Med. **322:** 941–949.
13. CONNOR, E.M., R.S. SPERLING, R. GELBER, *et al.* 1994. Reduction of maternal-infant transmission of human immunodeficiency virus type 1 with zidovudine treatment. Pediatric AIDS Clinical Trials Group Protocol 076 Study Group. N. Engl. J. Med. **331:** 1173–1180.
14. BARBARO, G., G. DI LORENZO & B. GRISORIO. 1998. Incidence of dilated cardiomyopathy and detection of HIV in myocardial cells of HIV-positive patients. Gruppo Italiano per lo Studio Cardiologico dei Pazienti Affetti da AIDS. N. Engl. J. Med. **339:** 1093–1099.
15. BARBARO, G. 1999. Dilated cardiomyopathy in the acquired immunodeficiency syndrome. Eur. Heart J. **20:** 629–630
16. DOMANSKI, M.J., M.M. SLOAS, D.A. FOLLMANN, *et al.* 1995. Effect of zidovudine and didanosine treatment on heart function in children infected with human immunodeficiency virus. J. Pediatr. **127:** 137–146.
17. CULNANE, M., M. FOWLER, S.S. LEE, *et al.* 1999. Lack of long-term effects of in utero exposure to zidovudine among uninfected children born to HIV-infected women. Pediatric AIDS Clinical Trials Group Protocol 219/076 Teams. JAMA **281:** 151–157.
18. LIPSHULTZ, S.E., K.A. EASLEY, E.J. ORAV, *et al.* 2000. Absence of cardiac toxicity of zidovudine in infants. Pediatric Pulmonary and Cardiac Complications of Vertically Transmitted HIV Infection Study Group. N. Engl. J. Med. **343:** 759–766.
19. LEWIS, W., SIMPSON J.F., R.R. MEYER, *et al.* 1994. Cardiac mitochondrial DNA polymerase-gamma is inhibited competitively and noncompetitively by phosphorylated zidovudine. Circ. Res. **74:** 344–348.
20. LEWIS, W. 2000. Mitochondrial toxicity: potential mechanism and experimental evidence. Collected abstracts of the 40th Interscience Conference on Antimicrobial Agents and Chemotherapy, Toronto, Ontario, Canada, no. 1372.
21. BRINKMAN, K., H.J. TER HOFSTEDE, D.M. BURGER, *et al.* 1998. Adverse effects of reverse transcriptase inhibitors: mitochondrial toxicity as common pathway. AIDS **12:** 1735–1744.
22. SKUTA, G., G.M. FISCHER, T. JANAKY, *et al.* 1999. Molecular mechanism of the short-term cardiotoxicity caused by 2',3'-dideoxycytidine (ddC): modulation of reactive oxygen species levels and ADP-ribosylation reactions. Biochem. Pharmacol. **58:** 1915–1925.
23. CARR, A., K. SAMARAS, S. BURTON, *et al.* 1998. A syndrome of peripheral lipodystrophy, hyperlipidaemia and insulin resistance in patients receiving HIV protease inhibitors. AIDS **12:** F51–F58.
24. CARR, A., K. SAMARAS, D.J. CHISHOLM, *et al.* 1998. Pathogenesis of HIV-1-protease inhibitor-associated peripheral lipodystrophy, hyperlipidaemia, and insulin resistance. Lancet **351:** 1881–1883.

25. BRINKMAN, K., J.A. SMEITINK, J.A. ROMIJN, *et al.* 1999. Mitochondrial toxicity induced by nucleoside-analogue reverse-transcriptase inhibitors is a key factor in the pathogenesis of antiretroviral-therapy-related lipodystrophy. Lancet **354:** 1112–1115.
26. MOYLE, G. & C. BALDWIN. 2000. Switching from a PI-based to a PI-sparing regimen for management of metabolic or clinical fat redistribution. AIDS Read. **10:** 479–485.
27. HENRY, K., H. MELROE, J. HUEBSCH, *et al.* 1998. Severe premature coronary artery disease with protease inhibitors. Lancet **351:** 1328.
28. CARR, A., K. SAMARAS, A. THORISDOTTIR, *et al.* 1999. Diagnosis, prediction, and natural course of HIV-1 protease-inhibitor-associated lipodystrophy, hyperlipidaemia, and diabetes mellitus: a cohort study. Lancet **353:** 2093–2099.
29. BEHRENS, G., A. DEJAM, H. SCHMIDT, *et al.* 1999. Impaired glucose tolerance, beta cell function and lipid metabolism in HIV patients under treatment with protease inhibitors. AIDS **13:** F63–F70.
30. WALLI, R., O. HERFORT, G.M. MICHL, *et al.* 1998. Treatment with protease inhibitors associated with peripheral insulin resistance and impaired oral glucose tolerance in HIV-1-infected patients. AIDS **12:** F167–F173.
31. PERIARD, D., A. TELENTI, P. SUDRE, *et al.* 1999. Atherogenic dyslipidemia in HIV-infected individuals treated with protease inhibitors. The Swiss HIV Cohort Study. Circulation **100:** 700–705.
32. GALLI, M., F. VEGLIA, G. ANGARANO, *et al.* 2000. Risk of developing metabolic and morphological alterations under antiretroviral therapy according to the drug combinations. Antiviral Ther. **5**(Suppl. 5): 58.
33. KOPPEL, K., G. BRATT, B. LUND, *et al.* 2000. Is hyperlipidemia the only cardiovascular risk factor that normalises when discontinuing protease inhibitors? AIDS **14**(Suppl. 4): S62.
34. BEHRENS, G., H. SCHMIDT, D. MEYER, *et al.* 1998. Vascular complications associated with use of HIV protease inhibitors. Lancet **351:** 1958.
35. GALLET, B., M. PULIK, P. GENET, *et al.* 1998. Vascular complications associated with use of HIV protease inhibitors. Lancet **351:** 1958–1959.
36. VITTECOQ, D., L. ESCAUT, J.J. MONSUEZ, *et al.* 1998. Vascular complications associated with use of HIV protease inhibitors. Lancet **351:** 1959.
37. CURRAN, S., S. CLARKE, C. FORKIN, *et al.* 2000. Myocardial infarction and protease inhibitors therapy: two case reports. AIDS **14**(Suppl. 4): S62.
38. MARY-CRAUSE, M., L. COTTE, A. SIMON-COUTELLIER, *et al.* 2000. Myocardial infarction (MI) in HIV seropositive men in the era of HAART treatments in France. Collected abstracts of the XIII International AIDS Conference, Durban, South Africa, WePe B4231 vol.2, p. 86.
39. DAVID, M.H. & C.J. FICHTENBAUM. 2000. A case-control study of cardiovascular risk in persons with HIV-infection. Collected abstracts of the 38th Annual IDSA Meeting, no. 355, p. 274.
40. MERCIE, P., R. THIÉBAUT, V. LAVIGNOLLE, *et al.* 2000. Intima-media thickness measures in HIV-1 infected patients with HAART lipodystrophy and metabolic disorders: The SUPRA study. AIDS **14** (Suppl. 4): S61.
41. MAGGI, P., G. SERIO, G. EPIFANI, *et al.* 2000. Premature lesions of the carotid vessels in HIV-1-infected patients treated with protease inhibitors. AIDS **14:** F123–F128.
42. WOLFE, F., D.M. MITCHELL, J.T. SIBLEY, *et al.* 1994. The mortality of rheumatoid arthritis. Arthritis Rheum. **37:** 481–494.
43. JONSONN, H., O. NIVED, G. STURFELT, *et al.* 1989. Outcome in systemic lupus erythematosus: a prospective study of patients from a defined population. Medicine **68:** 141–150.
44. BALLANTYNE, C.M., E.J. PODET, W.P. PATSCH, *et al.* 1989. Effects of cyclosporine therapy on plasma lipoprotein levels. JAMA **262:** 53–56.
45. DUBÉ, M.P., D. SPRECHER, W.K. HENRY, *et al.* 2000. Preliminary guidelines for the evaluation and management of dyslipidemia in adults infected with human immunodeficiency virus and receiving antiretroviral therapy: recommendations of the adult AIDS clinical trial group cardiovascular disease focus group. Clin Infect Dis. **31:** 1216–1224.

46. BALDINI, F., S. DI GIAMBENEDETTO, A. CINGOLANI, *et al.* 2000. Efficacy and tolerability of pravastatin for the treatment of HIV-1 protease inhibitor-associated hyperlipidaemia: a pilot study. AIDS **14:** 1660–1662.
47. DESPRES, J.P., B. LAMARCHE, P. MAURIEGE, *et al.* 1996. Hyperinsulinemia as an independent risk factor for ischemic heart disease. N. Engl. J. Med. **334:** 952–957.
48. EGGER, M. 2000. Cardiovascular complications of HAART: need for perspective. Collected abstracts of the 40th Interscience Conference on Antimicrobial Agents and Chemotherapy, Toronto, Ontario, Canada, no. 1374.
49. TASK FORCE ON THE DEFINITION AND CLASSIFICATION OF CARDIOMYOPATHIES. 1996. Report of the 1995 WHO/ISFC Circulation **93:** 841–842.
50. TAMARGO, J. 2000. Drug-induced torsade de pointes: from molecular biology to bedside. Jpn. J. Pharmacol. **83:** 1–19.
51. DE PONTI, F., E. POLUZZI & N. MONTANARO. 2000. QT-interval prolongation by noncardiac drugs: lessons to be learned from recent experience. Eur. J. Clin. Pharmacol. **56:** 1–18.
52. MOSS, A.J. 1999. The QT interval and torsade de pointes. Drug Saf. **21:** 5–10.
53. DRICI, M.D., B.C. KNOLLMANN, W.X. WANG, *et al.* 1998. Cardiac actions of erythromycin: influence of female sex. JAMA **280:** 1774–1776.
54. LEE, K.L., M.H. JIM, S.C. TANG, *et al.* 1998. QT prolongation and torsades de pointes associated with clarithromycin. Am. J. Med. **104:** 395–396.
55. KAMOCHI, H., T. NII, K. EGUCHI, *et al.* 1999. Clarithromycin associated with torsades de pointes. Jpn. Circ. J. **63:** 421–422.
56. GUELON, D., B. BEDOCK, C. CHARTIER & R.F. RITZ. 1986. QT prolongation and recurrent "torsades de pointes" during erythromycin lactobionate infusion. Am. J. Cardiol. **58:** 666.
57. SCHOENENBERGER, R.A., W.E. HAEFELI, P. WEISS, *et al.* 1990. Association of intravenous erythromycin and potentially fatal ventricular tachycardia with Q-T prolongation (torsades de pointes). BMJ **300:** 1375–1376.
58. WIENER, I., D.A. RUBIN, E. MARTINEZ, *et al.* 1981. QT prolongation and paroxysmal ventricular tachycardia occurring during fever following trimethoprim-sulfamethoxazole administration. Mt. Sinai J. Med. **48:** 53–55.
59. LOPEZ, J.A., J.G. HAROLD, M.C. ROSENTHAL, *et al.* 1987. QT prolongation and torsades de pointes after administration of trimethoprim-sulfamethoxazole. Am. J. Cardiol. **59:** 376–377.
60. SAMAHA, F.F. 1999. QTC interval prolongation and polymorphic ventricular tachycardia in association with levofloxacin. Am. J. Med. **107:** 528–529.
61. DEMOLIS, J.L., A. CHARRANSOL, C. FUNCK-BRENTANO, *et al.* 1996. Effects of a single oral dose of sparfloxacin on ventricular repolarization in healthy volunteers. Br. J. Clin. Pharmacol. **41:** 499–503.
62. LIPSKY, B.A., M.B. DORR, D.J. MAGNER, *et al.* 1999. Safety profile of sparfloxacin, a new fluoroquinolone antibiotic. Clin. Ther. **21:** 148–159.
63. MORGANROTH, J., T. HUNT, M.B. DORR, *et al.* 1999. The cardiac pharmacodynamics of therapeutic doses of sparfloxacin. Clin. Ther. **21:** 1171–1181.
64. BULL, P., L. MANDELL, Y. NIKI, *et al.* 1999. Comparative tolerability of the newer fluoroquinolone antibacterials. Drug Saf. **21:** 407–421.
65. STAHLMANN, R. & H. LODE. 1999. Toxicity of quinolones. Drugs **58:** 37–42.
66. MOREAU, A. & M.J. POSTAL. 1987. Episodes of torsade de pointe during infusion of amphotericin B in a malnourished patient. Presse Med. **16:** 1976.
67. ZIMMERMANN, M., H. DURUZ, O. GUINAND, *et al.* 1992 Torsades de pointes after treatment with terfenadine and ketoconazole. Eur. Heart J. **13:** 1002–1003.
68. HONIG, P.K., D.C. WORTHAM & R. HULL. 1993. Itraconazole affects single-dose terfenadine pharmacokinetics and cardiac repolarization pharmacodynamics. J. Clin. Pharmacol. **33:** 1201–1206.
69. POHJOLA-SINTONEN, S., M. VIITASALO & L. TOIVONEN. 1993. Itraconazole prevents terfenadine metabolism and increases risk of torsades de pointes ventricular tachycardia. Eur. J. Clin. Pharmacol. **45:** 191–193.
70. ALBENNGRES, E., H. LE LOUET & J.P.TILLEMENT. 1998. Systemic antifungal agents. Drug interactions of clinical significance. Drug Saf. **18:** 83–97.

71. SOLER, J.A., L. IBANEZ, J. ZUAZU, et al. 1993. Bradycardia after rapid intravenous infusin of amphotericin B. Lancet **341:** 372–373.
72. RINGDEN, O., V. JONSSON, M. HANSEN, et al. 1998. Severe and common side-effects of amphotericin B lipid complex. Bone Marrow Transplant. **22:** 733–734.
73. AGUADO, J.M., M. HIDALGO, J.M. MOYA, et al. 1993. Ventricular arrhythmias with conventional and liposomal amphotericin. Lancet **342:** 1239.
74. DORSEY, S.T. & L.A. BIBLO. 2000. Prolonged QT interval and torsades de pointes caused by the combination of fluconazole and amitriptyline. Am. J. Emerg. Med. **18:** 227–229.
75. POHJOLA-SINTONEN, S., M. VIITASALO, L. TOIVONEN, et al. 1993. Torsades de pointes after terfenadine-itraconazole interaction. BMJ **306:** 186.
76. ROMKES, J.H., C.L. FROGER & E.F. WEVER. 1997. Syncopes during simultaneous use of terfenadine and itraconazole. Ned. Tijdschr. Geneeskd. **141:** 950–953.
77. HOOVER, C.A., J.K. CARMICHAEL, P.E. NOLAN, et al. 1996. Cardiac arrest associated with combination cisapride and itraconazole therapy. J. Cardiovasc. Pharmacol. Ther. **1:** 255–258.
78. WASSMANN, S., G. NICKENIG & M. BOHM. 1999. Long QT syndrome and torsade de pointes in a patient receiving fluconazole. Ann. Intern. Med. **131:** 797.
79. PUJOL, M., J. CARRATALA, J. MAURI, et al. 1988. Ventricular tachycardia due to penta-midine isethionate. Am. J. Med. **84:** 980.
80. BIBLER, M.R., T.C. CHOU, R.J. TOLTZIS, et al. 1988. Recurrent ventricular tachycardia due to pentamidine-induced cardiotoxicity. Chest **94:** 1303–1306.
81. STEIN, K.M., H. HARONIAN, G.A. MENSAH, et al. 1990. Ventricular tachycardia and torsades de pointes complicating pentamidine therapy of *Pneumocystis carinii* pneu-monia in the acquired immunodeficiency syndrome. Am. J. Cardiol. **66:** 888–889.
82. EISENHAUER, M.D., A.H. ELIASSON & A.J. TAYLOR. 1994. Incidence of cardiac arrhyth-mias during intravenous pentamidine therapy in HIV-infected patients. Chest **105:** 389–95.
83. GIRGIS, I., J. GUALBERTI, L. LANGAN, et al. 1997. A prospective study of the effect of I.V. pentamidine therapy on ventricular arrhythmias and QTc prolongation in HIV-infected patients. Chest **112:** 646–653.
84. WHARTON, J.M., P.A. DEMOPULOS & N. GOLDSCHLAGER. 1987. Torsade de pointes dur-ing administration of pentamidine isethionate. Am. J. Med. **83:** 571–576.
85. MITCHELL, P., P. DODEK, L. LAWSON, et al. 1989. Torsades de pointes during intrave-nous pentamidine isethionate therapy. CMAJ **140:** 173–174.
86. DONNELLY, H., E.M. BERNARD, H. ROTHKOTTER, et al. Distribution of pentamidine in patients with AIDS. J. Infect. Dis. **157:** 985–989.
87. COHEN, A.J., B. WEISER, Q. AFZAL, et al. 1990. Ventricular tachycardia in two patients with AIDS receiving ganciclovir (DHPG). AIDS **4:** 807–809.
88. BROWN, D.L., S. SATHER & M.D.CHEITLIN. 1993. Reversible cardiac dysfunction asso-ciated with foscarnet therapy for cytomegalovirus esophagitis in an AIDS patient. Am. Heart J. **125:** 1439–1441.
89. COOPMAN, S.A., R.A. JOHNSON, R. PLATT, et al. 1993. Cutaneous disease and drug reactions in HIV infection. N. Engl. J. Med. **328:** 1670–1674.
90. SIMONS, F.E., W.T. WATSON & K.J. SIMONS. 1988. Lack of subsensitivity to terfena-dine during long-term terfenadine treatment. J. Allergy Clin. Immunol. **82:** 1068–1075.
91. WOOSLEY, R.L., Y. CHEN, J.P. FREIMAN, et al. 1993. Mechanism of the cardiotoxic actions of terfenadine. JAMA **269:** 1532–1536.
92. LINDQUIST, M. & I.R. EDWARDS. 1997. Risks of non-sedating antihistamines. 1997. Lancet **349:** 1322.
93. YAP, Y.G. & J. CAMM. 2000. Risk of torsades de pointes with non-cardiac drugs. Doc-tors need to be aware that many drugs can cause qt prolongation. BMJ **320:** 1158–1159.
94. YAP, Y.G. & A.J. CAMM. 1999. The current cardiac safety situation with antihista-mines. Clin. Exp. Allergy **29:** 15–24.

95. BAKER, B., P. DORIAN & P. SANDOR. 1997. Electrocardiographic effects of fluoxetine and doxepin in patients with major depressive disorder. J. Clin. Psychopharmacol. **17:** 15–21.
96. SWANSON, J.R., G.R. JONES, W. KRASSELT, *et al.* 1997. Death of two subjects due to imipramine and desipramine metabolite accumulation during chronic therapy: a review of the literature and possible mechanisms. J. Forensic Sci. **42:** 335–339.
97. WELCH, R. & P. CHUE. 2000. Antipsychotic agents and QT changes. J. Psychiatry Neurosci. **25:** 154–160.
98. BUCKLEY, N.A., I.M. WHYTE & A.H. DAWSON. 1995. Cardiotoxicity more common in thioradizine overdose than with other neuroleptics. J. Toxicol. Clin. Toxicol. **33:** 199–204.
99. JACKSON, T., L. DITMANNSONN & B. PHIBBS. 1997. Torsades de pointes and low-dose oral haloperidol. Arch. Intern. Med. **157:** 2013–2015.
100. KRIWISKY, M., G. Y. PERRY, D. TARCHITSKY, *et al.* 1998. Haloperidol-induced torsades de pointes. Chest **98:** 482–484.
101. LAWRENCE, K.R. & S.A. NASRAWAY. 1997. Conduction disturbances associated with administration of butyrophenone antipsychotics in the critically ill: a review of the literature. Pharmacotherapy **17:** 531–537.
102. DESTA, Z., T. KERBUSCH, D.A. FLOCKHART, *et al.* 1999. Effect of clarithromycin on the pharmacokinetics and pharmacodynamics of pimozide in healthy poor and extensive metabolizers of cytochrome. Clin. Pharmacol. **65:** 10–20.
103. VAN KAMMEN, D.P., J.P. MCEVOY, S.D. TARGUM, *et al.* 1996. A randomized, controlled, dose-ranging trial of sertindole in patients with schizophrenia. Psychopharmacology **124:** 168–175.
104. BROWN, G.R., J.R. RUNDELL, S.E. MCMANIS, *et al.* 1992. Prevalence of psychiatric disorders in early stages of HIV infection. Psychosom. Med. **54:** 588–601.
105. KHOUZAM, H.R., N.J. DONNELLY, N.F. IBRAHIM, *et al.* 1998. Psychiatric morbidity in HIV patients. Can. J. Psychiatry **43:** 51–56.
106. PERRETTA, P., H.S. AKISKAL, C. NISITA, *et al.* 1998. The high prevalence of bipolar II and associated cyclothymic and hyperthymic temperaments in HIV-patients. J. Affect. Disord. **50:** 215–224.
107. JOHNSON, J.G., J.G. RABKIN, J.D. LIPSITZ, *et al.* Recurrent major depressive disorder among human immunodeficiency virus (HIV)-positive and HIV-negative intravenous drug users: findings of a 3-year longitudinal study. Compr. Psychiatry **40:** 31–34.
108. GOULET, J.L., S. MOLDE, J. COSTANTINO, *et al.* 2000. Psychiatric comorbidity and the long-term care of people with AIDS. J. Urban Health **77:** 213–221.
109. MC DANIEL, J.S., E. FOWLIE, M.B. SUMMERVILLE, *et al.* 1995. An assessment of rates of psychiatric morbidity and functioning in HIV disease. Gen. Hosp. Psychiatry **17:** 346–352.
110. LEFRAK, E.A., J. PITHA, S. ROSENHEIM, *et al.* 1973. A clinicopathologic analysis of adriamicin cardiotoxicity. Cancer **32:** 302–314.
111. BUJA, L.M., V.J. FERRANS & R.J. MAYER. 1973. Cardiac ultrastructural changes induced by daunorubicin therapy. Cancer **32:** 771–778.
112. BRISTOW, M.R., J.W. MASON & M.E. BILLINGHAM. 1978. Doxorubicin cardiomyopathy: evaluation by phonocardiography, endomyocardial biopsy, and cardiac catheterization. Ann. Intern. Med. **88:** 168–175.
113. GRENIER, M.A. & S.E. LIPSHULTZ. 1998. Epidemiology of anthracycline cardiotoxicity in children and adults. Semin. Oncol. **25:** 72–85.
114. HORENSTEIN, M.S., R.S. VANDER HEIDE & T.J. L'ECUYER. 2000. Molecular basis of anthracycline-induced cardiotoxicity and its prevention. Mol. Genet. Metab. **71:** 436–444.
115. HACKER, M.P., J.S. LAZO & T.R. TRITTON. 1988. Organ directed toxicities of anticancer drugs. Martinus NiJhoff.The Hague.
116. SPEYER, J.L., M.D.GREEN, E. KRAMER, *et al.* 1988. Protective effect of the bispiperazinedione ICRF-187 against doxorubicin-induced cardiac toxicity in women with advanced breast cancer. N. Engl. J. Med. **319:** 745–752.

117. PAI, V.B. & M.C. NAHATA. Cardiotoxicity of chemotherapeutic agents: incidence, treatment and prevention. 2000. Drug Saf. **22:** 263–302.
118. SWAIN, S.M., F.S. WHALEY, M.C. GERBER, et al. 1997. Cardioprotection with dexrazoxane for doxorubicin-containing therapy in advanced breast cancer. J. Clin. Oncol. **15:** 1318–1332.
119. MARTIN, F. 1997. Pegylated liposomial doxorubicin: scientific rationale and preclinical pharmacology. Oncology **11:** 33–37.
120. NORTHFELT, D. 1997. Liposomial anthracycline chemotherapy in the treatment of AIDS-related Kaposi's sarcoma. Oncology **11:** 21–32
121. GOEDERT, J.J. 2000. The epidemiology of acquired immunodeficiency syndrome malignancies. Semin. Oncol. **27:** 390–401.
122. DUPONT, C., E. VASSEUR, A. BEAUCHET, et al. 2000. Long-term efficacy on Kaposi's sarcoma of highly active antiretroviral therapy in a cohort of HIV-positive patients. CISIH 92. Centre d'information et de soins de l'immunodeficience humaine. AIDS **14:** 987–993.
123. DEZUBE, B.J. 2000. Acquired immunodeficiency syndrome-related Kaposi's sarcoma: clinical features, staging, and treatment. Semin. Oncol. **27:** 424–430.
124. ALBERTS, D.S. & D.J. GARCIA. 1997. Safety aspects of pegylated liposomial doxorubicin in patients with cancer. Drugs **54:** 30–35.
125. BERRY, G., M. BILLINGHAM, E. ALDERMAN, et al. 1998. The use of cardiac biopsy to demonstrate reduced cardiotoxicity in AIDS Kaposi's sarcoma patients treated with pegylated liposomial doxorubicin. Ann. Oncol. **9:** 711–716.
126. TIRELLI, U., D. ERRANTE, M. SPINA, et al. 1996. Second-line chemotherapy in human immunodeficiency virus-related non-Hodgkin's lymphoma: evidence of activity of a combination of etoposide, mitoxantrone, and prednimustine in relapsed patient. Cancer **77:** 2127–2131.
127. KERSTEN, M.J., T.J. VERDUYN, P. REISS, et al. 1998. Treatment of AIDS-related non-Hodgkin's lymphoma with chemotherapy (CNOP) and r-hu-G-CSF: clinical outcome and effect on HIV-1 viral load. Ann. Oncol. **9:** 1135–1138.
128. WISEMAN, L. R. & C.M. SPENCER. 1997. Mitoxantrone. A review of its pharmacology and clinical efficacy in the management of hormone-resistant advanced prostate cancer. Drugs Aging **10:** 473–485.
129. VIAL, T. & J. DESCOTES. 1994. Clinical toxicity of interferons. Drug Saf. **10:** 115-50.
130. SONNENBLICK, M. & A. ROSIN. 1991. Cardiotoxicity of interferon. A review of 44 cases. Chest **99:** 557–561
131. DEYTON, L.R., R.E. WALKER, J.A. KOVACS, et al. 1989. Reversible cardiac dysfunction associated with interferon alpha therapy in AIDS patients with Kaposi's sarcoma. N. Engl. J. Med. **321:** 1246–1249.
132. EMERY, S., W.B. CAPRA, D.A. COOPER, et al. 2000. Pooled analysis of 3 randomized, controlled trials of interleukin-2 therapy in adult human immunodeficiency virus type 1 disease. J. Infect. Dis. **182:** 428–434.
133. KRUIT, W.H., K.J. PUNT, S.H. GOEY, et al. 1994. Cardiotoxicity as a dose-limiting factor in a schedule of high dose bolus therapy with interleukin-2 and alpha-interferon. An unexpectedly frequent complication. Cancer **74:** 2850–2856.
134. WHITE, R.L., D.J. SCHWARTZENTRUBER, A. GULERIA, et al. 1994. Cardiopulmonary toxicity of treatment with high dose interleukin-2 in 199 consecutive patients with metastatic melanoma or renal cell carcinoma. Cancer **74:** 3212–3222.
135. DU BOIS, J.S., J.E. UDELSON, M.B. ATKINS, et al. 1995. Severe reversible global and regional ventricular dysfunction associated with high-dose interleukin-2 immunotherapy. J. Immunother. Emphasis Tumor. Immunol. **18:** 119–123.
136. PISCITELLI, S.C., N. BHAT & A. PAU. 2000. A risk-benefit assessment of interleukin-2 as an adjunct to antiviral therapy in HIV infection. Drug Saf. **22:** 19–31.
137. DRESSER, G.K., J.D.SPENCE & D.G. BAILEY. 2000. Pharmacokinetic-pharmacodynamic consequences and clinical relevance of cytochrome P450 3A4 inhibition. Clin. Pharmacokinet. **38:** 41–57.
138. GUENGERICH, F.P. 1999. Cytochrome P-450 3A4: regulation and role in drug metabolism. Annu. Rev. Pharmacol. Toxicol. **39:** 1–17.

139. RICHEY, D.P. & A.D. BENDER. 1997. Pharmacokinetc consequences of aging. Annu. Rev. Pharmacol. Toxicol. **17:** 49–65.
140. HUNT, C.M., W.R. WESTERKAM & G.M. STAVE. 1992. Effect of age and gender on the activity of human hepatic CYP3A. Biochem. Pharmacol. **44:** 275–283.
141. IQBAL, S., C. VICKERS & E. ELIAS. 1990. Drug metabolism in end-stage liver disease. In vitro activities of some phase I and phase II enzymes. J. Hepatol. **11:** 37–42.
142. SLAIN, D., A. PAKYZ & D.S. ISRAEL. 2000. Variability in activity of hepatic CYP3A4 in patients infected with HIV. Pharmacotherapy **20:** 898–907.

Cardiovascular Disease Risk Factors in HIV-Infected Patients in the HAART Era

M. GALLI, A.L. RIDOLFO, AND C. GERVASONI

Institute of Infectious Diseases and Tropical Medicine, L.Sacco Hospital, University of Milan, 20157 Milan, Italy

ABSTRACT: HIV infection is accompanied by disturbances in lipid and glucose metabolism, which are further compounded by changes induced by antiretroviral drugs. There is increasing concern that these changes will lead to an epidemic of cardiovascular disease. Cardiovascular disease will no doubt increase, but current data indicate that the average absolute levels are likely to remain low, although patients with additional risks (smoking, hypertension, diabetes, age, family history, etc.) are certainly more susceptible. The complications of therapy need to be taken into account when deciding on the time of treatment, and reducing risk factors should become a routine aspect of the care of an HIV population that now lives longer as a result of highly active antiretroviral therapy.

KEYWORDS: cardiovascular disease; risk; HIV infection; metabolism; antiretroviral therapy

INTRODUCTION

The widespread use of HIV-1 protease inhibitors as components of highly active antiretroviral therapy (HAART) has greatly modified the natural history of HIV infection and led to a significant decline in the incidence of AIDS and related deaths.[1] However, at the same time, HIV+ patients have started to experience an increasingly frequent array of unexpected metabolic side effects, the most serious of which are characterized by body adipose tissue changes, hypertriglyceridemia, hypercholesterolemia, insulin resistance and overt type II diabetes mellitus.[2] Body changes and metabolic disorders are often associated in what is currently defined as lipodystrophy syndrome[3] (see TABLE 1). Despite the increasing awareness of the prevalence of this syndrome in patients treated with antiretroviral drugs, the underlying mechanism remains obscure and there seem to be multiple causes. It has been suggested that protease inhibitors (PI)-induced peripheral cellular lipolysis plays a key role[4] and, more recently, that nucleoside reverse transcriptase inhibitors (NRTI)-induced mitochondrial toxicity may further explain the wasting and accumulation of body fat.[5] The long-term consequences of these metabolic alterations is currently a critical issue. A matter of major concern is that some aspects of lipodystrophy syndrome resemble those of the so-called metabolic syndrome X, a combination of very similar abnormalities that are risk factors for the development of cardiovascular disease in the HIV− population.[6] Furthermore, vascular disorders, coronary artery disease and

Address for correspondence: Prof. Massimo Galli, Instituto di Malattie Infettive e Tropicali, L. Sacco Hospital, via G.B. Grassi 74, 20157, Milan, Italy. Voice: +39 02-329042583; fax: +39 02-3560805.

TABLE 1. Metabolic and morphologic changes associated with antiretroviral therapy

Metabolic changes	Morphologic changes
Glucose metabolism	Fat accumulation
Insulin resistance	Abdominal obesity
Impaired glucose tolerance	Buffalo hump
Hyperglycemia	Lipomatosis
Frank diabetes (rare)	Breast enlargement (in both men and women)
Lipid metabolism	Fat loss
Increased triglyceride levels	Upper and lower limbs
Increased cholesterol levels	Face
	Buttocks

myocardial infarction have recently been described in individual patients on long-term HAART[7–15] and, although anecdotal, these descriptions have drawn attention to the conditions that currently represent risk factors for coronary disease in the HIV+ population.

PREDISPOSING FACTORS FOR CARDIOVASCULAR AND HEART DISEASES IN THE PRE-HAART ERA

HIV Infection and Metabolic Alterations

Like many other infections, HIV infection is accompanied by metabolic disturbances. Serum lipid abnormalities have been reported during disease progression, with high density lipoprotein (HDL) cholesterol decreasing early, followed by decreases in low density lipoprotein (LDL) cholesterol.[16,17] Increased serum triglyceride levels have been described in association with the progression to AIDS[16,17] together with a decreased clearance and increased production of triglyceride-rich particles.[17,18] Furthermore, triglyceride levels have been correlated with increased levels of interferon-α,[18] and zidovudine monotherapy has been associated with a decline in both serum triglyceride and interferon-α levels.[19]

It is known that a decrease in HDL and the presence of hypertriglyceridemia increase susceptibility to atherosclerosis and are predictors of cardiovascular disease,[20,21] but the short life expectancy of HIV+ patients and their relatively young age did not raise serious concerns during the pre-HAART era. It is still not clear whether increased life expectancy will lead to a cardiovascular risk due to the chronicity of the infection regardless of treatment-induced metabolic alterations.

HIV, Endothelial Damage and Evidence of Cardiovascular Disease in the pre-HAART Era

Although coronary artery disease was thought to be uncommon during the course of HIV infection before the introduction of HAART, there is growing evidence that HIV affects the physiology of the endothelium. Endothelial dysfunction and/or injury is pivotal to the development of cardiovascular disease, and autopsy studies performed before the introduction of combined antiretroviral therapy revealed signs of vascular endothelial damage in children and young patients in the absence of the risk factors traditionally associated with coronary artery disease.[22,23] During the course of HIV infection, there is an elaboration of circulating markers of endothelial activation, such as soluble adhesion molecules and procoagulant proteins,[24–28] and endothelial activation may also be caused by cytokines secreted in response to virus-induced mononuclear or adventitial cell activation or by the endothelial effects of the secreted HIV-associated proteins, gp 120 and Tat.[29–31] It has also been found that HIV can infect endothelial cell lines *in vitro*,[32,33] although the *in vivo* significance of this finding in relation to vascular endothelial damage is unknown. Finally, HIV patients are frequently coinfected with cytomegalovirus and herpes simplex virus, which are believed to contribute to vascular endothelial damage.[34]

PREDISPOSING FACTORS FOR CARDIOVASCULAR AND HEART DISEASES IN THE HAART ERA

Glucose Metabolism Alterations

Shortly after the introduction of PIs into clinical practice, reports began to appear linking their use with the development of diabetes mellitus or the worsening of pre-existing diabetes.[35–38] Subsequent studies of HAART-treated HIV-patients have estimated that the overall incidence of new-onset diabetes mellitus type 2 is low (1–6%),[4,36,39] but insulin resistance and impaired glucose tolerance can be demonstrated in a considerable proportion of patients.[3,40–43] Walli *et al*.[40] have reported that more than 60% of PI-treated patients have abnormal oral glucose tolerance test results. Similarly, Beherens *et al*.[41] reported that 18 of 38 PI recipients (46%) had impaired glucose tolerance detected and 5 (13%) had diabetes detected by means of oral glucose tolerance testing, whereas only 4 of 17 PI-naive subjects (24%) had impaired glucose tolerance and none had detected diabetes. Prospective studies have shown the relatively rapid development of insulin resistance after the initiation of PI treatment,[43,44] but a higher than expected prevalence of impaired glucose tolerance has also been found among patients naive for antiretroviral drugs or receiving nucleoside analogue therapy without PIs,[41,45] thus suggesting that factors other than PI-therapy may play a role. In this regard, Hadigan *et al*.[46] found an association between elevated fasting insulin-to-glucose ratios and an increase in truncal adiposity but not protease inhibitor use in a group of HIV+ women.

The cause of insulin resistance among HIV+ patients is not known, but possible mechanisms include a direct metabolic effect of antiretroviral therapies,[4,47] metabolic dysfunction secondary to HIV disease itself, related cytokine and hormonal abnormalities, or a combination of all of these factors.

A possible direct role of therapy emerged in our recent prospective study of a consecutive series of patients who started HAART during primary HIV infection.[48] The cohort included 15 males with a median age of 35 years (range 23–62), who were followed for 36 months. None of the patients had a previous history of dyslipidemia or diabetes, or above normal serum cholesterol or triglyceride levels. The median glucose concentration in the cohort did not significantly change during the follow-up, but diabetes (fasting glycemia greater than 140 mg/dL in two or more consecutive tests) associated with hypertriglyceridemia occurred within 12 months of treatment in one patient, and within 18 months in a further two. Interestingly, these were the only three patients aged more than 50 years when starting antiretroviral therapy (ART). Although based on a small series of patients, these data suggest that metabolic abnormalities are caused by a mechanism that is largely independent of early infection and directly triggered by treatment. Moreover, the onset of overt diabetes in all of the patients aged more than 50 years a short time after beginning treatment suggests a possible limitation to the use of long-term ART in elderly subjects and raises concerns about early exposure to its potentially harmful effects.

Alterations in glucose metabolism have cardiovascular implications. Diabetes mellitus is associated with an increased risk of coronary artery and peripheral vascular disease, and insulin resistance per se is associated with a significant increase in cardiovascular diseases,[49,50] as well as with abnormalities in endothelial function, impaired nitric oxide production, and diminished vasodilation, which may contribute to an atherogenic environment. This raises the concern that long-lasting insulin resistance caused by antiretroviral therapy may contribute to atherosclerotic disease. Moreover, the extent to which this metabolic alteration and subsequent endothelial damage may be reversible is still unclear, although some reports have described a reversal of hyperglycemia and an improvement in insulin resistance after the discontinuation of PI therapy.[36,38,51]

A few initial studies in which protease inhibitors were substituted by a drug with a lesser tendency to induce insulin resistance (i.e., a non-NRTI [NNRTI] or NRTI) seem to show an improvement in the metabolic alteration: Martinez *et al.*[52] reported a significant improvement in insulin resistance after substituting nevirapine for PI in NNRTI-naive patients, and greater insulin sensitivity has also been reported with the substitution of efavirenz and abacavir.[53]

No controlled studies of diabetes mellitus treatment in HIV patients have been performed, but the reported cases have been typically non-ketotic and often treatable with oral hypoglycemic agents.[36,40,41] Although sulfanylurea agents are probably safe for diabetic HIV$^+$ patients, they do not directly affect insulin resistance and may exacerbate hyperinsulinemia.

There is some evidence that HIV$^+$ patients with insulin resistance may benefit from insulin-sensitizing agents such as metformin and glitazones,[54,55] which may be particularly useful because they can also lower triglyceride levels, increase subcutaneous fat and reduce visceral adiposity. However, both metformin and NRTI therapy may be associated with lactic acidosis,[56,57] and theoretical concerns exist about the concomitant use of NRTIs and metformin. Troglitazone has recently been withdrawn from the market in the United States after the observation of some cases of severe hepatotoxicity;[58] furthermore, the same drug induces CYP34A and may thus decrease the effectiveness of PIs. Rosiglitazone lacks the extensive CYP34A metabolism of triglitazone and can therefore be expected to have fewer interactions with PIs.[59] However, there are still insufficient data to consider insulin-sensitizing agents for routine use in HIV$^+$ patients on HAART, and controlled trials are needed.

Studies of diet and aerobic exercise, which are generally recommended for patients with diabetes, have not been performed in the case of insulin-resistant HIV patients, but a specific diet and regular exercise as a general health measure is one reasonable approach for improving insulin sensitivity and lipid profiles.

Lipid Metabolism Alterations

Dyslipidemia is a prevalent condition among patients receiving HAART. Carr *et al.*[4] found increased triglyceride or cholesterol levels in up to 74% of their patients receiving PI therapy, and significant increases in both have been associated with all of the available PIs.[3,43,60–63]

Data from the largest published series of PI-treated patients show an average increase in total cholesterol and triglyceride levels of respectively 28% and 96% in comparison with pre-treatment values or levels in cohorts of PI-naive HIV patients.[3,40,41,62]

The triglyceride increase occurs in both VLDL and LDL; PIs also induce a small increase in LDL cholesterol, whereas there is no change or may be a decrease in HDL levels.[3,43,64]

The hypertriglyceridemia associated with PI therapy may be very high (more than 1,000 mg/dl),[60,61] particularly in patients receiving ritonavir. Periard *et al.*[62] have estimated that patients receiving ritonavir are 19.6 times more likely to develop hypercholesterolemia than PI-naive patients, and the risk was 8.5 times with nelfinavir and 3.8 times with indinavir; furthermore, the administration of ritonavir (but not nelfinavir or indinavir) was associated with a 7.2-fold increase in the risk of developing high plasma triglyceride levels.

Despite the common association between PI therapy and hyperlipidemia, the degree of hyperlipidemia varies widely in patients treated with different PIs, thus suggesting that the mechanism of these effects is multifactorial.

Triglyceride and cholesterol levels are significantly higher among HIV+ patients with lipodystrophy syndrome.[3,65] Although hyperlipidemia may be a consequence of lipodystrophy and/or insulin resistance, it has also been observed in patients without any observable peripheral lipodystrophy or visceral lipohypertrophy, and in the absence of insulin resistance.[43,66]

A study of ritonavir therapy in healthy volunteers established that this PI can directly cause major increases in lipid levels within a period of two weeks[67]: total cholesterol increased by 24% and triglycerides by 137%. This suggests that PIs have a direct effect on triglyceride levels, but the underlying mechanism remains to be defined. It is interesting to note that increased lipid levels have also been described in patients receiving NNRTI,[68,69] and high triglyceride levels have been found in PI-naive patients treated with NRTIs.[70–72] The risk of hypertriglyceridemia in this setting seems to be greater in patients receiving combinations including stavudine, but there is still no convincing explanation for this.

Increased triglyceride levels and a high total cholesterol to HDL ratio are risk factors for coronary heart disease.[21,73,74] Another recent finding of greater concern is that PI therapy may increase the plasma levels of lipoprotein (a) by as much as 48%;[62] the importance of this finding lies in the fact that lipoprotein (a) has been associated with premature atherosclerosis regardless of cholesterol levels.[75] Lipid alterations in HIV+ subjects may have a particular atherogenic tendency when combined with other HIV- and treatment-associated metabolic abnormalities; furthermore, the cardiovascular risk in this population may be significantly higher in the presence of other risk factors such as smoking and hypertension.

The optimal treatment of ARV-associated hyperlipidemia is undefined. Discontinuing ARV therapy or replacing the PI with another antiretroviral agent may be beneficial, but raises problems in terms of HIV infection control.

Some studies have shown that substituting nevirapine for PI therapy in NNRTI-naive patients can improve their lipid profile,[52,76,77] but a number of studies have not found a beneficial effect of switching to efavirenz.[78–82] Various reports have described a trend toward an improvement in lipid levels after a switch to abacavir.[83–85] However, as many patients have already experienced NNRTI or NRTI therapy, the long-term virologic efficacy of switching may be problematical; furthermore, no studies have yet compared the effects of treatment switching with those of adding lipid-lowering agents to ongoing successful therapy.

Given the availability of cholesterol- and triglyceride-reducing agents, the treatment of hyperlipidemia is an area of active investigation. Preliminary reports suggest that dietary intervention has a modest effect on serum lipids, although extremely low fat diets may have a substantial effect in subjects with the highest triglyceride levels. Fibrates decrease serum triglyceride but not serum cholesterol concentrations, whereas the HMG CoA reductase inhibitors (statins) decrease both. However, the use of these hypolipidemic agents is complicated by their potential adverse drug interactions: pravastatin is the least susceptible, followed by atorvastatin; fluvastatin is an acceptable alternative, but lovastatin and simvastatin should be avoided. The combination of a fibrate and statin may be considered, but caution is required because of the increased risk of skeletal toxicity.

The Lipodystrophy Syndrome

Changes in body fat distribution (the so-called lipodystrophy syndrome) have been widely reported among HIV$^+$ patients receiving antiretroviral therapy: the alterations appear to be particularly pleiomorphic, including a large range of presentations ranging from generalized or localized lipoatrophy[3,86–88] to regional fat accumulation (periabdominal or intra-abdominal adiposity, breast enlargement or "buffalo hump"),[89–94] and combined forms of coexisting peripheral fat loss and truncal obesity have also been frequently described.[95,96] Patients with fat distribution alterations have significantly higher triglyceride and cholesterol levels, and insulin resistance indices, than those without lipodystrophy.[3] Longitudinal studies indicate that insulin resistance often precedes lipodystrophy, which suggests that insulin resistance may be the proximate cause of the syndrome; however, the timing of the various metabolic alterations and the degree of their correlation have not been clearly established, and some evidence suggests that they may be largely independent phenomena.[43,65]

Estimates of the frequency of body fat tissue changes are hampered by the lack of a consensual definition of the diagnostic criteria. The published reports concerning the prevalence of the symptoms of lipodystrophy syndrome vary widely: between 2% and 84% of the patients treated with antiretroviral drugs (reviewed in ref. 2). Although the initial identification of lipodystrophy syndrome coincided with the widespread use of PIs, the etiology of the abnormalities remains obscure: the first reports indicated a strict association with PI use,[3,86,87,89,90,93,94] but subsequent studies have shown that the same abnormalities may occur in NRTI- or NNRTI-treated patients.[72,88,92,95,97]

The two main pathogenetic hypotheses regarding the toxic mechanisms of the two principal ARV drug classes, protease inhibitors,[4] and nucleoside reverse transcriptase inhibitors,[5] remain unproved and have been recently refuted. Furthermore, there is growing evidence that lipodystrophy syndrome has a multifactorial origin including, in addition to direct drug effects, immune reconstitution,[98] altered cytokine production,[99,100] and hormonal interferences.[101,102]

The similarity between some aspects of lipodystrophy syndrome and metabolic X syndrome has raised serious concerns about the long-term consequences of the metabolic alterations and the accumulation of visceral fat in terms of the risk of coronary artery disease.

Hadigan et al.[65] have recently described metabolic abnormalities and cardiovascular disease risk parameters in men and women with HIV lipodystrophy by comparing their clinical characteristics with those of healthy participants in a population-based observational study of cardiovascular disease risk factors (the Framingham Offspring Study). They found that the risk of cardiovascular disease in the patients with lipodystrophy was higher than the expected risk in healthy individuals of similar age and weight. In particular, the risk factors of hypertriglyceridemia, hypercholesterolemia and low HDL were significantly more frequent among the HIV+ patients with lipodystrophy than in those without and in healthy controls.

Given that switching from PIs to other drugs does not reverse the morphologic alterations, it is probably not warranted: what is absolutely crucial is to identify the risk factors associated with these manifestations.

Evidence of Cardiovascular Disease and Risk Estimates

The impact of the HAART-related metabolic alterations discussed above on long-term cardiovascular health is not known but there is clearly cause for concern, as is demonstrated by the increasing number of reports of coronary artery disease in HAART-treated patients.[7–15]

In 1998, Henry et al.[7] first described two cases of severe premature coronary artery disease in HIV+ patients taking PIs: one had lipodystrophy and hypercholesterolemia in the absence of other known risk factors, the other presented clear risk factors such as i.v. cocaine use and cigarette smoking. Gallet et al.[8] reported three patients with ischemic cardiopathy, two of whom suffered a myocardial infarction. All of them were taking PIs, and two presented high lipid levels that were not present before the antiretroviral treatment. Similarly, Vittecoq et al.[9] described four young patients experiencing ischemic coronary events, three of which were myocardial infarctions. All but one of the patients were taking PIs; three showed major alterations in plasma lipid levels which, in two cases, were associated with smoking and genetic factors. Passalaris et al.[15] described six patients receiving PI-containing antiretroviral therapy with significant coronary artery disease, four of whom suffered an acute myocardial infarction: angiography revealed isolated thrombotic lesions in two, atherosclerotic lesions in two, and both in thrombotic and atherosclerotic disease in two.

Similar reports have appeared in the medical literature over the last few years,[10–14] but the epidemiological data supporting an association between antiretroviral therapy and a higher risk of coronary events are still limited and somewhat conflicting.

In a retrospective case-control study of 15 HIV⁺ patients with a recent cardiovascular event,[103] multivariate analysis identified only the traditional risk factors of smoking, hypertension, high cholesterol levels and family history, whereas HAART did not seem to be a risk factor. Moreover, a cross-protocol analysis of randomized phase III clinical trials examining treatment with various protease inhibitors[104] found no difference in the rate of myocardial infarction between the subjects receiving PIs and control subjects receiving only nucleoside analogues. On the other hand, a retrospective study of a cohort of 4993 HIV⁺ patients treated with different antiretroviral regimens[105] found that the incidence of myocardial infarction increased after the introduction of HAART, passing from 0.86 in 1983–86 to 3.41 in 1995–98: an age of more than 40 years and previous HAART were the factors significantly associated with myocardial infarction. Furthermore, a retrospective analysis by Jutte *et al.*[106] found a fivefold increased risk of myocardial infarction in PI-treated patients.

A number of long-term cohorts have been set up to monitor the development of cardiac events in HIV disease, but these will take many years to establish rates. In the meantime, the use of existing cohort databases may help to predict risk rates in clinical practice. To this end, Egger *et al.*[107] used data from Carr *et al.*[4] concerning the rates of cardiovascular risk factors in subjects with or without lipodystrophy and compared them with the rates in the Caerphilly Cohort, a large Welsh study of cardiovascular disease: they found that the more severe forms of HAART-related lipodystrophy can increase the risk of coronary artery disease by 3–4 times. Using the Framingham equation, they estimated the absolute risk of cardiovascular disease in the next five years for cases of HAART-induced lipodystrophy considering men and women aged 30 or 50 years and smokers or nonsmokers: the number of subjects-needed-to-treat before the next person is harmed in the population aged 30 years was respectively 71 and 217 for non-smoking men and women, and 40 and 100 for male and female smokers; in the population aged 50 years, the corresponding figures were 18 and 15 for nonsmokers, and 13 and 10 for smokers. Age and smoking led to a significantly worse potential outcome.

The above-mentioned epidemiological studies do not clarify the role of PIs in the development of ischemic heart disease, but it is worth pointing out that, in the presence of existing cardiovascular risk factors, the metabolic alterations induced by antiretroviral therapy in some patients, could significantly contribute towards the establishment of an atherosclerotic process, particularly in coronary circulation.

It is therefore now important to plan clinical trials with a longer follow-up with the aim of clarifying the role of these drugs in coronary and systemic atherogenesis.

Surrogate Markers of Subclinical Atherosclerosis in HIV⁺ Patients

Some studies have recently started to evaluate the role of surrogate markers of subclinical atherosclerosis in HAART-treated HIV⁺ patients by detecting alterations in the flows and walls of the common and internal carotid arteries. In a cross-sectional study, Sosman *et al.*[108] assessed endothelial function by means of flow-mediated vasodilation of the brachial artery in 22 non-smoking HIV⁺ subjects treated with PI-based therapy for at least six months and 10 treated with PI-free regimens for a similar period. They found that flow-mediated vasodilation was impaired in the subjects receiving PIs, but nitroglycerin-mediated vasodilation (which is not endothelial dependent) was normal in both groups. The subjects taking PIs had significantly higher total cholesterol and triglyceride levels.

It has been shown that an ultrasonographically measured increased in the thickness of the carotid artery wall is predictive of an increased risk of myocardial infarction. Depairon et al.[109] used B-mode ultrasonography of the femoral and carotid arteries to assess the thickness of the intima media in 131 subjects taking PI-based therapy for an average of 27 months and 27 HIV+ controls not taking protease inhibitors: 56% of the PI-treated subjects and 45% of the controls had atherosclerotic plaques (defined as an intima media thickness greater than 1.2 mm at any of the four studied sites), and multivariate analysis found that age and cigarette smoking but not PI therapy were independently associated with their presence. In another study by Maggi et al.,[110] acquired lesions of the vascular wall were found at ultrasonography in 29/55 PI-treated patients (52.7%), in 7/47 PI-naive patients (14.9%) and in 7/104 healthy controls (6.7%). A slightly significant correlation was found between the carotid lesions and age, male sex and hypercholesterolemia, whereas smoking, hypertriglyceridemia and HIV stage significantly increased the risk of a vascular lesion, and the use of PIs had the highest significance.

Lenormand et al.[111] found increased carotid intima media thickness (greater than 1 mm) with no hemodynamic stenosis in 10/29 HIV+ hyperlipemic subjects who had been treated with PIs for more than 12 months. Age and LDL cholesterol proved to be significant correlated factors, but not smoking, fat redistribution, triglyceride, cholesterol or HDL cholesterol levels, or the duration of PI therapy.

Talwani et al.[112] used coronary vessel electron beam computed tomography (EBCT) to quantify coronary artery calcium (CAC, a sensitive and established marker of subclinical coronary artery disease) in 60 HIV+ patients aged more than 40 years of age, who were ART-naive or had been on stable ART for at least six months, and a group of HIV− age-, sex-, and race-matched controls. There were no significant between-group differences in terms of detectable (EBCT score: greater than 0) or clinically relevant CAC (EBCT score: exceeding 100).

Overall, the indications are still very crude, and prospective studies are needed to give greater substance to the usefulness of these tests as surrogates for preventive purposes. It is nevertheless worth considering them in clinical practice in the case of patients at risk on the grounds of their family history or the long-term persistence of metabolic alterations.

CONCLUSIONS

The main goal in the past management of HIV patients was to improve their survival and quality of life, but the introduction of HAART now makes it necessary to consider the long-term adverse effects of both the infection and its therapy. In particular, clinicians must monitor patients for potential cardiovascular complications (by screening for cardiovascular risk factors such as family history, smoking, hypertension, menopausal status, physical inactivity, obesity, diabetes, and routinely measuring serum lipid levels), individualize therapy, and consider the risks and benefits of switching HAART and starting additional medications.

REFERENCES

1. PALELLA, F.J., Jr. *et al.* 1998. Declining morbidity and mortality among patients with advanced human immunodeficiency virus infection. HIV Outpatient Study Investigators. N. Engl. J. Med. **338:** 853–860.
2. SAFRIN, S. & C. GRUNFELD. 1999. Fat distribution and metabolic changes in patients with HIV infection. AIDS **13:** 2493–2505
3. CARR, A. *et al.* 1998. A syndrome of peripheral lipodystrophy, hyperlipidemia, and insulin resistance in patients receiving HIV protease inhibitors. AIDS **12:** F51–F58.
4. CARR, A. *et al.* 1998. Pathogenesis of HIV-1 protease-inhibitor associated peripheral lipodystrophy, hyperlipidaemia, and insulin resistance. Lancet **351:** 1881–1883.
5. BRINKMAN, K. *et al.* 1999. Mitochondrial toxicity induced by nucleoside-analogue reverse-transcriptase inhibitors is a key factor in the pathogenesis of antiretroviral-therapy-related lipodystrophy. Lancet **354:** 1112–1115.
6. TREVISAN, M. *et al.* 1998. Syndrome X and mortality: a population-based study. Risk Factor and Life Expectancy Research Group. Am. J. Epidemiol. **148:** 958–966.
7. HENRY, K. *et al.* 1998. Severe premature coronary artery disease with protease inhibitors. Lancet **351:** 1328.
8. GALLET, B. *et al.* 1998. Vascular complications associated with the use of HIV protease inhibitors. Lancet **351:** 1958–1959.
9. VITTECOQ, D. *et al.* 1998. Vascular complications associated with the use of HIV protease inhibitors. Lancet **351:** 1959.
10. BEHRENS, G. *et al.* 1998. Vascular complications associated with the use of HIV protease inhibitors. Lancet **351:** 1958.
11. KARMOCHKINE, M. & G. RAGUIN. 1998. Severe coronary artery disease in a young HIV infected man with no cardiovascular risk factors who was treated with indinavir. AIDS **12:** 2499.
12. ERIKSSON, U. *et al.* 1998. Is treatment with ritonavir a risk factor for myocardial infarction in HIV-infected patients? AIDS **12:** 2079–2080.
13. KOPPEL, K. *et al.* 1999. Sudden cardiac death in a patient on 2 years of highly active antiretroviral treatment: a case report. AIDS **13:** 1993–1994.
14. FLYNN, T.E. & L.A. BRICKER. 1999. Myocardial infarction in HIV infected men receiving protease inhibitors. Ann. Intern. Med. **131:** 548.
15. PASSALARIS, J.D. *et al.* 2000. Coronary artery disease and human immunodeficiency virus infection. Clin. Infect. Dis. **31:** 787–797.
16. GRUNFELD, C. *et al.* 1989. Hypertriglyceridemia in the acquired immunodeficiency syndrome. Am. J. Med. **86:** 27–31.
17. GRUNFELD, C. *et al.* 1992. Lipids, lipoproteins, triglyceride clearance, and cytokines in human immunodeficiency virus infection and the acquired immunodeficiency syndrome. J. Clin. Endocrinol. Metab. **74:** 1045–1052.
18. HELLERSTEIN, M.K. *et al.* 1993. Increased de novo hepatic lipogenesis in human immunodeficiency virus infection. J. Clin. Endocrinol. Metab. **76:** 559-565.
19. MILDVAN, D. *et al.* 1992. Endogenous interferon and triglyceride concentrations to assess response to zidovudine in AIDS and advanced AIDS-related complex. Lancet **339:** 453–456.
20. GORDON, D.J. *et al.* 1989. High density lipoprotein cholesterol and cardiovascular disease: four prospective American studies. Circulation **79:** 8–15.
21. ASSMANN, G. *et al.* 1998. The emergence of triglycerides as a significant independent risk in coronary artery disease. Eur. Heart J. **19** (Suppl. M): M8–M14.
22. JOSHI, V.V. *et al.* 1987. Arteriopathy in children with AIDS. Pediatr. Pathol. **7:** 261–275.
23. PATON, P. *et al.* 1993. Coronary artery lesions and human immunodeficiency virus infection. Res. Virol. **144:** 225–231.

24. BLANN, A. *et al.* 1998. The platelet and endothelium in HIV infection. Br. J. Haematol. **100:** 613–614.
25. LAFEUILLADE, A. *et al.* 1992. Endothelial cell dysfunction in HIV infection. J. Acquir. Immune Defic. Syndr. **5:** 127–131.
26. ZIETZ, C. *et al.* 1996. Aortic endothelium in HIV-1 infection. Am. J. Pathol. **149:** 1887–1898.
27. KAROCHKINE, M. *et al.* 1998. Plasma hypercoagulability is correlated to plasma HIV load. Thromb. Haemost. **80:** 208–209.
28. SEIGNEUR, M. *et al.* 1997. Soluble adhesion molecules and endothelial cell damage in HIV infected patients. Thromb. Haemost. **77:** 646–649.
29. CHI, D. *et al.* 2000. The effects of HIV infection on endothelial function. Endothelium **7:** 223–242.
30. ULLRICH, C.K. *et al.* 2000. HIV-1 gp120- and gp160-induced apoptosis in cultured endothelial cells is mediated by caspases. Blood **96:** 1438–1442.
31. HUANG, M.B. *et al.* 1999. Effect of extracellular human immunodeficiency virus type 1 glycoprotein 120 on primary human vascular endothelial cell cultures. AIDS. Res. Hum. Retroviruses **15:** 1265–1277.
32. CONALDI, P.G. *et al.* 1995. Productive HIV-1 infection of human vascular endothelial cells requires cell proliferation and is stimulated by combined treatment with interleukin-1 β plus tumor necrosis factor-α. J. Med. Virol. **47:** 355–363.
33. CORBEIL, J. *et al.* 1995. Productive in vitro infection of human umbilical vein endothelial cells and three colon carcinoma cell lines with HIV-1. Immunol. Cell. Biol. **73:** 140–145.
34. VALLENCE, P. *et al.* 1998. Infection, inflammation, and infarction: does acute endothelial dysfunction provide a link? Lancet **349:** 1391–1392.
35. AULT, A. 1997. FDA warns of potential protease-inhibitor link to hyperglycaemia. Lancet **349:** 1819.
36. DUBE, MP *et al.* 1997. Protease inhibitor associated hyperglycemia. Lancet **350:** 713–714.
37. VISNEGARWALA, F. *et al.* 1997. Severe diabetes associated with protease inhibitor therapy. Ann. Intern. Med. **127:** 349.
38. EASTONE, J.A. & C.F. DECKER. 1997. New-onset diabetes mellitus associated with use of protease inhibitor. Ann. Intern. Med. **127:** 948.
39. DEVER, L.L. *et al.* 2000. Hyperglycemia associated with protease inhibitors in an urban HIV-infected minority patient population. Ann. Pharmacother. **34:** 580–584.
40. WALLI, R. *et al.* 1998. Treatment with protease inhibitors associated with peripheral insulin resistance and impaired oral glucose tolerance in HIV-1 infected patients. AIDS **12:** F167–F73.
41. BEHRENS, G. *et al.* 1999. Impaired glucose tolerance and beta cell function and lipid metabolism in HIV patients under treatment with protease inhibitors. AIDS **13:** F63–F70.
42. YARASHESKI, K.E. *et al.* 1999. Insulin resistance in HIV protease inhibitor-associated diabetes. J. Acquir. Immune Defic. Syndr. **21:** 209–216.
43. MULLIGAN, K. *et al.* 2000. Hyperlipidemia and insulin resistance are induced by protease inhibitors independent of changes in body composition in patients with HIV infection. J. Acquir. Immune Defic. Syndr. **23:** 35–43.
44. DUBÉ, M.P. *et al.* 1999. Effect of initiating indinavir therapy on glucose metabolism in HIV-infected patients: results of minimal model analysis. Antiviral Ther. **4** (Suppl. 2): 34.
45. GLESBY, M. *et al.* 1998. Collected abstracts of 6th Conference on Retroviruses and Opportunistic Infections (Chicago, IL), no. 650. Foundation for Retroviruses and Human Health.
46. HADIGAN, C. *et al.* 1999. Fasting hyperinsulinemia and changes in regional body composition in human immunodeficiency virus infected women. J. Clin. Endocrinol. Metab. **84:** 1932–1937.
47. MURATA, H. *et al.* 2000. The mechanism of insulin resistance caused by HIV protease inhibitor therapy. J. Biol. Chem. **275:** 20251–20254.

48. RIDOLFO, A.L. *et al.* 2000. Incidence of lipodystrophy and metabolic alterations among patients receiving ART since primary HIV infection. Antiviral Ther. **5** (Suppl. 5): 68.
49. FESKENS, E.J. & D. KROMHOUT. 1992. Glucose tolerance and the risk of cardiovascular disease: the Zutphen Study. J. Clin. Epidemiol. **45:** 1327–1334.
50. JARRET, R.J. 1996. The cardiovascular risk associated with impaired glucose tolerance. Diabet. Med. **13** (Suppl. 2): S15–S19.
51. BOTELLA, J.I. *et al.* 2000. Complete resolution of protease inhibitor induced diabetes mellitus. Clin. Endocrinol. **52:** 241–243.
52. MARTINEZ, E. *et al.* 1999. Reversion of metabolic abnormalities after switching from HIV-1 protease inhibitors to nevirapine. AIDS **13:** 805–810.
53. GOEBEL, F.D. & R.K. WALLI. 2000. Collected abstracts of 7th Conference on Retroviruses and Opportunistic Infections (San Francisco, CA), no. 51. Foundation for Retroviruses and Human Health.
54. SAINT-MARC, T. & J.L. TOURAINE. 1999. Effects of metformin on insulin resistance and central adiposity in patients receiving effective protease inhibitor therapy. AIDS **13:** 1000–1002.
55. HADIGAN, C. *et al.* 2000. Metformin in the treatment of HIV lipodystrophy syndrome: a randomized controlled trial. JAMA **284:** 472–477.
56. PEARLMAN, B.L. *et al.* 1996. Metformin-associated lactic acidosis. Am. J. Med. **101:** 109–110.
57. CARR, A. *et al.* 2000. A syndrome of lipoatrophy, lactic acidaemia and liver dysfunction associated with HIV nucleoside analogue therapy: contribution to protease inhibitor-related lipodystrophy syndrome. AIDS **14:** F25–F32.
58. KOHLROSER, J. *et al.* 2000. Hepatotoxicity due to troglitazone: report of two cases and review of adverse events reported to the United States Food and Drug Administration. Am. J. Gastroenterol. **95:** 272–276.
59. BALFOUR, J.A. & G.L. PLOSKER. 1999. Rosiglitazone. Drugs **57:** 921–930.
60. DANNER, S.A. *et al.* 1995. A short-term study of the safety, pharmacokinetics, and efficacy of ritonavir, an inhibitor of HIV-1 protease. European-Australian Collaborative Ritonavir Study Group. N. Engl. J. Med. **333:** 1528–1533.
61. SULLIVAN, A.K. *et al.* 1998. Marked hypertriglyceridemia associated with ritonavir therapy. AIDS **12:** 1393–1394.
62. PERIARD, D. *et al.* 1999. Atherogenic dyslipidemias in HIV-infected individuals treated with protease inhibitors. Swiss HIV Cohort Study. Circulation **100:** 700–705.
63. ROBERTS, A.D. *et al.* 1999. Alterations in serum levels of lipids and lipoproteins with indinavir therapy for human immunodeficiency virus-infected patients. Clin. Infect. Dis. **29:** 441–443.
64. BONNET, F. *et al.* 2000. Increase of atherogenic plasma profile in HIV-infected patients treated with protease inhibitor-containing regimens. J. Acquir. Immune Defic. Syndr. **25:** 199–200.
65. HADIGAN, C. *et al.* 2001. Metabolic abnormalities and cardiovascular disease risk factors in adults with human immunodeficiency virus infection and lipodystrophy. Clin. Infect. Dis. **32:** 130–139.
66. PETIT, J.M. *et al.* 2000. HIV-1 protease inhibitors induce an increase of triglyceride level in HIV-infected men without modification of insulin sensitivity: a longitudinal study. Horm. Metab. Res. **32:** 367–372.
67. PURNELL, J.Q. *et al.* 2000. Effect of ritonavir on lipids and post-heparin lipase activities in normal subjects. AIDS **14:** 51–57.
68. DU PONT PHARMACEUTICALS. 1998. Sustiva (efavirenz capsules) [package insert]. Wilmington, DE.
69. MOYLE, G.J. & C. BALDWIN. 1999. Lipid elevations during non-nucleoside RTI (NNRTI) therapy: a cross-sectional analysis [abstract]. Antiviral Ther. **4** (Suppl. 2): 58.
70. SAINT-MARC, T. *et al.* 2000. Fat distribution evaluated by computed tomography and metabolic abnormalities in patients undergoing antiretroviral therapy: preliminary results of the LIPOCO study. AIDS **14:** 37–49.

71. GALLI, M. *et al.* 2000. Collected abstracts of 40th Interscience Conference on Antimicrobial Agents and Chemotherapy (Toronto, Ontario, Canada), no. 1292. American Society of Microbiology.
72. POLO, R. *et al.* 2000. Lipoatrophy, fat accumulation, and mixed syndrome in protease inhibitor-naive HIV-infected patients. J. Acquir. Immune Defic. Syndr. **25:** 284–286.
73. PYÖRÄLÄ, K. *et al.* 1994. Prevention of coronary heart disease in clinical practice. Recommendations of the Task Force of the European Society of Cardiology, European Atherosclerosis Society and European Society of Hypertension. Eur. Heart J. **15:** 1300–1331.
74. HAIM, M. *et al.* 1999. Elevated serum triglyceride levels and long-term mortality in patients with coronary heart disease: the Bezafibrate Infarction Prevention (BIP) Registry. Circulation **100:** 475–482.
75. ASSMANN, G. *et al.* 1996. Hypertriglyceridemia and elevated lipoprotein (a) are risk factors for major coronary events in middle-aged men. Am. J. Cardiol. **77:** 1179–1184.
76. RUIZ, L. *et al.* 2000. Collected abstracts of 7th Conference on Retroviruses and Opportunistic Infections (San Francisco, CA), no. 1292. Foundation for Retroviruses and Human Health.
77. TEBAS, P. *et al.* 2000. Collected abstracts of 7th Conference on Retroviruses and Opportunistic Infections (San Francisco, CA), no. 45. Foundation for Retroviruses and Human Health.
78. BONNET, E. *et al.* 2000. Collected abstracts of 7th Conference on Retroviruses and Opportunistic Infections (San Francisco, CA), no. 49. Foundation for Retroviruses and Human Health.
79. GHARAKHANIAN, S. *et al.* 2000. Collected abstracts of 7th Conference on Retroviruses and Opportunistic Infections (San Francisco, CA), no. 46. Foundation for Retroviruses and Human Health.
80. MARTINEZ, E. *et al.* 2000. Collected abstracts of 7th Conference on Retroviruses and Opportunistic Infections (San Francisco, CA), no. 50. Foundation for Retroviruses and Human Health.
81. MOYLE, G.J. *et al.* 1999. Changes in visceral adipose tissue and blood lipids in persons reporting fat redistribution syndrome switched from PI therapy to efavirenz. Antiviral Ther. **4** (Suppl. 2): 48.
82. ROZENBAUM, W. *et al.* 1999. Prospective follow-up of a PI substitution for efavirenz in patients with HIV-related lipodystrophy syndrome. Antiviral Ther. **4** (Suppl. 2): 55.
83. GOEBEL, F. & R.K. WALLI. 2000. Collected abstracts of 7th Conference on Retroviruses and Opportunistic Infections (San Francisco, CA), no. 51. Foundation for Retroviruses and Human Health.
84. OPRAVIL, M. *et al.* 2000. Collected abstracts of 7th Conference on Retroviruses and Opportunistic Infections (San Francisco, CA), no. 457. Foundation for Retroviruses and Human Health.
85. ROZENBAUM, W. *et al.* 2000. Collected abstracts of 7th Conference on Retroviruses and Opportunistic Infections (San Francisco, CA), no. 47. Foundation for Retroviruses and Human Health.
86. VIRABEN, R. & C. AQUILINA. 1998. Indinavir-associated lipodystrophy. AIDS **12:** F37–F39.
87. HO, T.T. *et al.* 1998. Abnormal fat distribution and use of protease inhibitors. Lancet **351:** 1736–1737.
88. SAINT-MARC, T. *et al.* 1999. A syndrome of peripheral fat wasting (lipodystrophy) in patients receiving long term nucleoside analogue therapy. AIDS **13:** 1659–1667.
89. HENGEL, R.L. *et al.* 1997. Benign symmetric lipomatosis associated with protease inhibitors. Lancet **350:** 1596.
90. HERRY, I. *et al.* 1997. Hypertrophy of the breasts in a patient treated with indinavir. Clin. Infect. Dis. **25:** 937–938.
91. LUI, A. *et al.* 1998. Another case of breast hypertrophy in a patient treated with indinavir. Clin. Infect. Dis. **26:** 1482.
92. LO, J.C. *et al.* 1998. "Buffalo hump" in men with HIV-1 infection. Lancet **351:** 867–870.

93. ROTH, V.R. *et al.* 1998. Development of cervical fat pads following therapy with human immunodeficiency virus type 1 protease inhibitors. Clin. Infect. Dis. **27:** 65–67.

94. MILLER, K.D. *et al.* 1998. Visceral abdominal-fat accumulation associated with use of indinavir. Lancet **351:** 871–875.

95. GERVASONI, C. *et al.* 1999. Redistribution of body fat in HIV-infected women undergoing combined antiretroviral therapy. AIDS **13:** 465–471.

96. DONG, K.L. *et al.* 1999. Changes in body habitus and serum lipid abnormalities in HIV-positive women on highly active antiretroviral therapy (HAART). J. Acquir. Immune Defic. Syndr. **21:** 107–113.

97. ALDEEN, T. *et al.* 1999. Lipodystrophy associated with nevirapine-containing antiretroviral therapies. AIDS **13:** 865–867.

98. WURTZ, R. & S. CEASER. 2000. Adipose redistribution in human immunodeficiency virus-seropositive patients: association with CD4 response. Clin. Infect. Dis. **31:** 1497–1498.

99. LEDRU, E. *et al.* 2000. Alteration of tumor necrosis factor-alpha T-cell homeostasis following potent antiretroviral therapy: contribution to the development of human immunodeficiency virus-associated lipodystrophy syndrome. Blood **95:** 3191–3198.

100. CLERICI, M. *et al.* 2000. Immunoendocrinologic abnormalities in human immunodeficiency virus infection. Ann. N.Y. Acad. Sci. **917:** 956–961.

101. YANOVSKI, J.A. *et al.* 1999. Endocrine and metabolic evaluation of human immunodeficiency virus-infected patients with evidence of protease inhibitor-associated lipodystrophy. J. Clin. Endocrinol. Metab. **84:** 1925–1931.

102. CHRISTEFF, N. *et al.* 1999. Lipodystrophy defined by a clinical score in HIV-infected men on highly active antiretroviral therapy: correlation between dyslipidaemia and steroid hormone alterations. AIDS **13:** 2251–2260.

103. DAVID, M.H. *et al.* 2000. Collected abstracts of 38th Annual Meeting of the Infectious Diseases Society of America (New Orleans, LA), no. 355.

104. COPLAN, P. *et al.* 2000. Collected abstracts of 7th Conference on Retroviruses and Opportunistic Infections: (San Francisco, CA), no. 34. Foundation for Retroviruses and Human Health.

105. RICKERTS, V. *et al.* 2000. Incidence of myocardial infarctions in HIV-infected patients between 1983 and 1998: the Frankfurt HIV-cohort study. Eur. J. Med. Res. **5:** 329–333.

106. JUTTE, A. *et al.* 1999. Increasing morbidity from myocardial infarction during HIV protease inhibitor treatment? AIDS **13:** 1796–1797.

107. EGGER, M. 2000. Collected abstracts of 40th Interscience Conference on Antimicrobial Agents and Chemotherapy (Toronto, Ontario, Canada), no. 1374. American Society for Microbiology.

108. SOSMAN, J.M. *et al.* 2000.Collected abstracts of 7th Conference on Retroviruses and Opportunistic Infections (San Francisco, CA), no. 29. Foundation for Retroviruses and Human Health.

109. DEPAIRON, M. *et al.* 2000. Collected abstracts of 7th Conference on Retroviruses and Opportunistic Infections (San Francisco, CA), no. 30. Foundation for Retroviruses and Human Health.

110. MAGGI, P. *et al.* 2000. Premature lesions of the carotid vessels in HIV-1-infected patients treated with protease inhibitors. AIDS **14:** F123–F128.

111. LENORMAND-WALCKENAER, C. *et al.* 2000. Collected abstracts of 40th Interscience Conference on Antimicrobial Agents and Chemotherapy (Toronto, Ontario, Canada), no. 1298. American Society for Microbiology.

112. TALWANI, R. *et al.* 2000. Collected abstracts of 40th Interscience Conference on Antimicrobial Agents and Chemotherapy (Toronto, Ontario, Canada): No. 1299. American Society for Microbiology.

Metabolic and Morphologic Disorders in Patients Treated with Highly Active Antiretroviral Therapy since Primary HIV Infection

PASQUALE NARCISO,[a] VALERIO TOZZI,[a] GIANPIERO D'OFFIZI,[a] GABRIELLA DE CARLI,[b] NICOLETTA ORCHI,[b] VINCENZO GALATI,[b] LAURA VINCENZI,[a] RITA BELLAGAMBA,[a] CHIARINA CARVELLI,[a] AND VINCENZO PURO[b]

[a]Clinical Department, IV Division, [b]Department of Epidemiology, National Institute for Infectious Diseases, "Lazzaro Spallanzani"—IRCCS, 00149 Rome, Italy

ABSTRACT: Our objective was to describe morphologic and metabolic disorders in patients treated with highly active antiretroviral therapy (HAART) since primary HIV infection (PHI). Our method was prospective evaluation of patients with PHI initiating HAART at the time of diagnosis. Outcome measures were: development of hyperglycemia, hypercholesterolemia, hypertriglyceridemia, and of body shape abnormalities indicative of lipodystrophy, assessed through self-reported questionnaires and physical examination. *Results:* From May 1997 to April 2001, 41 patients (35 males) with PHI presented at the National Institute for Infectious Diseases "Lazzaro Spallanzani" in Rome, Italy. A protease inhibitor-including regimen was started in 30 patients, and a nonnucleoside reverse transcriptase-inhibitor in 11. Median interval between enrollment and treatment initiation was 30 days (mean 39, range 10–150). Median HAART duration was 19 months (mean 21.2, range 3–47). Thirty-eight patients had undetectable (less than 80 cp/mL) HIV RNA after a median of 3 months (mean 4.1, range 1–15). Mean CD4 cells count increased from 632/mmc at baseline to 936/mmc at the last follow up. No cases of hyperglycemia (glucose level greater than 110 mg/dL) were observed. After a median of 6 months on HAART, 10 patients developed beyond grade 2 (greater than 240 mg/dL) hypercholesterolemia, 5 developed beyond grade 2 (greater than 400 mg/dL) hypertrygliceridemia, and two developed both. Body mass index did not change significantly. Five patients (12.2%) developed lipodystrophy after a median of 14.5 months (mean 15.3, range 2–30), with an incidence of 7.3 per 100 patient-years. *Conclusions:* Dyslipidemia and lipodystrophy can occur in patients treated with HAART since PHI. This risk of should be taken into account when considering this early antiretroviral treatment of HIV infection.

KEYWORDS: HIV; primary infection; antiretroviral agents; metabolic disorders; lipodystrophy

Address for correspondence: Pasquale Narciso, M.D., National Institute for Infectious Diseases, I.R.C.C.S. Lazzaro Spallanzani, IV Clinical Division, Via Portuense, 292, 00149 Rome, Italy. Voice: +39 06 55170400; fax: +39 06 5582825.
narciso@inmi.it

INTRODUCTION

Highly active antiretroviral therapy (HAART) for the treatment of HIV infection has been associated with morphologic abnormalities, known as HIV-associated lipodystrophy, and characterized by peripheral subcutaneous fat wasting, central adiposity, breast hypertrophy in women and dorsocervical fat pad ("buffalo hump").[1-3] These features are variably associated with insulin resistance and hyperglycemia, and with dyslipidemia, which generally consists of elevated triglyceride and total cholesterol levels.[1,4-6] Several potential mechanisms have been proposed, including the inhibition by protease inhibitors (PI) of host-cell proteins involved in lipid and carbohydrate metabolism,[7] and a direct mitochondrial toxicity of nucleoside reverse transcriptase inhibitors (NRTIs),[8] as well as a synergic effect of both these mechanisms.[9] This syndrome has been described extensively in chronically infected HIV+ patients, but only a few reports have focused on the development of lipodystrophy in patients treated with HAART since primary HIV infection (PHI).[10-12] Nevertheless, many experts would recommend antiretroviral therapy for all patients with PHI, but the potential benefits of an early treatment of PHI should be weighed against the potential risks,[13] which have not been fully explored.

Data collected from a cohort of 41 consecutive patients diagnosed with PHI presenting at the National Institute for Infectious Diseases "Lazzaro Spallanzani" in Rome, Italy, were analyzed in order to assess the risk of glucose and lipid alterations, and body shape abnormalities in the long-term treatment of patients who started HAART during, or shortly after, PHI diagnosis.

METHODS

Patients

Since the beginning of May 1997, all patients presenting at the Spallanzani Institute with PHI were enrolled in our prospective study on the efficacy and tolerability of a HAART regimen including two nucleoside reverse transcriptase inhibitors (NRTIs), plus a protease inhibitor (PI) or a nonnucleoside reverse transcriptase inhibitor (NNRTI).

The diagnosis of PHI was based on the presence of a positive plasma HIV RNA with either an evolving Western blot response plus clinical symptoms compatible with an acute retroviral syndrome (22 patients) or a documented seroconversion with a positive ELISA test and a negative HIV test in the previous 6 months, with (12 patients) or without (7 patients) a clinical history compatible with an acute retroviral syndrome.

Laboratory assessment and follow up visits were scheduled monthly in the first year, and every 2 and 4 months, respectively, thereafter. Among other routinely collected laboratory parameters (i.e., complete blood cell count, liver and kidney function tests), the following data were collected at baseline and follow up intervals: plasma HIV RNA, CD4 lymphocyte count, fasting glucose, triglyceride and, since October 1998, total cholesterol levels.

CD4 lymphocyte count was measured by flow cytometry, and plasma HIV-RNA levels by nucleic acid sequence based amplification (NASBA, Organon Teknika, Boxtel, The Netherlands). Fasting glucose, triglyceride, and total cholesterol levels were analyzed enzymatically. Our laboratory performed all measurements under standardized conditions, with internal quality control.

The Ethical Committee of the Institute approved the study, and informed consent was obtained from all patients.

Criteria and Outcomes

Hyperglycemia was defined as one or more fasting serum glucose values above 110 mg/dL obtained during follow up. Hypercholesterolemia was defined as one or more total cholesterol value between 200 and 239 mg/dL (grade 1), 240–299 mg/dL (grade 2), 300–400 mg/dL (grade 3), and above 400 mg/dL (grade 4). Hypertriglyceridemia was defined as at least one or more triglyceride value between 220 and 399 mg/dL (grade 1), 400–750 mg/dL (grade 2), 751–1200 mg/dL (grade 3), above 1200 mg/dL (grade 4).

Body mass index was calculated in all patients.

Patients' body shape abnormalities were assessed according to the criteria proposed by Carr, and co-workers:[4] fat wasting of the face, buttocks, arms or legs; increased muscle definition or prominent veins; fat accumulation in neck, buttocks, abdomen, and breasts in women. Apart from the routine examination performed during follow up visits, the assessment of body shape abnormalities was based on self-reported patients' questionnaires provided twice a year. For the purpose of this study, we defined lipodystrophy as body shape changes reported by the patient and confirmed by the doctor, or identified by the doctor and accepted by the patient. The onset of lipodystrophy was defined as the time in which the patient noticed the first manifestation of a body shape change that was confirmed by the doctor as a manifestation of the syndrome.

Statistical Analysis

Follow up of patients started at the date of HAART initiation and ended at the date of censoring. The censoring date was that of the last available visit or laboratory assessment. Other censoring reasons were patients lost to follow-up, or the development of an outcome. Since total cholesterol was only determined from October 1998 (23 patients), for those 18 patients for whom this value was not available at the time of HAART initiation, the first available total cholesterol value was used as baseline. The incidence of hypercholesterolemia and hypertrliglyceridemia were calculated including in the denominators those patients whose baseline or first available values were within the normal range, or at a lower grade, using a person-year analysis.

Cholesterol and triglyceride values of all patients at baseline were compared with their peak levels during follow up. Statistical analysis was performed using the SPSS for Windows statistical package V 9.0 (SPSS, Chicago, Illinois). Within each group, mean changes from baseline were analyzed using Student's t test; a two-sided p value less than 0.05 was considered significant.

RESULTS

Up to April 2001, 41 patients (35 men) fulfilling enrollment criteria were observed. The presumed route of exposure was self-reported: 24 were men who had sex with men, 14 had a sexual exposure to HIV$^+$ heterosexual partners, and the remaining 3 reported i.v. use of illicit drugs. Mean and median age at enrollment were 31 years (range 18–54); 34 patients (83%) had symptoms related to PHI. The median time between enrollment (i.e., the first positive plasma HIV RNA determination) and the initiation of treatment was 30 days (mean 38.9, range 10–150).

Initial HAART regimens were indinavir-zidovudine-lamivudine in 19 patients, nelfinavir-zidovudine-lamivudine in 8 patients, indinavir-stavudine-lamivudine in 3 patients, efavirenz-zidovudine-lamivudine in 10 patients, and nevirapine-zidovudine-lamivudine in 1 patient. The initial PI-including regimen was modified during the follow up by the treating physician in 8 patients, 4 of whom switched to a NNRTI-including regimen, and 4 to a different PI. These modifications were not taken into account in the analysis. Median HAART duration at the time of analysis was 19.0 months (mean 21.2, range 3–47). Only 1 patient was lost to follow up after 18 months of treatment.

Patients' plasma HIV RNA levels and lymphocytes CD4 cell counts at baseline and at the last follow up are reported in TABLE 1. Thirty-eight patients reached undetectable plasma HIV RNA levels (below 80 cp/ml) after a mean of 4.1 months (median 3, range 1–15). Three patients failed to reach undetectable viremia after 3, 18 and 26 months of HAART, respectively. Ten patients who had reached undetectable plasma HIV RNA had a viremic rebound after a median of 26.5 (range 12–40) months. From baseline to the last follow up, the mean CD4 cells count varied from 632 cells/mmc (median 597 cells/mmc) to 936 cells/mmc (median 796 cells/mmc).

Throughout the observation period, glucose levels remained within normal values (less than 110 mg/dL) in all cases. Total cholesterol and triglyceride baseline and peak levels reached during follow up are summarized in TABLE 2.

During the observation period 13 patients were prescribed dietary measures because of grade 1 or greater hypertrygliceridemia or hypercholesterolemia, and, among them, 2 patients also received drug therapy as a result of dyslipidemia.

TABLE 1. Baseline and follow up plasma HIV RNA value and lymphocyte cell counts in 41 patients who started HAART at the time of primary HIV infection

	Baseline	Follow-up
Months of HAART [mean (range)]	—	21.2 (3–47)
HIV RNA log cp/ml, mean	5.13	2.41
HIV RNA log cp/ml, median	5.15	1.90
HIV RNA log cp/ml, range	2.96–7.46	1.90–4.53
HIV RNA < 80 cp/ml, N patients	0	28
CD4/mmc, mean	632	936
CD4/mmc, median	597	796
CD4/mmc, range	200–1338	283–1965

TABLE 2. Total cholesterol and triglyceride baseline and peak levels observed during the follow-up on 41 patients who started HAART at the time of primary HIV infection

		Baseline N (%)	Follow-up Peak Value N (%)
Total cholesterol levels			
Normal value	<200 mg/dL	31 (75.6)	17 (41.5)
Grade 1	200–239 mg/dL	9 (22.0)	14 (34.1)
Grade 2	240–299 mg/dL	1 (2.4)	7 (17.1)
Grade 3	300–400 mg/dL	0	3 (7.3)
Grade 4	>400 mg/dL	0	0
Triglyceride levels			
Normal value	<220 mg/dL	33 (80.5)	25 (61.0)
Grade 1	220–399 mg/dL	8 (19.5)	11 (26.8)
Grade 2	400–750 mg/dL	0	4 (9.8)
Grade 3	751–1200 mg/dl	0	1 (2.4)
Grade 4	>1200 mg/dl	0	0

Among the 23 patients for whom a true baseline total cholesterol value was available, 7 had a grade 1 hypercholesterolemia at baseline, and 1 had grade 2. Of the remaining 18 patients for whom total cholesterol values at the time of starting HAART were not available, 2 had a grade 1 hypercholesterolemia (211 mg/dL, and

TABLE 3. Incidence of hypercholesterolemia and hypertriglyceridemia by grade in 41 patients who started HAART at the time of primary HIV infection

	Baseline	Follow-up			
	N	N/exposed	%	Months on HAART	Incidence/100 person years
Cholesterolemia					
Grade 1	9/41	14/31	45.0	599	28.00
Grade 2	1/41	9/40	22.5	668	16.20
Grade 3	0	3/41	7.3	674	5.34
Grade 4	0	0	0	674	0
Triglyceridemia					
Grade 1	8/41	9/33	27.3	555	19.46
Grade 2	0	5/41	12.2	642	9.34
Grade 3	0	1/41	2.4	642	1.87
Grade 4	0	0	0	642	0

TABLE 4. **Characteristics of the five patients treated with HAART since the diagnosis of PHI who developed lipodystrophy**

Patient number	Clinical presentation of PHI	Baseline HIV RNA log cp/ml	Baseline CD4 cells/mmc	Days between PHI and HAART	HAART regimen	HAART duration, months	HIV RNA, log cp/ml[*]	CD4 cells, /mmc[*]	Metabolic abnormality	Morphologic abnormality
5	Symptomatic	5.60	388	150	Indinavir, lamivudine, zidovudine	30	<1.90	800	Grade 2 hypercholesterolemia	Central obesity and limb wasting at month 15
11	Symptomatic	5.20	226	120	Indinavir, lamivudine, zidovudine	26	3.83	784	None	Central obesity at month 20
13	Symptomatic	5.73	462	120	Indinavir, lamivudine, zidovudine	27	<1.90	636	Grade 1 hypercholesterolemia	Central obesity at month 7
24	Symptomatic	5.89	507	20	Indinavir, lamivudine, zidovudine	19	<1.90	586	None	Central obesity and limb wasting at month 14
38	Symptomatic	6.54	543	30	Efavirenz, lamivudine, zidovudine	12	<1.90	1193	Grade 2 hypertrygliceridemia	Central obesity and Bichat fat pad atrophy at month 6

[*] At last evaluation.

215 mg/dL) at the first available determination performed after 3 and 6 months of HAART, respectively. Eight patients had a grade 1 hypertriglyceridemia at baseline.

TABLE 3 shows the incidence of hypercholesterolemia and of hypertriglyceridemia in the study population, by grade. Overall, among the study population the total cholesterol profile varied significantly from a mean of 174 ± 34 mg/dL (median 169, range 126–295) at baseline, to a mean peak value of 218 ± 47 mg/dL (median 208, range 133–359) during the follow up (Student's $t - 9.800$; $p < 0.001$).

Similarly, the triglyceride profile varied significantly from a mean of 146 ± 93 mg/dL (median 116, range 39–393), to a mean peak value of 245 ± 177 mg/dL (median 185, range 73–985) (Student's $t - 4.813$; $p < 0.001$).

Body mass index did not significantly change, averaging 23.1 at baseline (median 22.6, range 18.4–34.5), and 23.7 (median 22.7; range 19.8–37.6) at follow up.

Five patients (12.2%) developed lipodystrophy after a median of 14 months (mean 12.4, range 6–20) (see TABLE 4). From a clinical point of view the syndrome was judged as mild or moderate both by the patient and physician, in all these cases. The estimated incidence of lipodystrophy was 7.36 per 100 patient-years.

DISCUSSION

Our study confirms that lipodystrophy can occur even when HAART is begun during or shortly after PHI, and it provides a first estimate of its incidence: 7.36 per 100 patient-years. No efforts were made to measure body composition and fat content using objective techniques, such as dual energy x-ray adsorptiometry (DEXA), or computed tomography. Therefore, the incidence of actual fat redistribution could have been under- or even over-estimated. However, the patients' perception of altered body shape has been considered a method sufficiently sensible in patients with chronic HIV infection.[4–6] Moreover, in our cohort, the patients' perception was consistent with the physical examination by the physicians.

Reports estimating the prevalence of lipodystrophy in patients with chronic HIV infection vary widely.[1,4–6] In a prospective cohort study on antiretroviral-naive HIV$^+$ adults, Martinez et al. reported that the overall incidence of any lipodystrophy was 11.7 (95% CI 9.2–14.2) per 100 patient-years.[14] Thus, based on our data, the incidence of lipodystrophy in patients treated since the diagnosis of PHI seems a bit lower then the one reported in patients with chronic HIV infection. If confirmed, this finding could support the hypothesis that the duration of chronic HIV infection can contribute, at least partially, to the occurrence of metabolic and fat distribution abnormalities, once HAART is begun. Accordingly, a longer duration of HIV-1 infection, and concomitant immunological and metabolic changes, might be considered precipitating factors of the syndrome.[7] However, a direct effect of antiretroviral agents, in particular of protease inhibitors, on glucose[15] as well as lipid metabolism[16,17] has also been shown after a short course of drug exposure in healthy seronegative individuals.

A second finding of our study was the demonstration of the development of dyslipidemia in the treatment of patients starting HAART since the diagnosis of PHI, as shown in TABLES 2 and 3.

Again, the observed incidence of different grades of dyslipidemia could have been overestimated by the fact that we used, by definition, the first altered value observed, and did not take into account the high individual variability of lipid levels. However, if we consider only the incidence of grade 2 or greater dyslipidemia, that is less likely to be due to individual variability, we observed 10 patients developing hypercholesterolemia, and 3 hypertriglyceridemia, and 2 both. Of the 12 cases of hypercholesterolemia, 6 were treated with an efavirenz-including HAART regimen (total 29 months, mean 5, median 4.5, range 2–9), 4 with indinavir (total 60 months, mean 15, median 15, range 6–24) and 2 with nelfinavir (at month 6 and 9, respectively). Additionally, of the 5 cases of hypertriglyceridemia, 2 were treated with indinavir (3 and 12 months of treatment), one with nelfinavir (30 months), and the remaining 2 with efavirenz (6 months each).

Information on metabolic abnormalities and lipodystrophy occurrence in patients receiving antiretroviral treatment for PHI is very limited.

Our findings concur with the data from other cohorts of patients with PHI treated with HAART, in which the reported prevalence of lipodystrophy was 8%,[11] 16.7%,[12] and 20%.[10] A mild increase in triglyceride and cholesterol levels requiring dietary measures was noted by Capiluppi *et al.*[11] The discrepancy between studies may be the product of differences in cohort composition, and in the length of treatment or in the combination of antiretroviral agents used. For example, in Miller's cohort,[10] PHI was defined as seroconversion within 30 months prior to HAART treatment, and the results could therefore be interpreted as following an early treatment of chronic HIV infection, rather than the treatment of PHI.

The results of our study should be interpreted with caution, because of the relatively short follow-up, the small number of enrolled patients, and the lack of a control group. With all of the above mentioned limits, our study confirms and extends previous observations that both dyslipidemia and lipodystrophy can develop when HAART is begun during or shortly after PHI. Such risks should be taken into account when considering this early antiretroviral treatment of HIV infection.

ACKNOWLEDGMENTS

Partial funding for this project was provided by the Istituto Superiore di Sanità, II Programma di Ricerca Nazionale sull'AIDS, grant N. 319, and Ricerca Corrente IRCCS. We thank Lamberto Bolognesi, Graziella Cianca, Mirella Lupi, Daniela Menna, Cosima Vasile for nursing support with patients, Pierluca Piselli for his statistical suggestions, Zana Mariano for reviewing the text, and all patients for their collaboration.

REFERENCES

1. CARR, A., K. SAMARAS, S. BURTON, *et al.* 1998. A syndrome of peripheral lipodystrophy, hyperlipidaemia and insulin resistance in patients receiving HIV protease inhibitors. AIDS **12:** F51–F58.
2. MILLER, K.D., E. JONES, J.A. YANOVSKI, *et al.* 1998. Visceral abdominal-fat accumulation associated with use of indinavir. Lancet **351:** 871–875.
3. HO, T.T.Y., K.C.W. CHAN, K.H. WONG, *et al.* 1998. Buffalo hump and facial wasting in HIV. Lancet **351:** 1736–1737.

4. CARR, A., K. SAMARAS, A. THORISDOTTIR, *et al.* 1999. Diagnosis, prediction, and natural course of HIV-1 protease-inhibitor-associated lipodystropy, hyperlipidaemia, and diabetes mellitus: a cohort study. Lancet **353:** 2093–2099.

5. SAFRIN, S. & C. GRUNFELD. 1999. Fat distribution and metabolic changes in patients with HIV infection. AIDS **13:** 2493–2505

6. SAINT-MARC T., M. PARTISANI, I. POIZOT-MARTIN, *et al.* 2000. Fat distribution evaluated by computed tomography and metabolic abnormalities in patients undergoing antiretroviral therapy: preliminary results of the LIPOCO study. AIDS **14:** 37–49.

7. CARR, A., K. SAMARAS, D.J. CHISHOLM, *et al.* 1998. Pathogenesis of HIV-1-protease inhibitor-associated peripheral lipodystrohphy, hyperlipidaemia, and insuline resistance. Lancet **351:** 1881–1883.

8. BRINKMAN, K., J.A. SMEITINK, *et al.* 1999. Mitochondrial toxicity induced by nucleoside-analogue reverse-transcriptase inhibitors is a key factor in the pathogenesis of antiretroviral-therapy-related lipodystrophy. Lancet **354:** 1112–1115.

9. MALLAL, S.A, M. JOHN, C.B. MOORE, *et al.* 2000. Contribution of nucleoside analogue reverse transcriptase inhibitors to subcutaneous fat wasting in patients with HIV infection. AIDS **14:** 1309–1316.

10. MILLER, J., A. CARR, D. SMITH, *et al.* 2000. Lipodystrophy following antiretroviral therapy of primary HIV infection. AIDS **14:** 2406–2407.

11. CA LUPPI, B., D. CIUFFREDA, M. SCIANDRA, *et al.* 2000. Metabolic disorders in a cohort of patients treated with highly aggressive antiretroviral therapies during primary HIV-1 infection. AIDS **14:** 1861–1862.

12. GOUJARD, C., F. BOUFASSA, C. DEVEAU, *et al.* 2001. Incidence of clinical lipodystrophy in HIV-1-infected patients treated during primary infection. AIDS **15:** 282–284.

13. DEPARTMENT OF HEALTH AND HUMAN SERVICES (DHHS). Guidelines for the Use of Antiretroviral Agents in HIV-Infected Adults and Adolescents. Updated version: April 23, 2001. Available at www.hivatis.org.

14. MARTINEZ E, A. MOCROFT, M.A. GARCIA-VIEJO, *et al.* 2001. Risk of lipodystrophy in HIV-infected patients treated with protease inhibitors: a prospective cohort study. Lancet **357:** 592–598.

15. MUSTAFA A.N., J.C. LO, K. MULLIGAN, *et al.* 2001. Metabolic effects of indinavir in healthy HIV-seronegative men. AIDS **15:** 11–18.

16. PURNELL, J.Q., A. ZAMBON, R.H. KNOPP, *et al.* 2000. Effect of ritonavir on lipids and postheparin lipase activities in normal subjects. AIDS **14:** 51–57.1

17. PURO, V. for the ITALIAN REGISTRY OF ANTIRETROVIRAL POST-EXPOSURE PROPHYLAXIS. 2000. Effect of short-course of antiretroviral agents on serum triglycerides of healthy individuals. AIDS **14:** 2407–2408.

Clinical Manifestation of HIV-Related Pulmonary Hypertension

NICOLA PETROSILLO, ADRIANO M. PELLICELLI,
EVANGELO BOUMIS, AND GIUSEPPE IPPOLITO

Istituto Nazionale per le Malattie Infettive, "L. Spallanzani"—IRCCS, 00149 Rome, Italy

ABSTRACT: In recent years, much more thought has been given to the pathogenic role of HIV and to the clinical manifestations of HIV-related pulmonary hypertension (HRPH), which currently represents one of the most severe events during HIV disease. HRPH occurs in early and late stages of HIV infection and does not seem to be related to the degree of immune deficiency. Many of the symptoms in HRPH result from right ventricular dysfunction: the first clinical manifestation is effort intolerance and exertional dyspnea that will progress to the point of breathlessness at rest. The diagnosis of HRPH can be made only after all etiologies for pulmonary hypertension have been excluded. Echocardiography has been proven to be an extremely useful tool for diagnosing HRPH, and Doppler echocardiography can be used to estimate systolic pulmonary artery pressure and to monitor the effects of therapy. Assessment of hemodynamic measures by catheterization remains, however, the best test for evaluating response to therapy. Cardiac catheterization is mandatory to characterize the disease and exclude an underlying cardiac shunt as etiology. Vasodilators have been extensively used in the treatment of pulmonary hypertension, since vasoconstriction is a determinant characteristic of this disease. However, HRPH remains a progressive disease for which treatment is often unsatisfactory and there is no cure. As new, more efficient antiretroviral treatment are introduced, clinicians should expect to encounter an increasing number of cases of pulmonary hypertension in HIV⁺ patients in the future.

KEYWORDS: pulmonary hypertension; human immunodeficiency virus; echocardiography; cardiac catheterization; treatment

INTRODUCTION

Human immunodeficiency virus (HIV) has been implicated in several cardiopulmonary complications, both infectious and noninfectious. In the era of the new and potent antiretroviral treatments that have provided increased survival time and reduction of HIV-related opportunistic infections, much more attention is being given to noninfectious complications of HIV diseases, such as cardiomyopathy, pericardial effusion, and pulmonary hypertension. Some of them, such as pulmonary hypertension, were likely undetected in the previous era, owing to the short course of HIV infection and the abundance and severity of opportunistic infective manifestations.

Address for correspondence: Nicola Petrosillo, M.D., Istituto Nazionale per le Malattie Infettive, "Lazzaro Spallanzani"—IRCCS, Via Portuense, 292, 00149 Rome, Italy. Voice: +39 06 55170432; fax: +39 06 5594224.
    petrosillo@inmi.it

However, the first case of pulmonary hypertension in an HIV[+] subject was described in 1987.[1] The patient, a 40-year-old homosexual man, presented with progressive shortness of breath and pedal edema; chest radiograph revealed right ventricular enlargement, and prominent pulmonary arteries, and right side heart catheterization revealed a high right atrial pressure. The patient died three days after admission and autopsy revealed the presence of plexiform lesions in the pulmonary vessels.

In recent years, much more attention has been given to the pathogenic role of HIV and to the clinical manifestations of HIV-related pulmonary hypertension,[2–5] which currently represents one of the most severe events during the HIV disease.

Primary pulmonary hypertension is a rare disorder. Estimates of the incidence of primary pulmonary hypertension range from one to two cases per million people in the general population.[6,7] On the other hand, the incidence of pulmonary vascular disease appears to be higher among HIV[+] subjects. In a prospective study by Speich *et al.*, the incidence of PPH in the HIV[+] population was estimated to be 0.5% (6/1200).[8]

HIV-related pulmonary hypertension occurs in early and late stages of HIV infection and does not seem to be related to the degree of immune deficiency.[9] No specific risk factor for HIV infection is associated with this disease. Intravenous drug users, homosexuals, heterosexuals, and subjects who acquired HIV infection through transfusion have all been described among patients with HRPH.

In this article we describe the clinical manifestations of HIV-related pulmonary hypertension, and we review the literature pertaining to this disorder.

DEFINITION OF PRIMARY PULMONARY HYPERTENSION (PPH) AND HIV-RELATED PULMONARY HYPERTENSION (HRPH)

The diagnostic criteria of PPH are based on sustained elevations of pressure of the pulmonary artery without any demonstrable cause. In the National Institutes of Health (NIH) registry[10] diagnosis is based on a mean pulmonary artery pressure of more than 25 mm Hg at rest, or more than 30 mm Hg with exercise. Furthermore, diagnosis is based on the exclusion of known causes, including left-sided cardiac valvular disease, myocardial disease, congenital heart disease, and any significant respiratory, connective-tissue, or chronic thromboembolic diseases. Additionally, the use of drugs, especially cocaine inhalation, or appetite-suppressant agents should be ruled out in the diagnosis of PPH (see TABLE 1).

HRPH is a pulmonary vascular disease with clinical and pathological features, similar to those of PPH occurring in a patient with HIV infection. All other secondary causes of PH in patients with HIV infection should be ruled out. The role of intravenous drug use (IVDU) is controversial. Even though IVDU is frequently associated with PH in HIV[+] patients, only cocaine intravenous use seems to be a likely secondary cause of PH.[11]

Injection of small particles containing talc may cause granulomas within small pulmonary arteries and thereby lead to increased pulmonary vascular resistance, as evidenced in autoptic studies.[12] However, several studies conducted in the pre-AIDS era have extensively demonstrated that ordinary heroin does not contain enough

TABLE 1. Secondary causes of pulmonary hypertension

Congenital lung, thorax, pulmonary artery, or diaphragm abnormalities

Valvular heart disease

Primary myocardial disease

Pulmonary thromboembolic disease

Obstructive lung disease

Sickle cell anemia

Cocaine,amphetamine, or appetite suppressive agents' use

Collagen vascular disease

Interstitial pneumonia (including *Pneumocystis carinii* pneumonia, CMV pneumonia, lymphoid interstitial pneumonia, idiopathic fibrosis, sarcoidosis)

Granulomatous lung disease

crystalline debris to induce pulmonary angiothrombosis.[13] This observation was also confirmed by autoptic studies on injection drug users.[14]

CLINICAL PRESENTATION

The average age of HRPH patients is 33 years,[11,15] although the range can span from infancy to old age. The male-to-female ratio is about 1.5:1.[11] This ratio is different from the ratio of HIV⁻ patients with PPH, in whom the female-to-male ratio is 1.7:1.[16] This finding may reflect the higher frequency of HIV infection among male patients.

Among HRPH patients, the main risk factors associated with HIV infection include intravenous drug use (about one half of cases), homosexual behavior (about 20%), transfusion due to hemophilia or other causes (about 15%).[11,15]

Many of the symptoms in HRPH result from right ventricular dysfunction. Since the predominant symptom of HRPH is progressive shortness of breath, which can be present in many other clinical manifestations of HIV infection, the disease is typically diagnosed late in its course when the clinical and laboratory findings of severe pulmonary hypertension are generally present. Indeed, the first clinical manifestation is effort intolerance and exertional dyspnea that will progress to the point of breathlessness at rest.

Usually about six months elapse between the onset of symptoms and the establishment of HRPH.[15] This period is shorter than that evidenced for pulmonary hypertension in HIV⁻ individuals. In these patients this period is on average 2.5 years,[16] and in about 10% of patients the diagnosis is not established after 3 years of symptoms.[10,17] One likely explanation of this difference is the fact that HIV⁺ patients are more closely followed up starting from the time of the initial diagnosis of HIV infection. However, a more aggressive type of pulmonary hypertension in HIV⁺ patients can not be ruled out.

In a review of 131 cases of HRPH, Mehta *et al.* found that progressive shortness of breath was the most common presenting symptom (85% of cases), followed by pedal edema (30%), non-productive cough (19%), fatigue (13%), syncope or near syncope (12%), and chest pain (7%).[15]

Raynaud syndrome is a rare manifestation associated with severe HRPH.[18] Hoarseness, or breathy voice can be due to extrinsic compression of recurrent laryngeal nerve by dilated pulmonary artery. Hemoptysis is extremely rare.[11]

Pulmonary hypertensive pain may resemble angina in that it is precipitated by effort. The association of moderate or severe dyspnea and evidence of pulmonary hypertension are clues to the diagnosis. On physical examination the most frequent findings are increased intensity of P_2 with P_2 louder than A_2, right-sided S_3 and S_4 gallop, murmurs of tricuspid and pulmonic regurgitation, increased jugular venous pressure, and peripheral edema.[15] A pulmonary ejection sound can frequently be heard.

LABORATORY AND DIAGNOSTIC TESTS

The diagnosis of HRPH can be made only after all etiologies for pulmonary hypertension have been excluded. Specific information related to associated illnesses, use of cocaine or appetite suppressant drugs should be sought in the history.

Information about intravenous drug use should be also sought, because it may cause obstructive granulomas within small pulmonary arteries and thereby lead to increased pulmonary vascular resistance.[14] Moreover, the association of intravenous heroin and amphetamines is described.[19]

In a recent review by Pellicelli et al.[11] of 94 cases of pulmonary hypertension in HIV patients reported in the literature, only 77 satisfied the criteria for HRPH. Possible secondary causes were associated with pulmonary hypertension in the excluded 17 cases: pulmonary diffuse interstitial inflammation, Pneumocystis carinii pneumonia, cocaine and amphetamine use, pulmonary veno-occlusive disease, cytomegalovirus pneumonia, lymphoid interstitial pneumonia, pulmonary thromboembolic disease, pulmonary Kaposi's sarcoma, and pulmonary embolism due to talc in an intravenous drug user.[11]

Chest X-ray generally shows enlarged central pulmonary arteries and clear lung fields (see FIGURES 1 and 2); moreover, it is helpful in excluding some secondary causes of pulmonary hypertension, such as interstitial pneumonia. However, in the initial phases of the disorder, chest x-ray could not detect early changes of pulmonary arteries.

The electrocardiogram usually reveals right axis deviation and right ventricular hypertrophy. P waves are tall and most prominent in standard leads II, III, and VF because of right atrial enlargement. R waves are tall in V_1 with abnormal S waves in V_5 and V_6. Complete or incomplete right bundle branch block may be present.

Transthoracic echocardiography has been proved to be an extremely useful tool for diagnosis of HRPH; moreover, it is extremely helpful in ruling out congenital, valvular, and myocardial disease. The most frequent bidimensional echocardiographic features are: systolic flattening of the interventricular septum, an enlarged right atrium and ventricle (FIG. 2) and a reduction in both left ventricular systolic and diastolic dimensions (see FIGURE 3). Pericardial effusion and patent foramen ovale are also frequently detected by echocardiography. Doppler echocardiography may be used to estimate systolic pulmonary artery pressure (SPAP), by measuring regurgitant flow across the tricuspid valve using the Bernoulli formula, in absence of a stenotic pulmonary valve. Furthermore, Doppler echocardiography is able to demonstrate left ventricular diastolic dysfunction with marked dependence on atrial contraction for ventricular filling.

Echocardiography may be a useful, noninvasive way to monitor the effects of therapy; reductions in right chamber size and estimated pulmonary-artery systolic pressure may be observed in patients given long-term therapy with calcium-channel blockers.[20] Assessment of hemodynamic measures by catheterization remains, however, the best test for evaluating the response to therapy. Cardiac catheterization is mandatory to characterize the disease and exclude an underlying cardiac shunt as etiology. A right-to-left shunt might be attributable to a patent foramen ovale, but any left-to-right shunting implies the presence of a congenital defect.

In patients with HRPH, cardiac catheterization disclosed an increase of pulmonary artery pressure to levels three or more times normal, elevated right atrial pressure, and depressed cardiac output. Pressures on the left side of the heart are usually normal, although extreme dilatation of the right chambers can compress the left chambers to a degree that limits filling and produces small increases in diastolic pressures.

The pulmonary-capillary wedge pressure is usually normal, even in veno-occlusive disease and by definition, patients with HRPH should have a low or normal

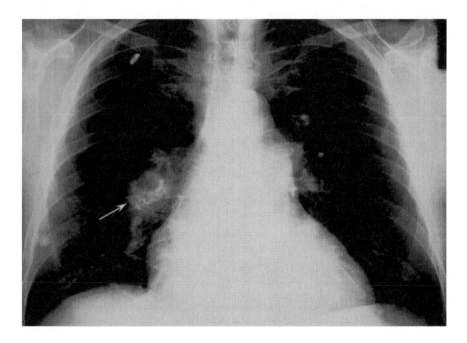

FIGURE 1. HIV-related pulmonary hypertension. Chest x rays show enlarged central pulmonary artery.

pulmonary capillary wedge pressure. However, when an increased wedge pressure is obtained, it must be correlated with left ventricular end-diastolic pressure.

It has been shown that left ventricular diastolic compliance becomes significantly impaired in HRPH, thus pulmonary capillary wedge pressure tends to rise slightly in the late stages of the disease. Furthermore, acute vasodilator testing is an important component of the hemodynamic assessment, since the responses to acute challenge with vasodilators is predictive of the long-term response to oral vasodilator therapy.

Pulmonary function test should be done to exclude significant parenchymal or airway disorders. Patients with severe HRPH may have a mild restrictive pattern or a low diffusion capacity, which does not correlate with the severity of pulmonary

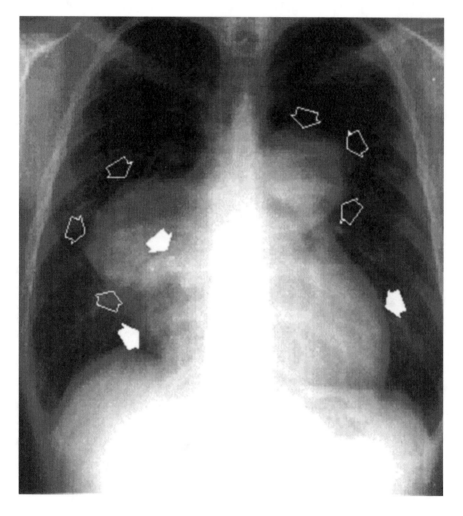

FIGURE 2. HIV-related pulmonary hypertension. Echocardiography shows enlargement of right atrium and ventricle.

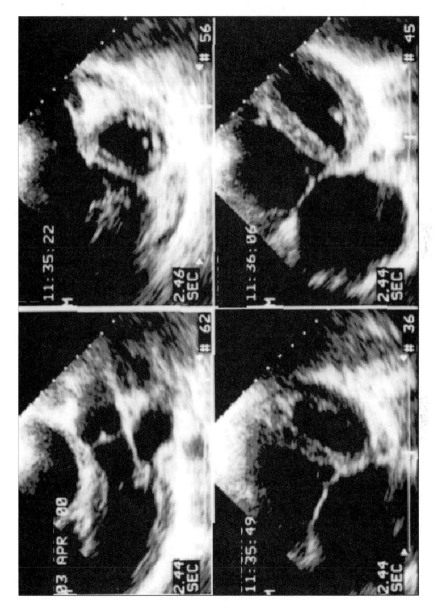

FIGURE 3. HIV-related pulmonary hypertension. Echocardiography shows reduction in both left ventricular systolic and diastolic dimension.

hypertension. Arterial blood gases can show a chronic respiratory alkalosis, and hypoxemia caused by ventilation-perfusion mismatching. Severe hypoxemia is caused by decreased cardiac output with ventilation-perfusion mismatching, or with intracardiac shunting through a patent foramen ovale.

The perfusion lung scan, done by the standard technique of injecting 3 mCi of ^{99}Tc-labeled microaggregate albumin into a vein in the peripheral arm, may be helpful in order to find secondary causes of pulmonary hypertension, such as pulmonary embolism. Specifically, only the normal and patchy distribution of tracer uptakes are considered as valid patterns. In particular, a normal lung perfusion scan is found in all the cases with a plexogenic arteriopathy, while a patchy distribution of the tracer is disclosed in patients with thromboembolic and veno-occlusive forms of HRPH.

A perfusion lung scan is useful not only as a diagnostic evaluation in a patient with suspected HRPH, but also to assess whether the patient should be treated with or without anticoagulation. Indeed, when a patchy distribution of the tracer is present, anticoagulation therapy could be advocated, whereas there is no indication to treat patients with normal lung perfusion scans.

Pulmonary angiography should be done when segmental or subsegmental perfusion defects suggest unresolved large vessel chronic thromboembolic disease. Pulmonary angiography will show characteristics pruning of distal vessels in patients with HRPH, rather then the webs, bands, and cut-offs of patients with chronic thromboembolic disease.

Lung biopsy is rarely necessary in the diagnosis of HRPH, and should only be used when the clinical diagnosis is unclear.

CLINICAL COURSE OF HRPH: RISK FACTORS

In a systematic review of cases of HRPH without any possible secondary cause, Pellicelli et al.[11] found that the mean CD4$^+$ cell counts in these patients were $0.30 \pm 0.25 \times 10 ^9$/L ($n = 56$ cases). In 30 patients, for all of whom CD4$^+$ cell counts and SPAP values were available, no correlation was found between SPAP level and CD4$^+$ cell count (Pearson $R = 0.043$; $p = 0.9$). The mean SPAP was not significantly different according to CD4$^+$ cells count, being 73 ± 13 mm Hg in 11 patients with low CD4$^+$ cells count (less than 0.2×10^9/L), 73.8 ± 11.4 mm Hg in 6 patients with CD4$^+$ between 0.2 and 0.4×10^9/L, and 70.5 ± 18 mm Hg in 13 patients with higher CD4$^+$ cells count (at least 0.4×10^9/L).

In 44 patients for whom CDC stage of AIDS and SPAP levels were available, a statistically significant difference was found between 12 patients with AIDS and 32 without AIDS, with regard to the degree of pulmonary hypertension. Indeed SPAP level was 85.4 ± 17 mm Hg in AIDS patients versus 71.8 ± 15 mm Hg in non-AIDS patients (95% CI: 2.98 to 24.22; $p = 0.013$). On the contrary, AIDS patients' SPAP levels were higher compared to those of asymptomatic and symptomatic HIV$^+$ patients, suggesting that higher levels of HIV viral load may play a role, likely indirect,[5] in the pathogenesis of HRPH.

In the review by Pellicelli et al.[11] liver cirrhosis was present in 11 (22.9%) out of 48 patients for whom this information was available. A higher mean SPAP value, that did not reach statistical significance, was found among patients with liver cirrhosis

(85 ± 21 mm Hg) versus those without cirrhosis (73.1 ± 15 mm Hg) (95% CI: −0.62 to 24.42; $p = 0.06$).

Several studies have described the association between pulmonary hypertension and portal hypertension.[21–23] Pulmonary hypertension is considerably more frequent than was previously estimated in patients with portal hypertension. In a large study, the prevalence of pulmonary hypertension in 507 patients, without HIV infection, hospitalized with portal hypertension but without known pulmonary hypertension who underwent cardiac catheterization was prospectively studied. Ten (2%) of these patients, six of whom were clinically asymptomatic, had primary pulmonary hypertension. Results of this study showed that the risk of developing pulmonary hypertension could increase with the duration of portal hypertension, without any clear relation to the degree of portal hypertension, hepatic failure, or amount of blood shunted.[24] It is likely that pulmonary hypertension can be caused or worsened by vasoactive substances, which bypass the liver in cirrhosis, causing damage to lung small vessels.[25]

TREATMENT OF HRHP

Treatment of HRPH is not substantially different from that used in case of primary pulmonary hypertension. Even though considerable progress in therapy has been made over the past few years, primary pulmonary hypertension and HRPH remain progressive diseases for which treatment is often unsatisfactory and there is no cure.

Vasodilators have been extensively used in the treatment of pulmonary hypertension, since vasoconstriction is a determinant characteristic of this disease. The aim of this treatment is to reduce pulmonary vascular resistance and to increase cardiac output without a reduction in the systemic arterial pressure. Indeed, maintenance of adequate systemic blood pressure is crucial for two reasons. First, pulmonary hypoperfusion due to low systemic blood pressure may worsen PH. Second, vasodilator drugs can provoke acute right ventricular ischemia due to the impairment of right ventricular coronary blood flow.

Patients' demographic or hemodynamic characteristics are not predictive of a response to vasodilators,[26] whereas an acute response to a vasodilator challenge is essential in identifying those patients who will respond to long-term oral therapy.[27] Infusion of epoprostenol (prostacyclin) during a right heart catheterization could be helpful in evaluating a beneficial effect. Patients who have a reduction in pulmonary-artery pressure, with a cardiac output increase and little or no change in systemic arterial pressure, are likely to respond and have sustained improvement.[20] Moreover, survival seems to be prolonged by high doses of calcium channel blockers.[28]

In patients in whom cardiac catheterization cannot be performed for technical reasons or is refused, echocardiographic parameters may be used to predict calcium-channel blocker hypotension.[29]

The response to a short-term vasodilator trial with epoprostenol in HRPH patients, and in HIV⁻ patients with primary pulmonary hypertension, has been evaluated by Petitpretz *et al.*[9] The authors ascertained that the percentage of responders to epoprostenol and the level achieved in pulmonary vasodilation were similar in the two groups.

Epoprostenol and other calcium-channel blockers have been administered in some of the reported cases of HRPH,[9,11,15, 30–33] with variable success. Epoprostenol is the most hopeful drug for PPH and HRPH; however, its principal limitation is its short half-life (i.e., 3–5 minutes after intravenous administration).

For this reason epoprostenol should be given by continuous intravenous infusion, through a portable infusion pump attached to a permanent indwelling central venous catheter. Its effectiveness in patients with PPH has been assessed in a randomized, prospective trial comparing this drug with conventional therapies.[34]

However, data examining the effects of long-term epoprostenol in HRPH are lacking. In a prospective study,[35] six patients with severe HIV-associated pulmonary hypertension were treated with continuous intravenous epoprostenol infusions. Acute infusion of epoprostenol resulted in a significant ($p < 0.05$) decrease in mean pulmonary artery pressure and pulmonary vascular resistance (PVR) of 16.4% and 32.7%, respectively, and a significant ($p < 0.05$) increase in the mean cardiac output of 36.9%.

At one year, mean pulmonary artery pressure and PVR had decreased by 21.7% and 54.9% ($p < 0.05$), respectively, and the mean cardiac output had increased by 51.4% ($p < 0.05$) when compared with baseline values. Repeat catheterizations of three patients at two years and one patient at 40 months demonstrated further improvement or maintenance of hemodynamics. In addition, NYHA functional class improved in all patients.[35]

However, some adverse effects of long-term therapy with epoprostenol should be considered. First, pump malfunction, central venous catheter-associated infections, and thrombosis could occur during the use of the pump system. Second, jaw pain, skin erythema, arthralgias, and diarrhea are directly induced by the drug. Third, if the infusion is interrupted the disease could suddenly worsen, and this event could be life-threatening.

The administration of an orally active prostacyclin, beraprost sodium (BPSB) may be helpful in the treatment of HRPH patients. In prospective studies on patients with pulmonary hypertension, BPSP improved the imbalance of thromboxane and prostacyclin biosynthesis and had the potential to prevent the progressive development of pathological changes in pulmonary vasculature.[36] It also had beneficial effects on the survival of outpatients with PPH, in comparison to conventional therapy alone.[37]

Finally, data on the efficacy of a beta-blocker, carvedilol, are still limited,[38] and symptomatic treatment with diuretics, oxygen or digoxin did not substantially improve the clinical course of the disease.[15] Anticoagulant therapy has also been advocated, based upon the evidence that thrombosis *in situ* is common.

The efficacy of antiretroviral treatment for HRPH is controversial. Opravil *et al.* prospectively followed 19 patients with HRPH and found that the right ventricular systolic pressure/right atrial pressure gradient decreased by 3.2 mm Hg for those six patients who received antiretroviral treatment, but increased by 19.0 mm Hg for untreated patients ($p = 0.026$).[33] This observation led the authors to recommend initiation of antiretroviral treatment in all patients with HRPH.[33]

In another prospective study, however, two patients with HRPH treated with antiretroviral agents including protease inhibitors had an accelerated course of pulmonary hypertension and a worsening of pulmonary artery systolic pressure, even though the HIV viral load was low. Indeed, the direct role of HIV in pulmonary hypertension is debatable; it is likely that the progression of the disease is due to high secretion of inflammatory mediators stimulated by unidentified pathogens different from HIV.[2] Moreover, the use of different therapeutic regimens is debatable.

In a retrospective study on 1042 HIV⁺ patients, cardiac involvement was noted in 284 of 544 (51.8%) patients treated with two nucleoside reverse transcriptase inhibitors (NRTI), whereas only 93 of 498 (18.6%) patients treated with highly active antiretroviral therapy (HAART) showed signs of cardiac involvement ($p < 0.0001$). However, the authors observed a significant increase of pulmonary hypertension in patients treated with HAART (2.0%) versus those treated with NRTI (0.7%) ($p = 0.048$).[39]

PROGNOSIS

Pulmonary hypertension seems to be more aggressive and lethal in patients with HIV or AIDS, than in those without HIV infection. In a cohort of 63 patients followed up by Mesa *et al.*[3] the one-year survival rate was 51% (32 of 63). This compares with a one-year survival rate of 68% for HIV⁻ patients with PPH.[7,16]

In their review of 131 cases, Mehta *et al.*[11] found that half of the patients died during the median follow-up period of 8 months. About two-thirds of the deaths were due to complications related to pulmonary hypertension, such as progressive right-sided heart failure, cardiogenic shock, and sudden death. Sudden death appears to be a late feature of the disease.

In the Swiss HIV Cohort Study, the 19 patients in whom HRPH was diagnosed were followed up for a median time of 1.3 years. Pulmonary hypertension was the cause of eight of 17 deaths. The probability of surviving was significantly decreased in patients with pulmonary hypertension in comparison with control subjects. Indeed, the probability of survival was reduced by half, the median survival being 1.3 years in HRPH patients versus 2.6 years among patients without pulmonary hypertension ($p < 0.05$).[33]

Finally, a slightly shorter median survival (300 days) was found among HRPH patients without any possible cause of secondary pulmonary hypertension.[11]

CONCLUSIONS

HRPH is a severe manifestation in the course of HIV disease. The occurrence of dyspnea in a patient with HIV infection which is unexplained after appropriate evaluation of infectious causes should prompt further evaluation of pulmonary hypertension, particularly if there is evidence of right ventricular dysfunction. Clinicians should be aware that the appearance and rapid progression of shortness of breath and other cardiopulmonary symptoms in HIV⁺ individuals should suggest HRPH.

As new, more efficient antiretroviral treatments are introduced we can expect to encounter an increasing number of cases of pulmonary hypertension in HIV⁺ patients in the future.

ACKNOWLEDGMENT

Work reported here was supported by Ricerca Corrente IRCCS, "L. Spallanzani".

REFERENCES

1. KIM, K.K. & S.M. FACTOR. 1987. Membranoproliferative glomerulonephritis and plexogenic pulmonary arteriopathy in a homosexual man with acquired immunodeficiency syndrome. Hum. Pathol. **18:** 1293–1296.
2. PELLICELLI, A.M. *et al.* 1998. Role of human immunodeficiency virus in primary pulmonary hypertension. Angiology **49:** 1005–1011.
3. MESA, R.A. *et al.* 1998. Human immunodeficiency virus infection and pulmonary hypertension: two new cases and a review of 86 reported cases. Mayo Clin. Proc. **73:** 37–45.
4. WEISS, J.R., G.G. PIETRA & S.M. SCHAFT. 1995. Primary pulmonary hypertension and the human immunodeficiency virus. Arch. Intern. Med. **155:** 2350–2354.
5. HUMBERT, M., G. MONTI & M. FARTOUKH. 1998. Platelet-derived growth factor expression in primary pulmonary hypertension: comparison of HIV seropositve and HIV seronegative patients. Eur. Respir. J. **11:** 554–559.
6. ABENHAIM, L. *et al.* 1996. Appetite-suppressant drugs and the risk of primary pulmonary hypertension. N. Engl. J. Med. **335:** 609–616.
7. RUBIN, L.J. *et al.* 1993. Primary pulmonary hypertension. Chest **104:** 236–250.
8. SPEICH, R. *et al.* 1991. Primary pulmonary hypertension in HIV infection. Chest **100:** 1268–1271.
9. PETITEPRETZ, P. *et al.* 1994. Pulmonary hypertension in patients with HIV infection. Circulation **89:** 2722–2727.
10. RICH, S. *et al.* 1987. Primary pulmonary hypertension: a national prospective study. Ann. Intern. Med. **107:** 216–223.
11. PELLICELLI, A.M. *et al.* 2001. Primary pulmonary hypertension in HIV patients: a systematic review. Angiology **52:** 31–41
12. KRINGSHOLM, B. & P. CHRISTOFFERSEN. 1987. The nature and the occurrence of birefringent material in different organs in fatal drug addiction. Forensic Sci. Int. **34:** 53–62.
13. OVERLAND, E. S., A. J. NOLAN & P.C. HOPEWELL. 1980. Alterations of pulmonary function in intravenous drug abusers: prevalence, severity and characterization of gas exchange abnormalities. Am. J. Med. **68:** 231–237.
14. TOMASHEFSKI, J.F. & C.S. HIRSH. 1980. The pulmonary vascular lesions of intravenous drug abuse. Hum. Pathol. **11:** 133–145.
15. MEHTA, N.J. *et al.* 2000. HIV-related pulmonary hypertension. Analytic review of 131 cases. Chest **118:** 1133–1141.
16. D'ALONZO, G.E. *et al.* 1991. Survival in patients with primary pulmonary hypertension: results from a national prospective registry. Ann. Intern. Med. **155:** 343–349.
17. RUBIN, L.J. 1997. Primary pulmonary hypertension. N. Engl. J. Med. **336:** 111–117.
18. AARONS, E.J. & F.J. NYE. 1991. Primary pulmonary hypertension and HIV infection. AIDS **5:** 1276–1277.
19. ROUVEIX, E. *et al.* 1989. Hypertension artérielle pulmonaire mortelle chez un toxicomane à l'heroine et aux amphétamines. Ann. Med. Interne (Paris) **140:** 153.
20. RICH, S. & B.H. BRUNDAGE. 1987. High-dose calcium channel-blocking therapy for primary pulmonary hypertension: evidence for long-term reduction in pulmonary arterial pressure and regression of right ventricular hypertrophy. Circulation **76:** 135–141.
21. HENKEL, M., K.J. PAQUET & U. RUHL. 1994. Correlation between pulmonary hypertension and portal hypertension. Two case reports of different forms of pre-sinusoidal portal hypertension. Leber. Magen. Darm. **24:** 10–14.
22. ARCANGELI, C., G. SQUILLANTINI & G. SANTORO. 1996. Association of pulmonary and portal hypertension. Minerva Cardioangiol. **44:** 343–352.

23. MURATA, K. *et al.* 1997. Asymptomatic primary pulmonary hypertension associated with liver cirrhosis. J. Gastroenterol. **32:** 102–104.
24. HADENGUE, A. *et al.* 1991. Pulmonary hypertension complicating portal hypertension: prevalence and relation to splanchnic hemodynamics. Gastroenterology **100:** 520–528.
25. GOSNEY, J.R. & M. RESL. 1995. Pulmonary endocrine cells in plexogenic pulmonary arteriopathy associated with cirrhosis. Thorax **50:** 92–93.
26. WEIR, E.K. *et al.* 1989. The acute administration of vasodilators in primary pulmonary hypertension: experience from the National Institutes of Health Registry on Primary Pulmonary Hypertension. Am. Rev. Respir. Dis. **140:** 1623–1630.
27. BARST, R.J. 1986. Pharmacologically induced pulmonary vasodilation in children and young adults with primary pulmonary hypertension. Chest **89:** 497–503.
28. RICH, S., E. KAUFMANN & P.S. LEVY. 1992. The effect of high doses of calcium-channel blockers in primary pulmonary hypertension. N. Engl. J. Med. **327:** 76–81.
29. RICCIARDI, M.J. *et al.* 1999. Echocardiographic predictors of an adverse response to a nifedipine trial in primary pulmonary hypertension. Chest **116:** 1218–1223.
30. POLOS, P.G. *et al.* 1992. Pulmonary hypertension and human immunodeficiency virus infection. Two reports and a review of the literature. Chest **101:** 474–478.
31. RHODES, J. *et al.* 1992. Severe pulmonary hypertension without significant pulmonary parenchymal disease in a pediatric patient with acquired immunodeficiency syndrome. Clin. Pediatr. **31:** 629–631.
32. PETUREAU, F. *et al.* 1998. Pulmonary artery hypertension in HIV seropositive drug addicts: apropos of 10 cases. Rev. Mal. Respir. **15:** 97–102.
33. OPRAVIL, M. *et al.* 1997. HIV-associated primary pulmonary hypertension. A case control study. Swiss HIV Cohort Study. Am. J. Respir. Crit. Care Med. **155:** 990–995.
34. BARST, R.J. *et al.* 1996. A comparison of continuous intravenous epoprostenol (prostacyclin) with conventional therapy for primary pulmonary hypertension. N. Engl. J. Med. **334:** 296–301.
35. AGUILAR, R.V. & H.W. FARBER. 2000. Epoprostenol (Prostacyclin) therapy in HIV-associated pulmonary hypertension. Am. J. Respir. Crit. Care Med. **162:** 1846–1850.
36. ICHIDA, F. *et al.* 1998. Chronic effects of oral prostacyclin analogue on thromboxane A2 and prostacyclin metabolites in pulmonary hypertension. Acta Paediatr. Jpn. **40:** 14–19.
37. NAGAYA, N. *et al.* 1999. Effect of orally active prostacyclin analogue on survival of outpatients with primary pulmonary hypertension. J. Am. Coll. Cardiol. **34:** 1188–1192.
38. VALENCIA ORTEGA, M.E. *et al.* 2000. Pulmonary hypertension in patients with human immunodeficiency virus infection. Study of 14 cases. Med. Clin. (Barc.) **115:** 181–184.
39. PUGLIESE, A. *et al.* 2000. Impact of highly active antiretroviral therapy in HIV-positive patients with cardiac involvement. J. Infection **40:** 282–284.

Cardiovascular Monitoring and Therapy for HIV-Infected Patients

STEVEN E. LIPSHULTZ,[a,d] STACY D. FISHER,[b,e] WYMAN W. LAI,[f,g] AND TRACIE L. MILLER[c,d]

[a]Division of Pediatric Cardiology, University of Rochester Medical Center and Strong Children's Hospital,[b]Cardiology Unit, University of Rochester Medical Center, [c]Division of Pediatric Gastroenterology and Nutrition, University of Rochester Medical Center and Strong Children's Hospital, [d]Department of Pediatrics and [e]Department of Medicine, University of Rochester School of Medicine and Dentistry, Rochester, New York 14642, USA

[f]Division of Pediatric Cardiology, Mt. Sinai Hospital and [g]Department of Pediatrics, Mt. Sinai School of Medicine, New York, New York 10032, USA

ABSTRACT: Cardiovascular complications are important contributors to morbidity and mortality in HIV-infected patients. These complications can usually be detected at subclinical levels with monitoring, which can help guide targeted interventions. This article reviews available data on types and frequency of cardiovascular manifestations in HIV[+] patients and proposes monitoring strategies aimed at early subclinical detection. In particular, we recommend routine echocardiography for HIV[+] patients, even those with no evidence of cardiovascular disease. We also review preventive and therapeutic cardiovascular interventions. For procedures that have not been studied in HIV[+] patients, we extrapolate from evidence-based guidelines for the general population.

KEYWORDS: HIV; AIDS; cardiovascular; congestive heart failure; atherosclerosis

INTRODUCTION

Cardiovascular abnormalities are common in HIV[+] individuals[1–4] but often go unrecognized or untreated, resulting in increased cardiovascular-related morbidity and mortality and reduced quality of life.[5] Clinicians may mistakenly attribute signs of cardiovascular abnormalities to pulmonary or infectious causes, an error that delays appropriate treatment.[6]

Routine cardiovascular monitoring can detect these abnormalities early enough to initiate therapy or preventive therapy. Such screening is associated with reductions in mortality. Clearly, such monitoring would be costly, and whether it would be cost-effective has not been directly studied. Nevertheless, in some situations, the evidence supporting cardiovascular monitoring in HIV[+] patients is strong.

Address for correspondence: Steven E. Lipshultz, M.D., Division of Pediatric Cardiology, University of Rochester Medical Center, 601 Elmwood Avenue, Box 631, Rochester, NY 14642. Voice: 716-275-6096; fax: 716-275-7436.
steve_lipshultz@urmc.rochester.edu

In this review, we will first discuss monitoring strategies for cardiovascular problems in HIV$^+$ patients, and then outline strategies for preventive and therapeutic treatment. Some of our recommendations are supported by research in HIV$^+$ populations. However, since relatively little evidence-based medicine and guideline development has been done on cardiovascular best practices in HIV$^+$ patients, some of our recommendations are drawn from research conducted in other patient groups.

CARDIOVASCULAR MONITORING IN HIV$^+$ PATIENTS

Routine physical examination is not as reliable a way of diagnosing cardiovascular problems in HIV$^+$ patients as in uninfected patients. Evidence supports the usefulness of a number of different monitoring modalities in HIV$^+$ patients. Some modalities, such as echocardiographic monitoring, may be appropriate for all HIV$^+$ patients, whereas others, such as electrocardiography, are probably useful only for a selected group. Screening and monitoring are essential for detecting early disease and targeting patients who require early intervention and aggressive early antiretroviral therapy.

Echocardiographic Monitoring

Serial echocardiography is useful for following HIV$^+$ patients over time. It can clearly identify three conditions that are common among HIV$^+$ adults and that are associated with poor outcomes: pericardial effusions,[7,8] valvular heart disease, and endocarditis.[9,10] Transesophageal echocardiography is more sensitive for detecting endocarditis than is conventional transthoracic echocardiography.

Echocardiography can also provide clear images of thrombi and masses within the myocardium, including sarcoma and lymphoma, both of which have been identified in the hearts of HIV$^+$ patients.[11] Clinicians can then initiate preventive strategies against pulmonary emboli or stroke or treatments for malignancy.

Echocardiography can provide information about pulmonary hypertension, which can focus attention on pulmonary interstitial disease or chronic upper airway obstruction, both of which are more common in this population than in healthy people.[12–15] Early treatment can reduce the chance of developing cor pulmonale.

Regional wall motion abnormalities may be helpful in identifying dyskinetic segments secondary to ischemia or infarction.

Echocardiography has been especially helpful at identifying left ventricular (LV) systolic dysfunction and inappropriately increased LV hypertrophy.[6,16] In previous multivariable analyses, we have reported that the development of either of these abnormalities in an HIV$^+$ infant or child is an independent predictor of all-cause mortality, even when wasting, encephalopathy, CD4 count, HIV viral load, and other risk factors are taken into account.[17] We have found that both of these abnormalities can be identified on echocardiography more than a year before death, which should allow ample time for preventive or therapeutic strategies to be initiated.

We have also found that LV diastolic dysfunction is common in HIV$^+$ children. The clinical significance of this dysfunction in these patients is not entirely clear, but in other patient groups, diastolic dysfunction is a primary or contributing cause of 30 to 60% of cases of congestive heart failure. The mechanisms regulating myocyte relaxation, passive stiffness, and early and late diastolic ventricular filling in HIV$^+$ patients have not been well studied. However, abnormalities of these basic mechanisms relate to the clinical diastolic dysfunction syndrome.

Recommendations for Use of Echocardiography

We recommend serial echocardiography in HIV$^+$ patients who do not have evidence of cardiac involvement. Cardiac abnormalities are common, and without echocardiography, health-care providers often cannot differentiate cardiac from noncardiac causes of symptoms. Echocardiography can identify patients at high risk for all-cause mortality, and these patients can be targeted for a more aggressive evaluation and preventive treatments. Intravenous immunoglobulin (IVIG) is available as a relatively simple treatment for HIV$^+$ patients at risk of heart disease; among our patients, those who received IVIG had less cardiac disease than those who did not.[18] An echocardiogram is the most cost-effective test in a patient with new onset cardiomyopathy and will often suggest a therapeutic approach. Diagnostically, the echocardiogram can help discriminate between a primary cardiomyopathy and a cardiomyopathy secondary to a valvular abnormality, ischemic heart disease, congenital heart defects, isolated right heart failure to pulmonary hypertension, diastolic dysfunction, infiltrative heart disease, and pericardial processes. In dilated cardiomyopathy, the LV size, wall thickness, regional wall motion abnormalities, and shortening or ejection fraction are important determinants of etiology, prognosis, and may help guide additional diagnostic testing.

Recommended Schedule for Echocardiography

On the basis of data from the pre-HAART era, we recommend a baseline echocardiographic evaluation at the time of diagnosis of HIV. Asymptomatic patients should then have a follow-up echocardiogram every 1 to 2 years. Patients with symptomatic HIV infection without cardiovascular abnormalities should have annual echocardiographic follow-up. When echocardiography identifies cardiovascular abnormalities, the follow-up should be guided by a cardiologist. Echocardiography should also be considered in patients with unexplained or persistent pulmonary symptoms and in those with viral coinfection (e.g., infection with cytomegalovirus [CMV], Epstein-Barr virus, or adenovirus).

Electrocardiography and Holter Monitoring

Conditions detectable by electrocardiography are common among HIV$^+$ patients, and such studies may be helpful in high-risk patients.

Abnormalities of intraventricular conduction and rhythm appear to be more common in HIV$^+$ individuals than the general population.[6] Autonomic dysfunction is also very common in this population.[19] Sinus tachycardia is frequently found in HIV$^+$ patients, and some studies suggest that the degree of abnormality affects the patient's outcome. In addition, many medications given to HIV$^+$ patients may result in QT prolongation, and ECG algorithms addressing the baseline QTc interval and change in the QTc interval with medications have been proposed to reduce the risk of developing pentamidine-associated torsades de pointes.[20,21]

Routine ECG or Holter monitoring of HIV$^+$ patients may not be indicated. However, it may be useful for HIV$^+$ patients with palpitations, syncope, near-syncope, unexplained stroke, or known autonomic dysfunction, and for those who are starting or receiving medications known to be arrhythmogenic or to affect repolarization.

Stress Testing

Stress testing may be helpful for HIV+ patients for three reasons.

First, stress testing may be used to determine whether exercise can be tolerated. Exercise is likely to be beneficial for HIV+ patients with asymptomatic LV dysfunction, because it is beneficial in similar HIV− patients. Exercise also has a beneficial effect on the immune system, which could be additionally helpful for HIV+ patients.

Second, an exercise stress test evaluation gives an indication of cardiac reserve. Baseline and serial monitoring will determine whether patients are maintaining maximal oxygen uptake (VO_2 max), deteriorating or progressing, assess the efficacy of medical therapy, and detect deconditioning or cardiomyopathy. This measurement is a surrogate for the maximal cardiac output a patient can generate with exercise and is an objective assessment of prognosis in patients with heart failure. Adult patients with a VO_2 max less than 14 ml/kg/m^2 have a significantly reduced one-year survival with medical therapy independent of resting cardiac output, pulmonary capillary wedge pressure or pulmonary pressures.

Third, premature atherosclerosis has been described in HIV+ patients, particularly those receiving HAART therapy, and stress testing may be helpful to screen for ischemia upon exertion. Noninvasive stress testing with dobutamine challenge can also be performed to detect focal ischemia, myocyte viability and residual ischemia.

Ultrafast Electron Beam Computerized Tomography

Ultrafast electron beam computerized tomography (EBCT) scans 3-mm sections of the coronary arteries to detect calcium accumulation, which correlates strongly with the severity of coronary atherosclerosis. This noninvasive test is used to calculate a coronary calcium score; these scores have about 90% sensitivity for detecting early coronary heart disease (CHD) and nearly 100% sensitivity for advanced disease.[22–24] The coronary calcium score gives a fairly good estimate of the total coronary plaque burden, which is a good predictor of future coronary events. The scores may be useful for assessing the risk of coronary plaque rupture, the cause of acute coronary syndromes such as myocardial infarction and unstable angina pectoris.

Coronary calcium measurements have several limitations. They have limited ability to identify obstructive coronary atherosclerosis (coronary artery disease), the cause of angina pectoris. It is also not clear whether coronary calcium scores predict CHD independently of standard risk factors such as cigarette smoking, hypertension, elevated low-density lipoprotein cholesterol (LDL-C), low high-density lipoprotein cholesterol (HDL-C), and family history of premature CHD.

Baseline and annual EBCT examinations may be useful in HIV+ patients on HAART therapy, but the clinical utility of EBCT screening in this population has not been tested. EBCT may assist with risk assessment in HIV+ patients on HAART; in these patients, the risk of CHD is not known, and high coronary calcium scores would identify patients who might benefit from more aggressive risk reduction interventions.

Other Tests of Subclinical Atherosclerosis

Early atheroscleosis involves the endothelium of many arteries[25,26] and information about peripheral arterial anatomy and function might be pertinent to the coronary circulation. Such information can be derived from vascular imaging studies such as studies of brachial artery reactivity and carotid intima medial thickness, or from the ankle-brachial blood pressure index. These tests might be used as indications or guides for preventive cardiology therapy in HAART-treated patients, but their application in clinical practice has been limited.

Recent reviews[25,26] of work in adults without HIV infection have concluded that flow-mediated dilation is abnormal in atherosclerotic vessels, and that abnormal dilation is associated with cardiovascular risk factors and may be a marker of preclinical disease. Treating atherosclerotic risk factors improves flow-mediated dilation, and some data suggest that vascular responsiveness is related to outcome. In these HIV⁻ patients, carotid intima medial thickness is associated with cardiovascular risk factors, and increased levels can predict myocardial infarction and stroke. Aggressive risk factor management can decrease intima medial thickness. The reviews concluded that brachial artery reactivity and carotid intima medial thickness are functional and structural markers of the atherosclerotic process.

The clinical use of brachial artery reactivity has been limited by varying reproducibility, concomitant illnesses such as diabetes mellitus or hypertension, and the influence of exogenous factors. This study may be more useful in patients who have no obstructive disease present because it will describe the physiologic state.

In contrast, carotid intima media thickness exhibits less variability. Measurements of carotid intima media may be more useful in patients with endothelial dysfunction and suspected thickening of the far wall of the common carotid when a cardiovascular risk factor is present. Studies of carotid intima medial thickness may be helpful in assessing the effects of antiatherosclerotic drug therapy. However, in patients without HIV infection, it has yet to be demonstrated that an improvement in response to treatment results in improvement in prognosis.

Unfortunately, the great vessels in HIV⁺ patients are more dilated than those in other subjects,[27] a phenomenon that creates problems in interpreting carotid artery intima medial thickness studies and diameter measured by B-mode sonography. Similarly, the use of brachial artery reactivity as a marker of endothelial function and a screen for premature coronary heart disease is confounded in HIV⁺ patients by autonomic abnormalities and endothelial HIV infection.

Cardiac magnetic resonance imaging has high sensitivity and specificity for *ex vivo* plaque characterization. Although it may be feasible in the clinical setting in the near future, it is currently experimental and expensive.[25,26] Early use of ultrasound plaque tissue characterization, another experimental technique, may help predict events by distinguishing soft plaques likely to rupture from calcified plaques unlikely to do so. Tissue characterization should be considered if there is plaque formation.

Intravascular ultrasound can provide detailed images of the artery and assess the volume, content, and vulnerability of coronary plaques.[28] However, the relationship between plaque volume and cardiovascular events has not yet been established,[28] and invasive studies for coronary artery disease are risky in HIV⁺ patients.

Nuclear Cardiology

Indium-111-antimyosin antibody scanning may be useful for detecting myocarditis in HIV[+] patients and for distinguishing acute coronary syndromes from myocarditis in patients with clinical symptoms.[29] Perfusion studies at rest or with exercise may help diagnose coronary artery disease in HIV[+] patients on HAART. Tagged white blood cell scans or nuclear stress evaluations may also be useful.

Catheterization and Biopsy

For HIV[+] patients with congestive heart failure of unclear etiology that has not responded to two weeks of anticongestive therapy, cardiac catheterization with endomyocardial biopsy may be indicated.[30–32] The finding of CMV inclusions or other histologic evidence of infection may direct therapy. The presence of abnormal mitochondria may suggest the need for a drug holiday from antiretroviral therapy. The presence of myocarditis may suggest immunomodulatory therapy.[33] Positive results on a viral polymerase chain reaction (PCR) may suggest myocardial infections not apparent histologically.[33] Angiography may be indicated for patients with suspected coronary artery disease.

Pericardiocentesis

Pericardiocentesis in an HIV[+] patient with a pericardial effusion leads to a diagnosis in about 50% of cases and may be useful diagnostically as well as therapeutically.[7,8] Patients with pericardial effusion without tamponade should be evaluated for treatable opportunistic infections such as tuberculosis and for malignancy. HAART should be initiated if it has not yet been. Repeat echocardiography is recommended after one month, or sooner if clinical symptoms of tamponade develop in the interim.

Tests for Treatable Nutritional and Biochemical Causes of Heart Failure

Deficiencies of micronutrients including selenium and carnitine are reversible causes of cardiomyopathy and should be considered in HIV[+] patients with LV dysfunction.[34,35] In patients with unexplained heart failure, the following tests may also be helpful: a complete blood count to determine anemia and other hematologic abnormalities, serum electrolytes for hypocalcemia, hypophosphatemia, hyponatremia, and hypokalemia, and albumin, thyroid-stimulating hormone measurements for hypothyroidism; measurement of iron and ferritin for iron overload or if hemochomatosis is a concern; measurement of serum angiotensin 1-converting enzyme activity is frequently elevated in sarcoid and gives an indication of granuloma load in the body; antinuclear antibody measurements, especially in young women; vanillymandelic acid measurements for pheochromocytoma; tests of amyloid, blood urea nitrogen (BUN), and creatinine, with urinalysis for renal failure; and assessment for hypogonadism and hepatic disease. Growth hormone deficiency can occur in HIV[+] patients and is a reversible cause of cardiomyopathy that can be assessed by blood testing. Consideration for a sleep study should be given if there is evidence of chronic upper airway obstruction or cor pulmonale.

Serum and Plasma Markers of Myocardial Injury and LV Dysfunction

Serum Cardiac Troponin T

For a patient with LV dysfunction, serum cardiac troponin T (cTnT), a biomarker of active myocardial injury, may help identify myocarditis, unstable angina, or acute myocardial infarction.[36,37] This may lead to additional testing such as endomyocardial biopsy for histology and viral PCR panel studies for suspected myocarditis, and stress, viability, and angiographic studies for suspected acute coronary syndromes. In some series, myocarditis was found in the majority of HIV+ adults.[4]

Plasma Brain Natriuretic Peptides

For HIV− patients, the assessment of brain natriuretic peptides (BNP) in the blood is becoming useful for detecting high risk for morbidity or mortality from LV dysfunction.[38–40] Pro-BNP and N terminal pro-BNP (NT-proBNP) can be commercially assayed to assess the severity of damage in congestive heart failure and help provide a differential diagnosis.[38–40] A number of diseases are associated with increases in natriuretic peptides including: acute or chronic systolic or diastolic heart failure; left ventricular hypertrophy; inflammatory cardiac disease (e.g., myocarditis, cardiac allograft rejection); systemic arterial hypertension with left ventricular hypertrophy; pulmonary hypertension; acute or chronic renal failure; ascitic liver cirrhosis; endocrine diseases (e.g., primary hyperaldosteronism, Cushing's syndrome); and paraneoplastic increases (e.g., small-cell lung cancer).

Blood Inflammatory Markers

Elevations of markers of inflammation have been shown to be predictive of increased subsequent coronary artery disease in HIV− patients. Inflammation has recently emerged as an important contributing factor to the formation of atherosclerotic plaques, and this mechanism may be an even greater contributor in HIV disease.[41] They have not been formally studied in HIV+ patients. Measurements of these substances may be confounded by coexisting health problems in HIV+ patients, and thus such measurements may be less useful than in other patients. Studies in this population would be useful.

General Inflammatory Markers

These include general inflammatory markers that are potential biochemical surrogates, such as highly sensitive C reactive protein (hsCRP), serum amyloid A, and fibrinogen. C-reactive protein is an acute phase protein produced by the liver in response to inflammation or infection, and inflammation is considered to be an etiologic factor in cardiovascular events such as myocardial infarction and stroke. Elevated hsCRP concentrations predict risk for first myocardial infarction, and recent studies[41–46] have shown that even minor elevations in hsCRP that are within the normal reference range are strongly associated with an increased risk of future myocardial infarction, stroke, and peripheral artery disease. The hsCRP may be linked to atherosclerosis by a direct vascular effect, a prothrombotic effect, a lipid peroxidation effect, a marker of environmental or infectious stimulus, a surrogate of interleukin-6 and cellular cytokines, a marker of monocyte and macrophage activity, or a generalized inflammation reflecting underlying endothelial dysfunction and degree of inflammation within the atherosclerotic lesion. In a recent study in postmenopausal women, high sensitivity CRP was the strongest single predictor of the risk of cardiovascular events.[44] The hsCRP elevations were predictive even in women with normal LDL levels.[44] The addition of hsCRP measurements to cholesterol screening may improve the ability to identify those at risk for cardiovascular events.[44] The peak hsCRP value is also associated with a greater risk of post-infarct morbidity and mortality. After the first infarct, elevated hsCRP is related to the incidence of subsequent cardiac events. Elevated hsCRP is associated with stroke and peripheral artery atherothrombotic disease.

Cytokines

Cytokines released from macrophages are considered probable promoters of inflammation because increases are associated with a general inflammatory response. Cytokines including tissue necrosis factor-alpha (TNF-α), TNF-α receptor, and interleukin-6 have also been studied as potential inflammatory biochemical surrogates.[41]

Endothelial Adhesion Molecules

Most intracellular adhesion molecules (ICAM) and vascular cellular adhesion molecules (VCAM) are cell-bound, but the soluble forms that leak into the plasma (sICAM and sVCAM) can be measured. These cellular adhesion molecules are thought to be play an important role in initiating atherosclerosis by assisting in both the adhesion of circulating leukocytes to endothelial cells and transendothelial migration. Levels of cellular adhesion molecules are increased by inflammatory cytokines such as interleukin-1, TNF, and interferon, and are expressed on the endothelial membrane. Found in many components of plaque, they may have a role in atherothrombosis and, along with e-selectin, have been studied as potential inflammatory biochemical surrogates.[41] ICAM has a direct, potentially critical role in early immune responses and is a direct mediator in inflammation response. There is a significant correlation between levels of ICAM and fibrinogen, suggesting that fibrinogen may mediate leukocyte adhesion to endothelium via a ICAM-mediated pathway. The risk of CAD in patients with elevated ICAM increases over time.

Lesion Lytic Enzymes

Lesion lytic enzymes include the matrix metalloproteinases (MMP) MMP-1, MMP-2, MMP-3, and MMP-9, are also potential inflammatory biochemical surrogates. Antibody staining shows high levels of MMP in both animal and human atherosclerotic lesions. These MMPs can also be measured in circulating plasma.[41]

Procoagulant and Fibrinolytic Biomarkers

These substances have been proposed as potential markers and possible targets for atherosclerotic interventions.[41] Potential procoagulant (thrombotic) biochemical surrogates include homocysteine, fibrinogen, factor VII (antigen/activity), activated protein C resistance, factor Xa, fibrinopeptide A, factor iX, fragments F1 and F2, and thrombin-antithrombin complex. Potential thrombolytic biochemical surrogates include tissue plasminogen activator antigen, plasminogen activator inhibitor antigen, D-dimer, and lipoprotein(a).

Lipoprotein-Associated Phospholipase A2

The enzyme lipoprotein-associated phospholipase A2 (Lp-PLA2) has recently been identified as a risk factor for coronary artery disease that is independent of classic risk factors. This molecule binds low-density lipoprotein and mediates LDL-associated vascular inflammation.[47] Lp-PLA2 is responsible for the release of highly bioactive products from oxidized LDL phospholipids that are chemoattractants for monocytes and play a role in proinflammatory LDL vascular wall injury, an antherosclerotic risk factor independent of the generalized inflammatory processes reflected in the blood levels of hsCRP.[48–50] Drugs that inhibit Lp-PLA2 are currently in clinical trials (SB-435495).

Lipid Profiles for Preventive Cardiology

Long-term therapy with protease inhibitors and HAART, although effective in prolonging life and disease-free survival, have deleterious effects on cardiovascular health. The mechanism of HAART-associated premature atherosclerosis is unclear, as is its incidence and severity.[51] Lipid profiles and other blood tests for preventive cardiology should be routine before and during HAART therapy. A number of biochemical surrogates have been targeted.

Before HAART is started, lipid profiles should be measured after an 8–12 hour fast to establish a baseline, and the measurements should be repeated routinely during the HAART therapy.[51] Serum glucose and hemoglobin A1C measurements are especially indicated for patients on HAART.

Fasting lipids and glucose should be measured before the initiation of protease inhibitors and at regular 3–6 month intervals thereafter.[51] For patients with elevated triglyceride levels at baseline, lipid measurements should be repeated within 1–2 months of starting HAART. If fasting triglyceride levels are above 400 mg/dL, then the calculated LDL-C level will be unreliable.[51]

Low-density lipoprotein cholesterol is currently the primary therapeutic target for cardiovascular disease, but other lipoproteins (HDL, apolipoprotein-B, and lipoprotein[a]) may also be useful for stratifying HIV⁻ patients by risk for cardiovascular disease.[52] Other potential biochemical lipid surrogates include triglycerides, HDL subfractions (HDL$_2$C/HDL$_3$C), LDL fractions (small, dense/pattern B), remnant particles, apolipoprotein A1, lipoprotein A1 particles, apolipoprotein CIII, lipoprotein CIII: Non-B (HDL apolipoprotein CIII). Nuclear magnetic resonance spectroscopy can identify small, dense low-density lipoprotein particles, which are important predictors of the risk of ischemic heart disease.[53,54] Other potential biochemical surrogates of CAD, as discussed above, include: lipid/apolipoprotein; procoagulant/fibrinolytic substances; inflammatory molecules; adhesion molecules; and lesion lytic enzymes.

Genetic Testing

Some aspects of genetic predisposition to heart disease can now be detected through commercially available assays, although the specific value of the results to HIV⁺ patients has not been studied.

The β$_2$-adrenergic receptor polymorphism plays a role in the pathogenesis of the failing ventricle. HIV⁻ patients with the 164Iie variant and heart failure may be candidates for earlier aggressive intervention or cardiac transplantation and this may be helpful in HIV$^+$ patients to identify a high-risk group for LV dysfunction.

Patients with non-HIV-associated cardiomyopathies may have any of a number of contractile protein gene abnormalities, many of which can be assessed.

Homozygous mutations (C677T and A1298C) of the MTHFR gene are responsible for increased plasma homocysteine levels, a risk factor for arteriosclerosis, vascular disease, and deep vein thrombosis.

Platelet glycoprotein IIIa PIA2 variant appears to be associated with premature atherosclerotic coronary artery disease, acute thrombotic complications, stroke, and sudden death of young individuals due to acute myocardial infarction.

The plasminogen activator inhibitor-1 gene 4G/5G polymorphism can be commercially measured and influences the plasma concentration of PAI-1, which is related to the extent of atherosclerosis in the vessel wall and is a reliable predictor of coronary events in patients with angina pectoris. Hyperinsulinemia was associated with increased levels of tissue plasminogen activator and PAI-1 in HIV$^+$ adults.

The interleukin-1 receptor antagonist gene encodes a protein that suppresses inflammation by blocking the actions of IL-1.[55] IL-1 polymorphisms include a variation that prevents restenosis in 48% of white Americans. This polymorphism can identify individuals with a 40 to 50% risk of restenosis at 6–9 months after a first procedure. The results of this test could identify patients who would benefit from aggressive follow-up after bypass surgery or could support a decision to select angioplasty instead.

Autoantibodies to oxidized palmitoyl aracidonoyl phosphocholine (phospholipid) are significantly higher in patients with hypertension and patients with previous infarction than in age- and sex-matched controls. These autoantibodies may serve as an autoimmune marker for the diagnosis of atherosclerosis.

The D/D genotype of the α_2B-adrenoceptor is a novel genetic risk factor for acute coronary events.[56] The angiotensin-1 converting enzyme D/D genotype is associated with consistently higher ACE activity, plaque instability, risk for plaque rupture, unstable angina, and premature myocardial infarction. This genotype is also associated with a significantly poorer transplant-free survival in patients with systolic dysfunction, especially in patients not treated with a β-blocker.[57,58]

Traditional Cardiovascular Risk Profiling

As with any patient, long-term cardiovascular risk factors must be addressed. Clinicians should identify risk factors such as a history of tobacco use, a family history of premature atherosclerosis, poor diet, high alcohol intake, lack of physical exercise, older age, diabetes, dyslipidemia, hypertriglyceridemia, hypertension, menopausal status, cocaine use, and heroin use. Other important risk factors are a family or patient history of hypothyroidism, renal disease, liver disease, or hypogonadism.

The global risk profile for coronary artery disease is based on seven factors identified from the Framingham study: age, sex, systolic or diastolic blood pressure, HDL cholesterol, total cholesterol, cigarette smoking, and diabetes.[59]

Commercially available, evidence-based programs are available to calculate risk for coronary artery disease, type II diabetes, and stroke from the patient's clinical signs and symptoms, results of laboratory tests, and family history. Although these products use only conventional risk factors, they may still be of use for HIV$^+$ patients.

Screening for Hypertension

Routine assessment of blood pressure in HIV$^+$ patients is important because these patients seem to be at higher risk of developing hypertension and of developing it at a younger age than the general population.[60] Predisposing conditions include such as vasculitis, acquired glucocorticoid resistance, acute and chronic renal failure, atherosclerosis, and drug interactions (e.g., the interaction between indinavir and stavudine-phenylproanolamine).[60] The true prevalence of hypertension in HIV$^+$ patients is unknown. Echocardiography is useful in assessing for increased LV mass in patients with systemic hypertension or to assess right ventricular pressure in a patient with suspected pulmonary hypertension.

PREVENTING AND TREATING CARDIOVASCULAR DISEASE IN HIV$^+$ PATIENTS

Preventing cardiovascular disease is always preferable to treating it after it has developed. Prevention is particularly important for HIV$^+$ patients, because full-blown cardiovascular disease is likely to coincide with symptomatic HIV disease, worsening the prognosis for both. No HIV-specific preventive or therapeutic strategies have been developed, but recommendations can be drawn from the evidence-based guidelines developed for the general population. However, medication interactions and side effects may change tolerance, and thus individualized therapy is essential in HIV$^+$ patients.

Cytokine Antagonist Therapy

Because inflammatory mediators, cytokines, and cytokine receptors are being recognized as important risk factors and surrogates in a number of cardiovascular diseases, cytokine antagonism is under active investigation in experimental therapeutic models of heart failure and reperfusion injury.[61] Etanercept, a recombinant TNF-α receptor that acts as a TNF antagonist, was recently tested in 47 HIV$^-$ patients with New York Heart Association class III to class IV heart failure who were already being treated with standard therapy.[62] The study showed a dose-related decline in end-systolic and end-diastolic volumes, a small increase in LV ejection fraction, and a trend toward clinical improvement in the treated patients compared with placebo.[62] Heart rate and blood pressure were not affected, and etanercept therapy was associated with an increase in IL-10 and an improved ratio of anti-inflammatory to pro-inflammatory cytokines.

Pentoxofylline and other modulators of cytokine levels may be effective in preventing or treating HIV-related cardiovascular disease. but they have not been studied in this population.

Immunomodulatory Therapy

Intravenous Immunoglobulin for Preventing
Abnormalities of LV Structure and Function

We have previously demonstrated that monthly IVIG infusion to HIV[+] children without congestive heart failure resulted in significantly less frequent echocardiographic abnormalities of LV structure and function (see FIGURE 1).[18] We continue to encourage use of this immunomodulatory therapy.

Intravenous Immunoglobulin for Treating
Congestive Heart Failure due to Myocarditis

FIGURE 2 illustrates how use of IVIG may also be beneficial in selected HIV[+] children with congestive heart failure refractory to conventional anticongestive therapy. The young child had persistent congestive heart failure of unclear etiology while taking anticongestive therapy. An endomyocardial biopsy revealed myocarditis. Intravenous immunoglobulin therapy was associated with resolution of congestive heart failure. Nine months later the patient died of noncardiac infectious complications, and an autopsy found no evidence of myocarditis or significant fibrosis.

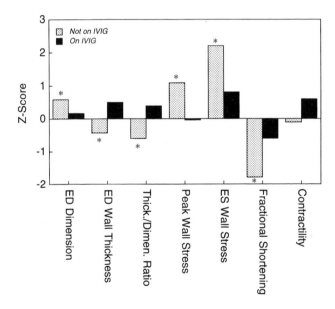

FIGURE 1. Monthly intravenous immunoglobulin (IVIG) therapy is associated with more normal left ventricular structure and function in HIV-infected patients without congestive heart failure.[18] Echocardiographic measurements of left ventricular structure and function in HIV[+] patients without heart failure who received monthly IVIG therapy (*black bars*) and who did not receive IVIG therapy (*shaded bars*). Z-scores indicate number of standard deviations above or below normal (*z*-score = 0) for each parameter. *Asterisks* indicate that the parameter was significantly different from normal. ED, end-diastolic; ES, end-systolic; thick., left ventricular thickness; dimen., left ventricular dimension.

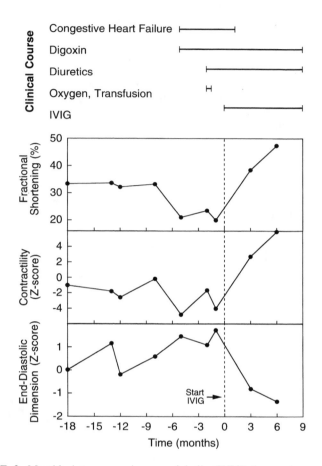

FIGURE 2. Monthly intravenous immunoglobulin (IVIG) therapy is associated with more normal left ventricular structure and function and resolution of congestive heart failure in a HIV⁺ patient with congestive heart failure due to myocarditis. This child with symptomatic HIV infection had serial echocardiographic evaluations that indicated normal left ventricular structure and function for one year prior to developing congestive heart failure. The development of congestive heart failure was associated with a fall in left ventricular fractional shortening, a measure of left ventricular systolic performance, a fall in left ventricular contractility, a measure of the health of the left ventricular myocytes, and an increase in left ventricular dimension, indicating the development of dilated cardiomyopathy. Digoxin was begun at that time without an improvement in symptoms or echocardiographic parameters. Diuretics, oxygen, and blood transfusion therapies were utilized to reduce congestive heart failure without success. A cardiac catheterization with endomyocardial biopsy was performed at time zero that indicated that dilated cardiomyopathy was due to histologically proven myocarditis. At that time monthly IVIG therapy (2 g/kg) was initiated. Clinical congestive heart failure resolved within one week and normalization of the previously documented echocardiographically determined left ventricular structure and function abnormalities occurred at three months on therapy and was sustained on follow-up at six months on therapy. The patients died nine months on IVIG therapy of an opportunistic infection. At autopsy there was no evidence of active myocarditis. In fact, the myocardium was notable for how normal it appeared. There was only trace fibrosis present.

Other Immunomodulatory Options

Some of the immunomodulatory therapies that have been suggested or shown to be useful in non-HIV myocarditis in children include steroids, cyclosporine, azathioprine, and OKT3 (muromonab), an Ig2a immunoglobulin that recognizes, binds, and blocks the CD3 complex of T cell receptors and is thought to block T cell–mediated myocardial injury.[63] Clinical trials would be helpful but are not likely to be done in this population.

Vesnarinone, which reduces TNF-α levels, has both immunomodulatory and anticongestive effects. In one study, it reduced mortality from non-HIV heart failure, but in a larger study, it increased non-HIV heart failure mortality.[64,65] It has also been associated with reduced HIV viral replication and may still be worth studying in an HIV$^+$ population.

In the future, inducing antigen-specific peripheral immune tolerance may be an effective approach for treating myocarditis with autoimmune involvement, as is often found in HIV$^+$ patients.[66]

Nutritional deficiencies, which are common in HIV$^+$ patients, also affect both immune function and LV function. Nutritional supplementation may improve LV function, especially if there are selenium or carnitine deficiencies.[34,35]

Antiinfective Therapy

We have found that viral coinfections increase the risk of symptomatic heart disease in HIV$^+$ patients and that viral DNA is detectable within the hearts of HIV$^+$ patients with congestive heart failure.[5,33] For HIV$^+$ patients with heart failure and evidence of viral coinfection, drugs for non-HIV viral infection may be useful.[67] Intravenous acyclovir is the drug of choice for treatment of serious infections caused by herpes simplex virus or varicella-zoster virus, but famciclovir or valacyclovir may be useful alternatives. Both amantadine and rimantadine are 70 to 90% effective in preventing influenza when started before exposure. Whether these drugs decrease the incidence of influenza-related cardiovascular complications is unknown. Oseltamivir and zanamivir can also decrease the severity and duration of symptoms caused by either influenza A or B. Ribavirin may decrease morbidity with respiratory syncytial virus.

Cytomegalovirus is particularly problematic in HIV heart failure. Cidofovir can delay progression of CMV retinitis and may be considered for CMV-associated heart failure in an HIV$^+$ patient. Fomivirsen is also approved for CMV retinitis in HIV$^+$ patients who cannot tolerate or have not responded to other drugs, but should not be given within 2 to 4 weeks of cidofovir. Foscarnet is effective in acyclovir-resistant HSV and VZV infections and in CMV retinitis, including cases caused by ganciclovir-resistant strains, but has been associated with arrhythmias. Ganciclovir has also been effective in the treatment of CMV infections in AIDS but has also been associated with arrhythmias. Interferon alpha has been useful in hepatitis B and C, but in high doses has been associated with cardiomyopathy.

Heart Failure Therapy

A May 2000 critical review of available evidence for the care of heart failure[68] contains much information that is applicable to HIV$^+$ patients.

Non-Drug Treatments, Including Exercise

Multidisciplinary care addressing nutrition, patient counseling, and patient education reduces hospital admissions for heart failure, may improve quality of life, and enhance patient knowledge.[69] However, other data suggest that multidisciplinary follow-up increases readmission rates.[69]

Prescribed exercise training improved functional capacity and quality of life, and reduced the rate of adverse cardiac events.[70-73] Patients should start slowly and gradually work to a goal of 20 to 30 minutes of medium to hard work. Exercise to the ventilatory threshold is sufficient. However, low-intensity training such as walking around the block is still beneficial both physiologically and in terms of quality of life.

Heart failure patients should be given diuretics to reduce volume overload as much as possible before exercising.

A stress test will establish the patient's baseline and may provide confidence that the exercise can proceed safely. Serial exercise tests are recommended. Patients whose VO_2 does not improve have a poorer prognosis. Tolerance of training may be assessed by serum cardiac troponin measurements.

When heart failure patients start exercising, those with the lowest LV ejection fractions achieve the greatest percentage increase in peak VO_2, suggesting that these patients should be the first to start exercise training. People with systolic dysfunction can undergo exercise training safely without exacerbation of arrhythmia and other problems, and American Heart Association endorsement of exercise for these patients is expected.

The benefits of exercise programs including improved work capacity, oxygen uptake, peripheral vascular resistance, peripheral blood flow, neural hormones, and efficiency of ventilation. Exercise also decreases pressure product and ventilatory threshold, lowers heart rate, and improves symptom scores. Patients who stop exercising lose these benefits. Exercise also has added noncardiac benefits such as gastrointestinal motility, improved respiration, better affect, and reduced risk of osteoporosis. Such improvements seem likely to reduce mortality, protect against arrhythmias, and improve vagal control and autonomic reflex activity.

Drug and Invasive Treatments

Pharmacotherapy for heart failure shifts the survival curve to the right, but patients continue to deteriorate over time. Not every drug that helps initially is necessarily a good long-term treatment. Five agents that are components of standard polypharmacy therapy for heart failure are: digoxin, loop diuretics, ACE inhibitors, aldosterone antagonists, and β-blockers.

Diuretics reduce volume overload and symptoms of dyspnea, but the effect of diuretics on mortality has not been studied. Angiotensin-converting enzyme inhibitors reduce mortality, admission to the hospital for heart failure, and ischemic events in people with heart failure.[74-78] Relative benefits are similar in different groups of people, but absolute benefits are greater in people with severe heart failure.[74-78]

There is no evidence that using ACE inhibitors to treat heart failure due to AIDS is beneficial, but the point can probably be taken on trust in view of the universal benefit of these agents in most other forms of heart failure. Angiotensin II receptor blockers and ACE inhibitors do not seem to differ in their effects on functional capacity and symptoms.[79–82] Angiotensin II receptor blockers have been determined to be at least as good as ACE inhibitors for reducing clinical events (death or admission to the hospital).[79–82] Adding an angiotensin-receptor blocker on top of an ACE inhibitor did not further reduce mortality, although it did reduce the hospitalization rate.[79–82] However, in patients receiving both an ACE inhibitor and a beta-blocker, the addition of an angiotensin-receptor blocker did not lead to any additional benefit. In fact, recent subgroup analysis suggested that it increased mortality. HIV$^+$ patients with nephropathy should receive extra care when treated with ACE inhibitor therapy.

Positive inotropic drugs improve symptoms but do not reduce mortality.[83–85] Many of the non-digoxin-positive inotropic drugs may actually increase mortality.[83–85] Of the positive inotropic agents, only digoxin has been found to improve morbidity in people already receiving diuretics and ACE inhibitors.[83–85] Adding a beta blocker to an ACE inhibitor regimen decreases the rate of death and admission to the hospital.[86–88] Beta blockers may also improve exercise capacity and reduce all-cause mortality.[86–88] Bisoprolol, carvedilol, and metoprolol have been shown to decrease the risk of hospitalization and to lower mortality in patients with mild, moderate, or severe heart failure.[89]

There is no evidence to support the use of calcium channel blockers in heart failure.[90] For patients with severe heart failure, adding an aldosterone receptor antagonist (spironolactone) to ACE inhibitor treatment reduced mortality compared with ACE inhibitors alone.[91] Only weak evidence suggests that amiodarone may reduce mortality in people with heart failure.[92,93] Data extrapolated from people treated after a myocardial infarction suggests that non-amiodarone antiarrhythmic drugs may increase mortality in people with heart failure. Good evidence exists that the implantable cardiac defibrillator reduces mortality in people with heart failure who have experienced a cardiac arrest, but there is conflicting evidence for prophylactic implantation of these devices in people at risk of arrhythmia.[92–98]

The best way to treat heart failure is to prevent it. In people with asymptomatic left ventricular systolic dysfunction, ACE inhibitors delay the onset of symptomatic heart failure and reduce cardiovascular events.[99,100] The HOPE study suggests that in asymptomatic patients with risk factors, such as HIV$^+$ patients on HAART therapy, the ACE inhibitor ramapril may be cost-effective, clinically useful, and worth considering for the prevention of ventricular dysfunction.[101]

HIV$^+$ patients with LV dysfunction should be evaluated and treated for deficiencies in selenium, carnitine, protein, thiamine, thyroid hormone, and growth hormone.

New therapies have been proposed: angiotensin-receptor blockers; neutral endopeptidase inhibitors; endothelin antagonists; cytokine antagonists; vasopressin antagonists; new diuretics; valve repair and high-risk coronary bypass surgery; defibrillators and multisite pacing; left ventricular assist devices; antiremodeling surgery; and gene therapy. Other new therapeutic approaches that may become common in the future include hemodynamic-guided therapy with intermittent and chronic monitoring, LV reduction therapy, cardiac resynchronization, ventricular assist devices, and cellular transplantation.[102,103] These will have to show incremental benefits above standard therapy to be considered useful.

Primary Prevention of Coronary Heart Disease

Aggressive modification of risk factors is recommended for patients without HIV infection who are at high risk of developing CHD.[104] However, the situation for

AIDS patients might be completely different. For example, it would be irresponsible to recommend aggressive statin therapy in such patients without evidence that it is effective.

In this section, we have listed recommendations for primary prevention in patients without HIV infection. Clinicians will have to determine the relative strengths of particular therapies in HIV$^+$ patients.

Preventing Cardiovascular Disease by Exercising[105–153]

Moderate to strenuous physical activity reduces the risk of coronary heart disease and stroke. Sudden death after strenuous exercise is rare, is more common in sedentary people, and does not outweigh the benefits of exercise. Regular exercise programs decrease rates of cardiovascular disease,[154] decrease the frequency of osteoporosis in women,[155] improve function in rheumatoid arthritis,[156] and lower the risk of diabetes.[157]

The effects of exercise on the immune system vary with its intensity. Moderate activity stimulates the immune system, but strenuous activity suppresses NK-cell function, lymphocyte proliferation, immunoglobulin production, and cytokine cascade activation.[158–160] Prolonged strenuous exercise, such as long-distance running, causes a leukocytosis, with an increase in neutrophils and depression of lymphocytes that can persist for up to 6 hours.[161] In many clinical conditions, the biologic effect of exercise on the immune system is unclear, but it appears to be safe in controlled training situations.[162] Exercise should be intense enough and should last long enough to provide benefits for the heart, lungs, and skeletal muscle, but must not be so strenuous as to induce injury.

Chronic illness, such as HIV, is likely to result in decreased physical activity, poor muscle strength, decreased aerobic capacity, and overall deconditioning. Pulmonary function studies of adults with HIV infection have shown lower workload, lower anaerobic threshold, and decreased oxygen utilization compared to an age-matched control group.[163] These conditions appear to be reversible; oxygen utilization improves with aerobic training in HIV$^+$ adults.[164] A retrospective study self-reported exercise patterns in 415 adults with HIV and controls suggested that exercise 3 to 4 times per week had a significant protective effect on HIV disease progression.[165] Studies of progressive resistance and aerobic training in HIV$^+$ adults have been limited, but current data show that exercise helps patients gain lean weight.[166–167] Furthermore, controlled training programs in HIV$^+$ patients have not produced decreases in CD4 lymphocyte counts or increased cytokine activation.[168–170] Strength-resistance training can decrease truncal adiposity, which is part of the fat redistribution syndrome that develops in many HAART-treated patients. In a small pilot study of 10 men, 16 weeks of resistance training significantly improved strength and decreased fat mass, particularly in the trunk.[171]

Encouraging life-long physical activity programs would appear to be even more important as HIV infection becomes a chronic disease. Because HAART may predispose patients to the chronic problems of abnormal lipid metabolism, fat redistribution, insulin resistance, and premature cardiovascular disease, it will be important to determine if exercise programs that benefit people without HIV infection are practical and effective in patients with HIV.

Encouraging a Healthy Diet[172–216]

High consumption of fruits and vegetables is associated with a reduced incidence of ischemic vascular disease. There is no evidence that beta carotene supplements are effective, and in fact they may be harmful. There is insufficient evidence for anti-oxidant supplements in healthy people.

Smoking Cessation[217–226]

There is a strong association between smoking and overall mortality and ischemic vascular disease. The increased risk associated with smoking falls after patients stop smoking, so smoking cessation should be encouraged.

Managing Hypertension[227–259]

Lifestyle interventions reduce blood pressure, but the evidence that these inter-ventions reduce mortality or morbidity is insufficient. Drug treatment reduces blood pressure, and does so more than lifestyle changes. The main determinant of benefit of treatment for hypertension is the pretreatment absolute cardiovascular disease risk. The evidence of beneficial effects on mortality and morbidity is strongest for diuretics and then for beta blockers. Diuretics alone and together with beta blockers have been shown in large-scale clinical trials to decrease mortality in patients with hypertension.

The best tolerated drugs for treatment of hypertension are diuretics (particularly in low doses) and angiotensin II receptor antagonists. β-Adrenergic blockers, ACE inhibitors, and calcium-channel blockers generally have mild adverse effects. Some have recommended that calcium channel blockers should be reserved for patients who do not respond to or cannot tolerate diuretics, beta blockers, ACE inhibitors, or angiotensin II receptor antagonists. ACE inhibitors may be particularly useful in patients with diabetes, especially those with nephropathy, and for patients with heart failure or left ventricular dysfunction. A beta blocker without intrinsic sympathomi-metic activity should be considered for hypertensive patients with angina pectoris, myocardial infarction, or migraine. For patients with hyperlipidemia, an ACE inhib-itor, alpha blocker, or calcium-channel blocker would be potentially useful. In Afri-can-Americans, diuretics and calcium-channel blockers are often more effective than beta blockers, ACE inhibitors, or angiotensin II receptor antagonists. If a drug from one class is ineffective or poorly tolerated, a drug from another class is substi-tuted. If more than one drug is needed the second drug is usually a diuretic.

There is no direct evidence on the effects of lowering blood pressure below 140/80 mm Hg. In people over age 60 with systolic blood pressures higher than 160 mm Hg, lowering systolic blood pressure decreased total mortality and fatal and non-fatal cardiovascular events.

In HIV[+] patients with hypertension, standard treatment based on guidelines from the Joint National Commission (JNC) should be followed as there are no specific sub-population studies at this time.

Antithrombotic Drugs[260–265]

There is insufficient evidence to identify which asymptomatic individuals would benefit overall and which would be harmed by regular treatment with aspirin. The benefits and harms of oral anticoagulation among individuals without symptoms of cardiovascular disease are finely balanced, and net effects are uncertain. Recent studies with clopidogrel antiplatelet therapy indicate that it is more effective compared with aspirin. The CURE study has recently suggested that clopidogrel is useful in unstable angina to prevent recurrent ischemic events.

Lowering Cholesterol[266-280]

Lipid abnormalities in HIV$^+$ patients predate HAART therapy and have included increases in serum triglyceride and cholesterol levels.[51] HIV infection is associated with low HLD-C and LDL-C, lower triglyceride clearance, increased lipoprotein(a), and higher LDL-B phenotype (small, dense LDL-C). Zidovudine has lowered serum triglyceride levels. Protease inhibitors and nonnucleoside reverse transcriptase inhibitor therapy are both associated with increased serum triglyceride and cholesterol levels. In one study, HAART therapy was associated with 47% of patients having serum cholesterol levels in the elevated but treatable range. The chronic abnormalities in lipids and other cardiovascular risk factors associated with HAART may mean the therapy is linked to premature cardiovascular events, but definitive studies showed a link are lacking.

Because pharmacologic treatment to reduce cholesterol in HIV$^+$ patients is complicated by drug interactions, nondrug therapies such as modification of CHD risk factors should be emphasized.[51] The 1994 National Cholesterol Education Program (NCEP) guidelines were recommended as a starting point for HIV$^+$ patients.[51] More recent NCEP guidelines have been published and are important to review (www.nhlbi.nih.gov and JAMA 2001; **285:** 2486–2497). The new guidelines place increased emphasis on therapy for "metabolic syndrome" that is obesity, physical inactivity, high blood pressure, high triglycerides, high blood sugar, high concentrations of LDL-C, low concentrations of HDL-C, insulin resistance, and diabetes. The "metabolic syndrome" is as strong a contributor to early heart disease as cigarette smoking and should be treated with intensive lifestyle changes including weight control, physical activity, and medication. The Guidelines define low HDL-C as less than 40 mg.dL and LDL-C less than 100 mg/dL as optimal.

Because LDL-C calculated values are unreliable in patients with a serum triglyceride level above 400 mg/dL, for patients with serum triglyceride levels above 400 mg/dL, a total cholesterol level above 240 mg/dL or an HDL cholesterol level below 35 mg/dL should prompt dietary interventions. In patients with established CHD or total cholesterol above 400 mg/dL, drug therapy should be considered as a concomitant initial therapy. If HIV-associated wasting is also present, it should be treated before dyslipidemia is treated. Beneficial therapies include dietary and exercise interventions, smoking cessation, obesity reduction, increased physical activity, and treatment of diabetes mellitus and hypertension. Estrogen replacement therapy should be used with caution because of the risk of thrombosis.

In asymptomatic members of the general public, reducing cholesterol concentration lowers the rate of cardiovascular events. However, there is no evidence that cholesterol reduction by any method reduces the overall death rate in people at low baseline risk of cardiovascular events. The combined use of a cholesterol-lowering diet and lipid-lowering drugs reduces cholesterol concentration more than lifestyle interventions alone. In the HIV$^+$ population, a bile acid sequestrant may have fewer side effects than HMG Co-A reductase inhibitors because it is less likely to cause drug interactions. However, cholestyramine and colestipol may be associated with increased triglyceride levels, and their effect on antiviral drug absorption has not been studied. Colesevelam lowers plasma LDL cholesterol and has an additive effect when taken with a statin.[278] It has fewer gastrointestinal side effects and less interference with intestinal absorption of vitamins and drugs compared with other sequestrants.

When exercise, colesevelam, and diet are not enough, certain statin drugs may be added to a diet regimen to: lower LDL cholesterol; raise HDL cholesterol; extend life by reducing the frequency of first and second heart attacks and of bypass surgery and angioplasty; and reduce the risk of stroke and slow progression of atherosclerosis for people with heart attacks or coronary heart disease. Unfortunately, the use of these agents is problematic in HIV$^+$ patients because of their side effects, which include muscle weakness, muscle pain, and elevated hepatic enzymes and because they may interact with protease inhibitors.

Statins may also have immunomodulatory effects. In human endothelial cells and macrophages, atorvastatin, lovastatin, and pravastatin suppressed the induction of major histocompatibility complex class II expression by interferon gamma in a dose-dependent fashion. In addition, statin pretreatment of human endothelial cells and monocyte-macrophages reduced subsequent proliferation of T lymphocytes, suggesting that statins can modulate T-cell activation.[279,280]

For HIV$^+$ patients with dyslipidemia, drug therapy to lower cholesterol may be useful if antiretroviral therapy cannot be changed, interrupted, or delayed.

Preliminary recommendations for the management of dyslipidemia in patients with HIV infection have been devised by the US-based Adult AIDS Clinical Trial Group Cardiovascular Disease Focus Group.[51] For PI-treated HIV$^+$ patients with hypercholesterolemia, treatment with low-dose pravastatin (initial dosage 20 mg/day) or atorvastatin (10 mg/day) is recommended. Careful monitoring of virologic status and creatine kinase values is recommended for patients on these therapies. Fluvastatin and cerivastatin are acceptable alternatives, but data are not available on potential interactions with protease inhibitors. Lovastatin or simvastatin therapy should be avoided because of interactions with protease inhibitors. When treatment with HMG CoA reductase inhibitors (statins) is not appropriate or when patients do not respond to these agents, gemfibrozil (600 mg twice daily) or fenofibrate (200 mg once daily) are reasonable alternatives. Concomitant use of fibrates and statins may increase the risk of skeletal muscle toxicity.

Lowering Triglycerides

Nondrug therapy (diet and exercise) is recommended for patients with fasting serum triglyceride levels of above 200 mg/dL.[51] Dietary and exercise interventions have been successful at reducing serum triglyceride in HIV$^+$ patients. Recommended actions include consulting a dietician, smoking cessation, regular aerobic exercise, weight reduction, decreasing fat intake without excess increases in carbohydrate intake, and replacing some saturated fat with monounsaturated fat. Severe hypertriglyceridemia requires a very low-fat diet, avoidance of free sugars, and decreased alcohol intake. Omega-3-fatty acids as oil or supplements may be helpful.

The cutoff at which isolated hypertriglyceridemia in this population should be treated with drugs is not known. In the absence of CHD risk factors or hypercholes-

TABLE 1. **Cardiovascular actions/ interactions of drugs commonly used in HIV therapy (table continued on next three pages)**

Class	Cardiac Drug Interactions	Cardiac Side Effects
Anti-retroviral		
A) Nucleoside Reverse Tran-scriptase Inhibitors	Zidovudine and dipyridamole	Rare–Lactic acidosis hypotension. Zidovudine: skeletal muscle myopathy, myocarditis, dilated cardi-omyopathy. Zalcitabine: Short-term free radical cardiotoxicity.
B) Non-Nucleoside Reverse- Tran-scriptase Inhibitors	calcium channel blockers, warfarin, beta-blockers, nifedipine, quini-dine, steroids, theophylline. Delavirdine can cause serious toxic effects if given with antiarrhyth-mic drugs and calcium channel blockers.	Delavirdine and vasocontrictors can cause ischemia.
C) Protease Inhibi-tors	Metabolized by cytochrome p-450 and interact with: antimycobacteri-als, antifungals, macrolide and quinolone antibacterials, anti-hista-mines, psychotropic drugs, anti-arrhythmics, cisapride, statins, antiepileptics, anti-neoplastic alkaloids to produce cardiotoxic effects including QT prolongation and torsades de pointes. Sildenafil, amio-darone, lidocaine, quinadine, warfarin (increased levels), 3-hydroxy-3-methylglutaryl coenzyme A reductase inhibitors (HMG co-A reduc-tase inhibitors – lovastatin and simvastatin). Bepridil and PIs should be avoided. Potentially dangerous interactions that require close monitor-ing or dose adjustment can occur between PIs and amiodarone, disopy-ramide, flecainide, lignocaine, mexiletine, propafenone, and quinidine. Co-administration of PIs with astemizole, terfenadine or cisapride is contraindicated due to life-threatening arrhythmias. Many anti-psychotic, antidepressant and anticonvulsant drugs interact with PIs. Some of these interactions are clinically relevant and contra-indicate concomitant use or require dose adjustment. Ritonavir is most potent cytochrome activity (CYP3A) inhibitor and is most likely to interact. Indivavir, amprenavir, and nelfinavir are moderate. Saquinavir has the lowest probability. Some: calcium channel blockers, prednisone, quinine, beta blockers (1.5-3x increase). Decreases theophylline concentrations	Implicated in premature atherosclerosis, dyslipidemia, insulin resis-tance, diabetes mellitus, fat wasting and redistribution.

TABLE 1/continued-1.

Class	Cardiac Drug Interactions	Cardiac Side Effects
Anti-infective		
A) Antibiotics	Rifampin: reduces digoxin therapeutic effect by induction of intestinal P-glycoprotein. Erythromycin: Cytochrome p-450 metabolism and drug interactions. Trimethoprim/ sulfamethoxazole (Bactrim) increases warfarin effects.	Erythromycin: Orthostatic hypotension, ventricular tachycardia, bradycardia, torsades (with drug interactions). Clarithromycin: QT prolongation and torsades de pointes. Trimethoprim/ sulfamethoxazole: Orthostatic hypotension, anaphy-laxis, QT prolongation, torsades de pointes, hypokalemia. Sparfloxacin (fluoroquinolones): QT prolongation
B) Antifungal agents	Amphotericin B: Digoxin toxicity. Ketoconazole or itraconazole: Cytochrome p-450 metabolism and drug interactions—increases levels of sildenafil, warfarin, HMG co-A reductase inhibitors, nifedipine, digoxin.	Amphotericin B: Hypertension, arrhythmia, renal failure, hypokalemia, thrombophlebitis, bradycardia, angioedema, dilated cardiomyopathy. Liposomal formulations still have the potential for electrolyte imbalance and QT prolongation. Ketoconazole, Fluconazole, Itraconazole: QT prolongation and torsades de pointes.
C) Antiviral agents	Ganciclovir: Zidovudine.	Foscarnet: Reversible cardiac failure, electrolyte abnormalities. Ganciclovir: ventricular tachycardia, hypotension
D) Anti-parasitic		Pentamidine: hypotension, QT prolongation, arrhythmias (torsades de pointes), ventricular tachycardia, hyperglycemia, hypoglycemia, sudden death. These effects are enhanced by hypomagnesemia and hypokalemia.

TABLE 1/continued-2.

Class	Cardiac Drug Interactions	Cardiac Side Effects
Chemotherapy agents	Vincristine, Doxorubicin: decrease digoxin level.	Vincristine: arrhythmia, myocardial infarction, cardiomyopathy, cardiac autonomic neuropathy. Recombinant Human Interferon-$\alpha\alpha$: Hypertension, hypotension, tachycardia, ischemic heart disease, acute coronary events including myocardial infarction, dilated cardiomyopathy, ventricular and supraventricular arrhythmias, sudden death, atrioventricular block, periperal vasodilation, increased cardiac work load. Contraindicated in patients with unstable angina or myocardial infarction. Interleukin-2: hypotension, arrhythmia, sudden death, myocardial infarction, dilated cardiomyopathy, cardiac failure, myocardial stunning, capillary leak, thyroid alterations Anthracyclines (Doxorubicin, Daunorubicin, Mitoxantrone): myocarditis, cardiomyopathy, cardiac failure. Liposomal Anthracyclines: As above for doxorubicin but also vasculitis.

TABLE 1/continued-3.

Class	Cardiac Drug Interactions	Cardiac Side Effects
Other		
A) systemic corticosteroids	Corticosteroids: decrease salicylate levels and increase gastric ulceration in combination with salicylates.	Corticosteroids: ventricular hypertrophy, cardiomyopathy, hyperglycemia.
B) Pentoxifylline		Pentoxifylline: decreased triglyceride levels, arrhythmias, chest pain.
C) Growth hormone		Growth hormone: ventricular hypertrophy, activation of the renal angiotension system (hypertension).
D) Megace		Megace: edema, thrombophlebitis, hyperglycemia.
E) Epoetin alpha		Epoetin alpha (erythropoetin): Hypertension, ventricular dysfunction, thrombotic events including myocardial infarction.
F) Anti-histamines: Terfenadine, Astemizole		Terfenidine, Astemizole: QT prolongation, torsades de pointes, sudden death.
G) Cisapride		Cisapride: torsades de pointes.
H) Tricyclic Anti-depressants (Amitriptyline, Doxepine, Desipramine, Imipramine, Clomipramine)		Tricyclic Anti-depressants: QT prolongation in all. Sudden death in desipramine, clomipramine, and imipramine.
I) Antipsychotic Agents (Butyrophenone and Phenotiazine Classes including thioridazine, chlorpromazine, pimozide, sertindole, haloperidol)		Antipsychotic Agents: QT prolongation and torsades de pointes.

terolemia, elevations of above 1000 mg/dL should be considered for treatment to reduce the risk of pancreatitis. This threshold may be even lower in a patient with a history of pancreatitis. Fibric acid analogs such as gemfibrozil and fenofibrate decrease serum triglycerides. These agents individually or in combination have been tested only in a preliminary fashion in HIV$^+$ patients with dyslipidemia but seem effective. Gemfibrozil (in adults 600 mg twice a day 30 minutes before the morning and evening meals) and micronized fenofibrate (in adults, 200 mg once daily) are recommended for patients with hypertriglyceridemia who require drug therapy, and these agents are also considered reasonable initial treatment choices for patients with combined hyperlipidemia. Statins are not generally recommended as first-line therapy for isolated hypertriglyceridemia, but cautious trial addition of a statin may be considered when fibrate therapy does not adequately lower triglyceride levels or when low density lipoprotein-cholesterol levels remain elevated.[51] Niacin, although likely to be effective at reducing elevated triglycerides, is not recommended as a first-line agent because of the frequency of side effects such as cutaneous flushing, pruritus, and insulin resistance.

Impact of Medical Therapy and Revascularization on Atherosclerotic Heart Disease in HIV$^+$ Patients

Although these interventions have been performed in HIV$^+$ patients, their impact has not been formally assessed.

Cardiovascular Complications of Therapeutic Drugs in HIV$^+$ Patients

More than 50 drugs are known to be associated with for the type of ventricular arrhythmia called torsades de pointes (www.torsades.org). This condition places patients at very high risk for sudden arrhythmic death. It can be caused by drugs that delay cardiac repolarization and lengthen the QT interval, usually by blocking cardiac potassium channels. In the last 3 years, terfenadine, astemizole, cisapride, mibefradil, and grepafloxacin were removed from the market because of link with torsades de pointes. Therapies used in HIV$^+$ patients that have been associated with torsades de points include pentamidine, foscarnet, and trimethoprim sulfamethoxazole, among other anti-infective therapies.

TABLE 1 illustrates cardiovascular side-effects and drug intereactions of drugs used to treat HIV$^+$ patients.[281–286]

SUMMARY

Because cardiovascular disease is common in HIV$^+$ patients, and because physical examination is not reliable for diagnosis, baseline and serial echocardiographic monitoring may be essential in detecting early disease and targeting patients who would benefit from early intervention and aggressive early antiretroviral therapy.

Preventing cardiovascular disease in HIV$^+$ patients is preferred to treating cardiovascular disease in symptomatic HIV disease. No HIV-specific preventive cardiovascular strategies have been developed, but evidence-based recommendations can be extrapolated from those in the general population. However, because of medication interactions and side effects, HIV$^+$ patients should receive individualized therapy.

ACKNOWLEDGMENTS

Work reported here was supported in part by research grants from the National Institutes of Health, Bethesda, MD [HL53392, HL59837, HL07937, HD34568, CA68484, CA79060, HD34568].

REFERENCES

1. STARC, T.J. *et al.* 1999. Cardiac complications in children with human immunodeficiency virus infection. Pediatrics **104**(2): e14.
   (9 pages URL:http://www.pediatrics.org/cgi/content/full/104/2/e14; HIV, cardiac disease, pediatrics
2. BARBARO, G. *et al.* 1998. Cardiac involvement in the acquired immunodeficiency syndrome: a multicenter clinical-pathological study. AIDS Res. **14**(12): 1071–1077.
3. ACIERNO, L.J. 1989. Cardiac complications in acquired immunodeficiency syndrome (AIDS): a review. J. Am. Coll. Cardiol. **13**(5): 1144–1154.
4. RERKPATTANAPIPAT, P. *et al.* 2000. Cardiac manifestations of acquired immunodeficiency syndrome. Arch. Intern. Med. **160**: 602–608.
5. LUGINBUHL, L.M. *et al.* 1993. Cardiac morbidity and related mortality in children with HIV infection. JAMA **269**(22): 2869–2875.
6. BARBARO, G. *et al.* 1996. early impairment of systolic and diastolic function in asymptomatic HIV-positive patients: a multicenter echocardiographic and echo-doppler study. AIDS Res. **12**(16): 1559–1563.
7. HEIDENREICH, P.A. *et al.* 1995. Pericardial effusion in AIDS. Incidence and survival. Circulation **92**: 3229–3234.
8. SILVA-CARDOSO, J. *et al.* 1999. Pericardial involvement in human immunodeficiency virus infection. Chest **115**: 418–422.
9. CURRIE, P.F. *et al.* 1995. A review of endocarditis in acquired immunodeficiency syndrome and human immunodeficiency virus infection. Eur. Heart J. **16**(B): 15–18.
10. NAHASS, R.G. *et al.* 1990. Infective endocarditis in intravenous drug users: a comparison of human immunodeficiency virus type 1-negative and -positive patients. J. Infect. Dis. **162**: 967–970.
11. JENSON, H.B. & B.H. POLLOCK. 1998. Cardiac cancers in HIV-infected patients. *In* Cardiology in AIDS. S.E. Lipshultz, Ed.: 255–263. Chapman & Hall. New York.
12. SAIDI, A. & J.T. BRICKER. 1998. Pulmonary hypertension in patients infected with HIV. *In* Cardiology in AIDS. S.E. Lipshultz, Ed.: 187–193. Chapman & Hall. New York.
13. HIMELMAN, R.B. *et al.* 1989. Severe pulmonary hypertension and cor pulmonale in the acquired immunodeficiency syndrome. Am. J. Cardiol. **64**: 1396–1399.
14. AARONS, E.J. & F.J. NYE. 1991. Primary pulmonary hypertension and HIV infection. AIDS **5**: 1276–1277.
15. COPLAN, N.L. *et al.* 1990. Primary pulmonary hypertension associated with human immunodeficiency viral infection. Am. J. Med. **89**: 96–99.
16. LIPSHULTZ, S.E. *et al.* 1998. Left ventricular structure and function in children infected with human immunodeficiency virus. The Prospective P^{2}C^2 HIV Multicenter Study. Circulation **97**: 1246–1256.
17. LIPSHULTZ, S.E. *et al.* 2000. Cardiac dysfunction and mortality in HIV-infected children. The Prospective P^{2}C^2 HIV Multicenter Study. Circulation **102**: 1542–1548.
18. LIPSHULTZ, S.E. *et al.* 1995. Immunoglobulins and left ventricular structure and function in pediatric HIV infection. Circulation **92**(8): 2220–2225.

19. FREEMAN, R. *et al.* 1990. Autonomic function and human immunodeficiency virus infection. Neurology **40**(4): 575–580.
20. WHARTON, J.M. *et al.* 1987. Torsades des pointes during administration of pentamidine isethionate. Am. J. Med. **83**: 571–576.
21. EISENHAUER, M.D. *et al.* 1994. Incidence of cardiac arrhythmias during intravenous pentamidine therapy in HIV-infected patients. Chest **105**: 389–395.
22. ARAD, Y. *et al.* 2000. Prediction of coronary events with electron beam computed tomography. J. Am. Coll. Cardiol. **36**: 1253–1260.
23. HECHT, H.S. & H. R. SUPERKO. 2001. Electron beam tomography and national cholesterol education program guidelines in asymptomatic women. J. Am. Coll. Cardiol. **37**: 1506–1511.
24. GRUNDY, S.M. 2001. Coronary calcium as a risk factor: role in global risk assessment. J. Am. Coll. Cardiol. **37**: 1512–1515.
25. FATHI, R. & T.H. MARWICK. 2001. Noninvasive tests of vascular function and structure: why and how to perform them. Am. Heart J. **141**: 694–703.
26. BARTH, J.D. 2001. Which tools are in your cardiac workshop? Carotid ultrasound, endothelial function, and magnetic resonance imaging. Am. J. Cardiol. **87**(suppl): 8A–14A.
27. LAI, W.W. *et al.* 2001. Dilation of the aortic root in children infected with human immunodeficiency virus type 1: The Prospective P^2C^2 HIV Multicenter Study. Am. Heart J. **141**: 661–670.
28. NISSEN, S. 2001. Coronary angiography and intravascular ultrasound. Am. J. Cardiol. **87**(Suppl.): 15A–20A.
29. SARDA, L. *et al.* 2001. Myocarditis in patients with clinical presentation of myocardial infarction and normal coronary angiograms. J. Am. Coll. Cardiol. **37**: 786–792.
30. MOORTHY, L.N. & S.E. LIPSHULTZ. 1998. Cardiovascular monitoring of HIV-infected patients. *In* Cardiology in AIDS. S.E. Lipshultz, Ed.: 345–386. Chapman and Hall. New York.
31. GIANTRIS, A. & S.E. LIPSHULTZ. 1998. Cardiac therapeutics in HIV-infected patients. *In* Cardiology in AIDS. S.E. Lipshultz, Ed.: 387–422. Chapman and Hall. New York.
32. GIANTRIS, A. & S.E. LIPSHULTZ. 1999. Cardiac Disease. *In* AIDS Therapy. R. Dolin, *et al.*, Eds.: 680–698. Churchill Livingston, Inc. New York.
33. BOWLES, N.E. *et al.* 1999. The detection of viral genomes by polymerase chain reaction in the myocardium of pediatric patients with advanced HIV disease. J. Am. Coll. Cardiol. **34**: 857–865.
34. HOFFMAN, M. *et al.* 1999. Malnutrition and cardiac abnormalities in the HIV-infected patient. *In* Nutritional Aspects of HIV Infection. T.L. Miller & S. Gorbach, Eds.: 133–139. Arnold. London.
35. MILLER, T.L. *et al.* 1997. Nutritional status and cardiac mass and function in children infected with the human immunodeficiency virus. Am. J. Clin. Nutr. **66**: 660–664.
36. LIPSHULTZ, S.E. *et al.* 1997. Predictive value of cardiac troponin T in pediatric patients at risk for myocardial injury. Circulation **96**: 2641–2648.
37. OTTLINGER, M. *et al.* 1998. New developments in the biochemical assessment of myocardial injury in children: troponin T and I as highly sensitive and specific markers of myocardial injury. Prog. Pediatr. Cardiol. **8**: 71–81.
38. MAIR, J. 2001. The utility of brain natriuretic peptides in patients with heart failure and coronary artery disease. *In* Markers in Cardiology: Current and Future Clinical Applications. J.E. Adams *et al.*, Eds.: 235–262. Futura Publishing Co. Armonk, NY.
39. CHEN, H.H. & J.C. BURNETT. 1999. The natriuretic peptides in heart failure: diagnostic and therapeutic potentials. Proc. Assoc. Am. Physicians **111**: 406–416.
40. TSUTAMOTO, T. *et al.* 1999. Plasma brain natriuretic peptide level as a biochemical marker of morbidity and mortality in patients with asymptomatic or minimally symptomatic left ventricular dysfunction. Eur. Heart J. **20**: 1799–1807.
41. STEIN, E. 2001. Laboratory surrogates for anti-atherosclerotic drug development. Am. J. Cardiol. **87**(Suppl.): 21A–26A.

42. RIDKER, P.M. 2001. High-sensitivity C-reactive protein: a novel inflammatory marker for predicting the risk of coronary artery disease. *In* Markers in Cardiology: Current and Future Clinical Applications. J.E. Adams *et al.*, Eds.: 173–184. Futura Publishing Co. Armonk, NY.

43. RIDKER, P.M. *et al.* 1997. Inflammation, aspirin, and the risk of cardiovascular disease in apparently healthy men. N. Engl. J. Med. **336:** 973–979.

44. RIDKER, P.M. *et al.* 2000. C-reactive protein and other markers of inflammation in the prediction of cardiovascular disease in women. N. Engl. J. Med. **342:** 836–843.

45. RIFAI, N. *et al.* 1999. Clinical efficacy of an automated high-sensitivity C-reactive protein assay. Clin. Chem. **45:** 2136–2141.

46. HAVERKATE, F. *et al.* 1997. Production of C-reactive protein and risk of coronary events in stable and unstable angina. Lancet **349:** 462–466.

47. PACKARD, C.J. *et al.* 2000. Lipoprotein associated phospholipase A2 as an independent predictor of coronary heart disease. N. Engl. J. Med. **343:** 1148–1155.

48. HAKKINEN, T. *et al.* 1999. Lipoprotein-associated phospholipase A(2), platelet–activating factor acetylhydrolase, is expressed by macrophages in human and rabbit atherosclerotic lesions. Arterioscler. Thromb. Vasc. Biol. **19:** 2909–2917.

49. TEW, D.G. *et al.* 1996. Purification, properties, sequencing, and cloning of a lipoprotein-associated, serine-dependent phospholipase involved in the oxidative modification of low-density lipoproteins. Arterioscler. Thromb. Vasc. Biol. **16:** 591–599.

50. MACPHEE, C.H. *et al.* 1999. Lipoprotein-associated phospholipase A2, platelet-activating factor acetylhydrolase, generates two bioactive products during the oxidation of low-density lipoprotein: use of a novel inhibitor. Biochem. J. **338:** 479–487.

51. DUBE, M.P. *et al.*, ADULT AIDS CLINICAL TRIAL GROUP CARDIOVASCULAR DISEASE FOCUS GROUP. 2000. Preliminary guidelines for the evaluation and management of dyslipidemia in adults infected with human immunodeficiency virus and receiving antiretroviral therapy: recommendations of the Adult AIDS Clinical Trial Group Cardiovascular Disease Focus Group. Clin. Infect. Dis. **31:** 11216–11224.

52. ORLOFF, D.G. 2001. Use of surrogate endpoints: a practical necessity in lipid-altering and antiatherosclerosis drug development. Am. J. Cardiol. **87**(Suppl.): 35A–41A.

53. OTVOS, J.D. 2000. Measurement of lipoprotein subclass profiles by nuclear magnetic resonance spectroscopy. *In* Handbook of Lipoprotein Testing, 2nd edit. N. Rifai, Ed.: 609–623. AACC. Washington, DC.

54. LAMARCHE, B. *et al.* 1997. Small, dense low-density lipoprotein particles as a predictor of the risk of ischemic heart disease in men. Prospective results from the Quebec Cardiovascular Study. Circulation **95:** 69–75.

55. KASTRATI, A. *et al.* 2000. Protective role against restenosis from an interleukin-1 receptor antagonist gene polymorphism in patients treated with coronary stenting. J. Am. Coll. Cardiol. **36:** 2168–2173.

56. SNAPIR, A. *et al.* 2001. An insertion/deletion polymorphism in the alpha$_{2B}$-adrenergic receptor gene is a novel genetic risk factor for acute coronary events. J. Am. Coll. Cardiol. **37:** 1516–1522.

57. MCNAMARA, D.M. *et al.* 2001. Pharmacogenetic interactions between beta-blocker therapy and the angiotensin-converting enzyme deletion polymorphism in patients with congestive heart failure. Circulation **103:** 1644–1648.

58. RODEN, D.M. & N.J. BROWN. 2001. Preprescription genotyping. Not yet ready for prime time, but getting there. Circulation **103:** 1608–1610.

59. WILSON, P.W.F. *et al.* 1998. Prediction of coronary heart disease using risk factor categories. Circulation **97:** 1837–1847.

60. AOUN, S. & E. RAMOS. 2000. Hypertension in the HIV-infected patient. Curr. Hypertension Rep. **2:** 478–481.

61. PARMLEY, W.W. 2001. How many medicines do patients with heart failure need? Circulation **103:** 1611–1612.

62. BOZKURT, B. *et al.* 2001. Results of targeted anti-TNF therapy with Etanercept (ENBREL) in patients with advanced heart failure. Circulation **103:** 1044–1047.

63. AHDOOT, J. *et al.* 2000. Use of OKT3 for acute myocarditis in infants and children. J. Heart. Lung. Transplant. **19:** 1118–1121.

64. FELDMAN, A.M. *et al.* 1993. Effects of vesnarinone on morbidity and mortality in patients with heart failure. N. Engl. J. Med. **329:** 149–155.
65. COHN, J.N. *et al.*, for the Vesnarinone Trial Investigators. 1998. A dose-dependent increase in mortality with vesnarinone among patients with severe heart failure. N. Engl. J. Med. **339:** 1810–1816.
66. GODSEL, L.M. *et al.* 2001. Prevention of autoimmune myocarditis through the induction of antigen-specific peripheral immune tolerance. Circulation **103:** 1709–1714.
67. ANONYMOUS. 1999. Drugs for non-HIV viral infections. Med. Lett. **41:** 113–120.
68. MCKELVIE, R. 2000. Heart failure. Clinical Evidence **4:** 34–50.
69. RICH, M.W. 1999. Heart failure disease management: 1 critical review. J. Card. Fail. **5:** 64–75.
70. MILLER, T.D. *et al.* 1997. Exercise and its role in the prevention and rehabilitation of cardiovascular disease. Ann. Behav. Med. **19:** 220–229.
71. DRACUP, K. *et al.* 1994. Management of heart failure. II. Counseling, education and lifestyle modification. JAMA **272:** 1442–1446.
72. EUROPEAN HEART FAILURE TRAINING GROUP. 1998. Experience from controlled trials of physical training in chronic heart failure. Protocol and patient factors in effectiveness in the improvement in exercise tolerance. Eur. Heart. J. **19:** 466–475.
73. BELARDINELLI, R. *et al.* 1999. Randomized, controlled trial of long-term moderate exercise training in chronic heart failure. Effects on functional capacity, quality of life, and clinical outcomes. Circulation **99:** 1173–1182.
74. GARG, R. *et al.* for the COLLABORATIVE GROUP ON ACE INHIBITOR TRIALS. 1995. Overview of randomized trials of angiotensin-converting enzyme inhibitors on mortality and morbidity in patients with heart failure. JAMA **273:** 1450–1456.
75. GHEORGHIADE, M. *et al.* 1997. Pharmacotherapy for systolic dysfunction; a review of randomized clinical trials. Am. J. Cardiol. **80**(Suppl. 8B): 14–27H.
76. YUSUF, S. *et al.* 1992. Effect of enalapril on myocardial infarction and unstable angina in patients with low ejection fractions. Lancet **340:** 1173–1178.
77. PACKER, M. *et al.*, on behalf of the ATLAS STUDY GROUP. 1999. Comparative effects of low and high doses of the angiotensin-converting enzyme inhibitor, lisinopril, on morbidity and mortality in chronic heart failure. Circulation **100:** 2312–2318.
78. SOLVD INVESTIGATORS. 1991. Effect of enalapril on survival in patients with reduced left ventricular ejection fractions and congestive heart failure. N. Engl. J. Med. **325:** 293–302.
79. SHARMA, D. *et al.*, and the LOSARTAN HEART FAILURE MORTALITY META-ANALYSIS STUDY GROUP. 2000. Meta-analysis of observed mortality data from all-controlled, double blind, multiple-dose studies of losartan in heart failure. Am. J. Cardiol. **85:** 187–192.
80. RIEGGER, G.A.J. *et al.*, for the SYMPTOM, TOLERABILITY, RESPONSE TO EXERCISE TRIAL OF CANDESARTAN CILEXETIL IN HEART FAILURE (STRETCH) INVESTIGATORS. 1999. Improvement in exercise tolerance and symptoms of congestive heart failure during treatment with candesartan cilexetil. Circulation **100:** 2224–2230.
81. MCKELVIE, R. *et al.*, for the RESOLVD INVESTIGATORS. 1999. Comparison of candesartan, enalapril, and their combination in congestive heart failure: randomized evaluation of strategies for left ventricular dysfunction (RESOLVD pilot study). Circulation **100:** 1056–1064.
82. HAMROFF, G. *et al.* 1999. Addition of angiotensin II receptor blockade to maximal angiotensive-converting enzyme inhibition improves exercise capacity in patients with severe congestive heart failure. Circulation **99:** 990–992.
83. KRAUS, F. *et al.* 1993. Wirksamkeit von Digitalis bei Patienten mit chronischer Herzinsuffizienz und Sinusrhythmus. Herz **18:** 95–117.
84. DIGITALIS INVESTIGATION GROUP. 1997. The effect of digoxin on mortality and morbidity in patients with heart failure. N. Engl. J. Med. **336:** 525–533.
85. PACKER, M. *et al.*, for the PROMISE STUDY RESEARCH GROUP. 1991. Effect of oral milrinone on mortality in severe chronic heart failure. N. Engl. J. Med. **325:** 1468–1475.
86. CIBIS-II INVESTIGATORS AND COMMITTEES. 1999. The cardiac insufficiency bisoprolol study II (CIBIS-II): a randomised trial. Lancet **353:** 9–13.

87. MERIT-HF STUDY GROUP. 1999. Effect of metroprolol CR/XL in chronic heart failure: metoprolol CR/XL randomised intervention trial in congestive heart failure. Lancet **353**: 2001–2007.
88. LECHAT, P. *et al.* 1998. Clinical effects of β-adrenergic blockade in chronic heart failure. A meta-analysis of double-blind, placebo-controlled, randomized trials. Circulation **98**: 1184–1191.
89. ANONYMOUS. 2001. Which beta-blocker? Med. Lett. **43**: 9–11.
90. PACKER, M. *et al.*, for the PROSPECTIVE RANDOMIZED AMIODIPINE SURVIVAL EVALUATION STUDY GROUP. 1996. Effect of amiodipine on morbidity and mortality in severe chronic heart failure. N. Engl. J. Med. **335**: 1107–1114.
91. PITT, B. *et al.*, for the RANDOMIZED ALDACTONE EVALUATION STUDY INVESTIGATORS. 1999. The effects of spironolactone on morbidity and mortality in patients with severe heart failure. N. Engl. J. Med. **341**: 709–717.
92. PIEPOLI, M. *et al.* 1998. Overview and meta-analysis of randomised trials of amiodarone in chronic heart failure. Int. J. Cardiol. **66**: 1–10.
93. AMIODARONE TRIALS META-ANALYSIS INVESTIGATORS. 1997. Effect of prophylactic amiodarone on mortality after acute myocardial infarction and in congestive heart failure: meta-analysis of individual data from 6500 patients in randomised trials. Lancet **350**: 1417–1424.
94. THE ANTIARRHYTHMIC VERSUS IMPLANTABLE DEFIBRILLATORS (AVID) INVESTIGATORS. 1997. A comparison of antiarrhythmic-drug therapy with implantable defibrillators 1 patients resuscitated from near-fatal ventricular arrhythmias. N. Engl. J. Med. **337**: 1576–1583.
95. MOSS, A.J. *et al.* 1996. Improved survival with an implanted defibrillator in patients with coronary disease at high risk for ventricular arrhythmia. N. Engl. J. Med. **335**: 1933–1940.
96. BIGGER, J.T., for the CORONARY ARTERY BYPASS GRAFT (CABG) PATCH TRIAL INVESTIGATORS. 1997. Prophylactic use of implanted cardiac defibrillators in patients at high risk for ventricular arrhythmias after coronary-artery bypass graft surgery. N. Engl. J. Med. **337**: 1569–1575.
97. TEERLINK, J.R. *et al.* 2000. Ambulatory ventricular arrhythmias in patients with heart failure do not specifically predict an increased risk of sudden death. Circulation **101**: 40–46.
98. CONNOLLY, S.J. 1999. Prophylactic antiarrhythmic therapy for the prevention of sudden death in high-risk patients: drugs and devices. Eur. Heart. J. (Suppl. C): 31–35.
99. SOLVD INVESTIGATIONS. 1992. Effect of enalapril on mortality and the development of heart failure in asymptomatic patients with reduced left ventricular ejection fractions. N. Engl. J. Med. **327**: 685–691.
100. RUTHERFORD, J.D. *et al.* 1994. Effects of captopril on ischaemic events after myocardial infarction. Circulation **90**: 1731–1738.
101. THE HEART OUTCOME PREVENTION EVALUATION STUDY INVESTIGATORS. 2000. Effects of an angiotensin-converting-enzyme inhibitor, ramipril, on cardiovascular events in high-risk patients. N. Engl. J. Med. **342**: 145–153.
102. KOCHER, A.A. *et al.* 2001. Neovascularization of ischemic myocardium by human bone-marrow-derived angioblasts prevents cardiomyocyte apoptosis, reduces remodeling and improves cardiac function. Nat. Med. **7**: 430–436.
103. ORLIC, D. *et al.* 2001. Bone marrow cells regenerate infracted myocardium. Nature **410**: 701–705.
104. FOSTER, C., M. MURPHY, A. NESS, *et al.* 2000. Primary prevention. Clinical Evidence **4**: 51–82.
105. HELLER, R.F. *et al.* 1984. How well can we predict coronary heart disease? Findings of the United Kingdom heart disease prevention project. BMJ **288**: 1409–1411.
106. TUNSTALL-PEDOE, H. *et al.* 1996. Sex differences in myocardial infarction and coronary deaths in the Scottish MONICA population of Glasgow 1985 to 1991: presentation, diagnosis, treatment, and 28-day case fatality of 3991 events in men and 1551 events in women. Circulation **93**: 1981–1992.
107. ANDERSON, K.V. *et al.* 1991. Cardiovascular disease risk profiles. Am. Heart J. **121**: 293–298.

108. NATIONAL HEART COMMITTEE. 1993. Guidelines for the management of mildly raised blood pressure in New Zealand. Wellington Ministry of Health http://www.nzgg.org.nz/library/gl_complete/bloodpressure/table1.cfm

109. POWELL, K.E. *et al.* 1987. Physical activity and the incidence of coronary heart disease. Ann. Rev. Public Health **8:** 253–287.

110. BERLIN, J.A. & G.A. COLDITZ. 1990. A meta-analysis of physical activity in the prevention of coronary heart disease. Am. J. Epidemiol. **132:** 612–628.

111. EATON, C.B. 1992. Relation of physical activity and cardiovascular fitness to coronary heart disease. Part 1: A meta-analysis of the independent relation of physical activity and coronary heart disease. J. Am. Board Fam. Pract. **51:** 31–42.

112. FRASER, G.E. *et al.* 1992. Effects of traditional coronary risk factors on rates of incident coronary events in a low-risk population: the Adventist health study. Circulation **86:** 406–413.

113. LINDSTED, K.D. *et al.* 1991. Self-report of physical activity and patterns of mortality in Seventh-Day Adventist men. J. Clin. Epidemiol. **44:** 355–364.

114. FOLSOM, A.R. *et al.* 1997. Physical activity and incidence of coronary heart disease in middle-aged women and men. Med. Sci. Sports. Exerc. **29:** 901–909.

115. JENSEN, G. *et al.* 1991. Risk factors for acute myocardial infarction in Copenhagen II: smoking, alcohol intake, physical activity, obesity, oral contraception, diabetes, lipids and blood pressure. Eur. Heart. J. **12:** 293–308.

116. SIMONSICK, E.M. *et al.* 1993. Risk due to inactivity in physically capable older adults. Am. J. Public Health **83:** 1443–1450.

117. HAAPANEN, N. *et al.* 1997. Association of leisure time physical activity with the risk of coronary heart disease, hypertension and diabetes in middle-aged men and women. Int. J. Epidemiol. **26:** 739–747.

118. SHERMAN, S.E. *et al.* 1994. Does exercise reduce mortality rates in the elderly? Experience from the Framingham heart study. Am. Heart J. **128:** 965–972.

119. RODRIGUEZ, B.L. *et al.* 1994. Physical activity and 23-year incidence of coronary heart disease morbidity and mortality among middle-aged men: the Honolulu heart program. Circulation **89:** 2540–2544.

120. EATON, C.B. *et al.* 1995. Self-reported physical activity predicts long-term coronary heart disease and all-cause mortalities: 21-year follow-up of the Israeli ischemic heart disease study. Arch. Fam. Med. **4:** 323–329.

121. STENDER, M. *et al.* 1993. Physical activity at work and cardiovascular disease risk: results from the MONICA Augsburg study. Int. J. Epidemiol. **22:** 644–650.

122. LEON, A.S. *et al.* 1997. Leisure time physical activity and the 16-year risks of mortality from coronary heart disease and all-causes in the multiple risk factor intervention trial (MRFIT). Int. J. Sports Med. **18**(Suppl. 3): 208–315.

123. ROSOLOVA, H. *et al.* 1994. Impact of cardiovascular risk factors on morbidity and mortality in Czech middle-aged men: Pilsen longitudinal study. Cardiology **85:** 61–68.

124. LUOTO, R. *et al.* 1998. Impact of unhealthy behaviors on cardiovascular mortality in Finland, 1978-1993. Prev. Med. **27:** 93–100.

125. WOO, J. *et al.* 1998. Cardiovascular risk factors and 18-month mortality and morbidity in an elderly Chinese population aged 70 years and over. Gerontology **44:** 51–55.

126. GARTSIDE, P.S. *et al.* 1998. Prospective assessment of coronary heart disease risk factors: The NHANES I epidemiologic follow-up study (NHEFS) 16-year follow-up. J. Am. Coll. Nutr. **17:** 263–269.

127. DOM, J.P. *et al.* 1999. World and leisure time physical activity and mortality in men and women from a general population sample. Ann. Epidemiol. **9:** 366–373.

128. HAKIM, A.A. *et al.* 1999. Effects of walking on coronary heart disease in elderly men: the Honolulu heart program. Circulation **100:** 9–13.

129. EATON, C.B. 1992. Relation of physical activity and cardiovascular fitness to coronary heart disease, part II: cardiovascular fitness and the safety and efficacy of physical activity prescription. J. Am. Board Fam. Pract. **5:** 157–165. Search date not stated; primary sources Medline and hand searches.

130. BLAIR, S.N. *et al.* 1995. Changes in physical fitness and all-cause mortality: a prospective study of healthy and unhealthy men. JAMA **273:** 1093–1098.

131. SACCO, R.L. *et al.* 1998. Leisure-time physical activity and ischemic stroke risk: the Northern Manhattan stroke study. Stroke **29:** 380–387.
132. SHINTON, R. 1997. Lifelong exposures and the potential for stroke prevention: the contribution of cigarette smoking, exercise, and body fat. J. Epidemiol. Community Health **51:** 138–143.
133. GILLUM, R.F. *et al.* 1996. Physical activity and stroke incidence in women and men. The NHANES I epidemiologic follow-up study. Am. J. Epidemiol. **143:** 860–869.
134. KIELY, D.K. *et al.* 1994. Physical activity and stroke risk: the Framingham study. Am. J. Epidemiol. **140:** 608–620. [correction appears in Am. J. Epidemiol. 1995. **141:** 178].
135. ABBOTT, R.D. *et al.* 1994. Physical activity in older middle-aged men and reduced risk of stroke: the Honolulu heart program. Am. J. Epidemiol. **139:** 881–883.
136. HAHEIM, L.L. *et al.* 1993. Risk factors of stroke incidence and mortality: a 12-year follow-up of the Oslo study. Stroke **24:** 1484–1489.
137. WANNAMETHEE, G. *et al.* 1992. Physical activity and stroke in British middle aged men. BBMJ **304:** 597–601.
138. MENOTTI, A. *et al.* 1990. Twenty-year stroke mortality and prediction in twelve cohorts of the seven countries study. Int. J. Epidemiol. **19:** 309–315.
139. LINDENSTROM, E. *et al.* 1993. Risk factors for stroke in Copenhagen, Denmark. II. Lifestyle factors. Neuroepidemiology **12:** 43–50.
140. LINDENSTROM, E. *et al.* 1993. Lifestyle factors and risk of cerebrovascular disease in women: the Copenhagen City heart study. Stroke **24:** 1468–1472.
141. FOLSOM, A.R. *et al.* 1990. Evidence of hypertension and stroke in relation to body fat distribution and other risk factors in older women. Stroke **21:** 701–706.
142. NAKAYAMA, T. *et al.* 1997. A 15.5 year follow-up study of stroke in a Japanese provincial city; the Shibata study. Stroke **28:** 45–52.
143. LEE, I.M. *et al.* 1999. Exercise and risk of stroke in male physicians. Stroke **30:** 1–6.
144. EVENSON, K.R. *et al.* 1999. Physical activity and ischemic stroke risk: the atherosclerosis in communities study. Stroke **30:** 1333–1339.
145. MITTLEMAN, M.A. *et al.* 1993. Triggering of acute myocardial infarction by heavy physical exertion. Protection against triggering by regular exertion: determinants of myocardial infarction onset study investigators. N. Engl. J. Med. **329:** 1677–1683.
146. WILLICH, S.N. *et al.* 1993. Physical exertion as a trigger of acute myocardial infarction: triggers and mechanisms of myocardial infarction study group. N. Engl. J. Med. **329:** 1684–1690.
147. PATE, R.R. *et al.* 1995. Physical activity and public health. A recommendation from the Center for Disease control and prevention and the American College of Sports Medicine. JAMA **273:** 402–407.
148. THOMPSON, P.D. 1996. The cardiovascular complications of vigorous physical activity. Arch. Intern. Med. **156:** 2297–2302.
149. OBERMAN, A. 1985. Exercise and the primary prevention of cardiovascular disease. Am. J. Cardiol. **55:** 10–20.
150. ANDERSEN, R.E. *et al.* 1999. Effects of lifestyle activity vs. structured aerobic exercise in obese women: a randomized trial. JAMA **281:** 335–340.
151. DUNN, A.L. *et al.* 1999. Comparison of lifestyle and structured interventions to increase physical activity and cardiorespiratory fitness: a randomized trial. JAMA **281:** 327–434.
152. PEREIRA, M.A. *et al.* 1998. A randomized walking trial in postmenopausal women: effects on physical activity and health 10 years later. Arch. Intern. Med. **158:** 1695–1701.
153. DEBUSK, R.F. *et al.* 1990. Training effects of long versus short bouts of exercise in healthy subjects. Am. J. Cardiol. **65:** 1010–1013.
154. ERIKSSEN, G. *et al.* 1988. Changes in physical fitness and changes in mortality. Lancet **352:** 759–762.
155. SHANGOLD, M.M. 1990. Exercise in the menopausal woman. Obstetrics & Gynecology **75**(Suppl): 53S–58S.

156. BELL, M.J. *et al.* 1998. A randomized controlled trial to evaluate the efficacy of community based physical therapy in the treatment of people with rheumatoid arthritis. J. Rheumatol. **25:** 231–237.
157. AGURS-COLLINS, T.D. *et al.* 1997. A randomized controlled trial of weight reduction and exercise for diabetes management in older African-American subjects. Diabetes Care **20:** 1503–1511.
158. SHEPARD, R.J. & P.N. SHEK. 1996. Impact of physical activity and sport on the immune system. **11:** 133–137.
159. CANNON, J.G. *et al.* 1989. Increased interleukin-1b in human skeletal muscle after exercise. Am. J. Physiol. **257:** R451–R455.
160. BOAS, S.R. *et al.* 1996. Effects of anaerobic exercise on the immune system in eight to seventeen year old trained and untrained boys. J. Pediatr. **129:** 846–855.
161. NIEMAN, D.C. 1997. Immune response to heavy exertion. J. Appl. Physiol. **82:** 1385–1394.
162. OSTERBACK, L. & Y. QVARNBERG. 1987. A prospective study of respiratory infections in 12 year old children actively engaged in sports. Acta Pediatr. Scand. **76:** 73–27.
163. JOHNSON, J.E. *et al.* 1990. Exercise dysfunction in patients seropositive for the human immunodeficiency virus. Am. Rev. Resp. Dis. **141:** 618–622.
164. MACARTHUR, R.D. *et al.* 1993. Supervised exercise training improves cardiopulmonary fitness in HIV-infected persons. Med. Sci. Sports Exercise **25:** 684–688.
165. MUSTAFA, T. *et al.* 1999. Association between exercise and HIV disease progression in a cohort of homosexual men. Ann. Epidemiol. **9:**127–131.
166. SPENCE, D.W. *et al.* 1990. Progressive resistance exercise: effect on muscle function and anthropometry of a select AIDS population. Arch. Phys. Med. Rehabil. **71:** 644–648.
167. ROUBENOFF, R. *et al.* 1997. Feasibility of increasing lean body mass in HIV-infected adults using progressive resistance exercise [abstract]. Nutrition **13:** 271.
168. RIGSBY, L.W. *et al.* 1992. Effects of exercise training on men seropositive for the human immunodeficiency virus-1. Med. Sci. Sports Exercise **24:** 6–12.
169. LAPIERRE, A. *et al.* 1991. Aerobic exercise training in an AIDS risk group. Int. J. Sports Med. **12:** S53–S57.
170. MOSHER, P.E. *et al.* 1998. Aerobic circuit training: effect on adolescents with well-controlled insulin-dependent diabetes mellitus. Arch. Phys. Med. Rehabil. **79:** 652–657.
171. ROUBENOFF, R. *et al.* 1999. A pilot study of exercise training to reduce trunk fat in adults with HIV-associated fat redistribution. AIDS **13:** 1373–1375.
172. NESS, A.R. & J.W. POWLES. 1997. Fruit and vegetables and cardiovascular disease: a review. Int. J. Epidemiol. **26:** 1–13. Search date 1995; primary sources Medline, Embase, and hand searches of personal bibliographies, books, reviews and citations in located reports.
173. LAW, M.R. & J.K. MORRIS. 1998. By how much does fruit and vegetable consumption reduce the risk of ischaemic heart disease? Eur. J. Clin. Nutr. **52:** 549–556. Search date not stated; primary sources Medline, Science Citation Index, and hand searches of review articles.
174. KLERK, M. *et al.* 1998. Fruits and vegetables in chronic disease prevention. Wageningen: Grafisch Bedrijf Ponsen and Looijen. Search date 1998; primary sources Medline, Current Contents, and Toxline.
175. KEY, T.J.A. *et al.* 1996. Dietary habits and mortality in 11,000 vegetarians and health conscious people: results of a 17 year follow up. BMJ **313:** 775–779.
176. PIETINEN, P. *et al.* 1996. Intake of dietary fibre and risk of coronary heart disease in a cohort of Finnish men. Circulation **94:** 2720–2727.
177. MANN, J.I. *et al.* 1997. Dietary determinants of ischaemic heart disease in health conscious individuals. Heart **78:** 450–455.
178. GELEIJNSE, M. 1997. Consumptie van groente en fruit en het risico op myocardinfarct. Basisrapportage, Rotterdam: Erasmus Universiteit (cited in appendix XIII of review by Klerk[174]).

179. TODD, S. *et al.* 1999. Dietary antioxidant vitamins and fiber in the etiology of cardiovascular disease and all-cause mortality: results from the Scottish heart health study. Am. J. Epidemiol. **150:** 1073–1080.
180. BAZZANO, L. *et al.* 2000. Fruit and vegetable intake reduces cardiovascular mortality; results from the NHANES I epidemiologic follow-up study (NHEFS), 40th Annual conference Cardiovascular Epidemiology and Prevention [abstract] Circulation 8-8.
181. LUI, S. *et al.* 2000. Fruit and vegetable intake and risk of cardiovascular disease. 40th Annual Conference Cardiovascular Epidemiology and Prevention [abstract] Circulation 30–31.
182. LUI, S. *et al.* 2000. Vegetable consumption and risk of coronary heart disease in men: results from the physicians health study. 40th Annual Conference Cardiovascular Epidemiology and Prevention [abstract] Circulation 30–31.
183. KNEKT, P. *et al.* 1994. Antioxidant vitamin intake and coronary mortality in a longitudinal population study. Am. J. Epidemiol. **139:** 1180–1189.
184. KELI, S.O. *et al.* 1996. Dietary flavonoids, antioxidant vitamins, and incidence of stroke. Arch. Intern. Med. **156:** 637–642.
185. DAVIGLUS, M.L. *et al.* 1997. Dietary vitamin C, beta-carotene and 30 year risk of stroke: results from the Western Electric study. Neuroepidemiology **16:** 69–77.
186. ASCHERIO, A. *et al.* 1997. Prospective study of potassium intake and risk of stroke among US men. Can. J. Cardiol. **13:** 44B.
187. YOCHUM, L. *et al.* 1999. Dietary flavonoid intake and risk of cardiovascular disease in postmenopausal women. Am. J. Epidemiol. **149:** 943–949.
188. KNEKT, P. *et al.* 2000. Quercetin intake and the incidence of cerebrovascular disease. Eur. J. Clin. Nutr. **54:** 415–417.
189. JOSHIPURA, K.U. *et al.* 1999. Fruit and vegetable intake in relation to risk of ischemic stroke. JAMA **282:** 1233–1239.
190. NESS, A.R. & J.W. POWLES. 1996. Does eating fruit and vegetables protect against heart attack and stroke? Chem. Indus. 792–794.
191. NESS, A.R. & J.W. POWLES. 1997. Dietary habits and mortality in vegetables and health conscious people: several uncertainities exist. BMJ **314:** 148.
192. SERDULA, M.K. *et al.* 1996. The association between fruit and vegetable intake and chronic disease risk factors. Epidemiology **7:** 161–165.
193. LONN, E.M. & S.YUSUF. 1997. Is there a role for antioxidant vitamins in the prevention of cardiovascular disease? An update on epidemiological and clinical trials data. Can. J. Cardiol. **13:** 957–965. Search date not stated: primary sources Medline, science citation index, handsearching.
194. JHA, P. *et al.* 1995. The antioxidant vitamins and cardiovascular disease: a critical review of epidemiologic and clinical trial data. Ann. Intern. Med. **123:** 860–872.
195. ROXRODE, K.M. & J.E. MANSON. 1996. Antioxidants and coronary heart disease: observational studies. J. Cardiovasc. Risk **3:** 363–367.
196. EGGER, M. *et al.* 1998. Spurious precision? Meta-analysis of observational studies. BMJ **316:** 140–144.
197. GAZIANO, J.M. 1996. Randomized trials of dietary antioxidants in cardiovascular disease prevention and treatment. J. Cardiovasc. Risk **3:** 368–371.
198. NESS, A.R. *et al.* 1997. Vitamin C and cardiovascular disease—a systemic review. J. Cardiovasc. Risk **3:** 513-521. Search date 1996; primary sources Medline, Embase and hand searches of personal bibliographies, books, reviews and citations in located reports.
199. KLIPSTEIN-GROBUSCH, K. *et al.* 1999. Dietary antioxidants and risk of myocardial infarction in the elderly: the Rotterdam study. Am. J. Clin. Nutr. **69:** 261–266.
200. ASCHERIO, A. *et al.* 1999. Relation of consumption of vitamin E, vitamin C and carotenoids to risk for stroke among men in the United States. Ann. Intern. Med. **130:** 963–970.
201. LI, J. *et al.* 1993. Nutrition intervention trials in Linxian, China: multiple vitamin/mineral supplementation, cancer incidence, and disease-specific mortality among adults with esophageal dysplasia. J. Natl. Cancer Inst. **85:** 1492–1498.
202. MARK, S.D. *et al.* 1996. Lowered risks of hypertension and cerebrovascular disease after vitamin/mineral supplementation. Am. J. Epidemiol. **143:** 658–664.

203. MARK, S.D. *et al.* 1998. Do nutritional supplements lower the risk of stroke or hypertension? Epidemiology **9:** 9–15.
204. LOSONCZY, K.G. *et al.* 1996. Vitamin E and vitamin C supplement use and risk of all-cause and coronary mortality in older persons: the established populations for epidemiologic studies of the elderly. Am. J. Clin. Nutr. **64:** 190–196.
205. SAHYOUN, N.R. *et al.* 1996. Carotenoids, vitamin C and E and mortality in an elderly population. Am. J. Epidemiol. **144:** 501–511.
206. KELI, S.O. *et al.* 1996. Dietary flavonoids, antioxidant vitamins, and incidence of stroke. Arch. Intern. Med. **156:** 637–642.
207. NEVE, J. 1996. Selenium as a risk factor for cardiovascular disease. J. Cardiovasc. Risk **3:** 42–47.
208. HERTOG, M.G.L. *et al.* 1993. Dietary antioxidant flavonoids and risk of coronary heart disease: The Zutphen Elderly Study. Lancet **342:** 1007–1011.
209. KNEKT, P. *et al.* 1996. Flavonoid intake and coronary mortality in Finland: a cohort study. BMHJ **12:** 478–481.
210. RIMM, E.B. *et al.* 1996. Relation between intake of flavonoids and risk for coronary heart disease in male health professionals. Ann. Intern. Med. **125:** 384–389.
211. HERTOG, M.G.L. *et al.* 1997. Antioxidant flavonoids and ischemic heart disease in a Welsh population of men: The Caerphilly Study. Am. J. Clin. Nutr. **65:** 1489–1494.
212. DOERING, Q.V. 1996. Antioxidant vitamins, cancer, and cardiovascular disease. N. Engl. J. Med. **335:** 1065.
213. PIETRZIK, K. 1996. Antioxidant vitamins, cancer and cardiovascular disease. N. Engl. J. Med. **335:** 1065–1066.
214. HENNEKENS, C.H. *et al.* 1995. Antioxidant vitamin cardiovascular disease hypothesis is still promising, but still unproven; the need for randomised trials. Am. J. Clin. Nutr. **62**(suppl): 1377–1380.
215. BATES, C.J. *et al.* 1991. Biochemical markers for nutrient intake. *In* Design Concepts in Nutritional Epidemiology. B.M. Margetts & M. Nelson, Eds. Oxford Medical Publications. Oxford, UK.
216. THE ALPHA-TOCOPHEROL BETA CAROTENE CANCER PREVENTION STUDY GROUP. 1994. The effect of vitamin E and beta carotene on the incidence of lung cancer and other causes in male smokers. N. Engl. J. Med. **330:** 1029–1035.
217. US DEPARTMENT OF HEALTH AND HUMAN SERVICES. 1990. The health benefits of smoking cessation: a report of the Surgeon General. US Department of health and Human Services, Public Health Service, Centers for Disease Control. Rockville, MD. DHHS Publication (CDC) 90-8416.
218. ROYAL COLLEGE OF PHYSICIANS. 1971. Smoking and health now. Pitman Medical and Scientific Publishing. London.
219. DOLL, R. *et al.* 1994. Mortality in relation to smoking: 40 years' observations on male British doctors. BMJ **309:** 901–911.
220. KAWACHI, I. *et al.* 1993. Smoking cessation in relation to total mortality rates in women: a prospective cohort study. Ann. Intern. Med. **119:** 992–1000.
221. ROSENBERG, L. 1985. The risk of myocardial infarction after quitting smoking in men under 55 years of age. N. Engl. J. Med. **313:** 1511–1514.
222. ROSENBERG, L. 1990. Decline in the risk of myocardial infarction among women who stop smoking. N. Engl. J. Med. **322:** 213–217.
223. ROSE, G. 1982. A randomised controlled trial of anti-smoking advice: 10-year results. J. Epidemiol. Community Health **36:** 102–108.
224. SHINTON, R. & G. BEEVERS. 1989. Meta-analysis of relation between cigarette smoking and stroke. BMJ **298:** 789-794. Search date 1988: primary source index references from three studies on cigarette smoking and stroke on medicine 1965–1988.
225. ROGOT, E. & J.L. MURRAY. 1980. Smoking and causes of death among US veterans: 16 years of observation. Public Health Rep. **95:** 213–222.
226. WANNAMETHEE, S.G. *et al.* 1996. History of parental death from stroke or heart trouble and the risk of stroke in middle-aged men. Stroke **276:** 1492–1498.
227. Drugs for hypertension. 2001. Med. Lett. **43:** 17–22.

228. HALBERT, J.A. *et al.* 1997. The effectiveness of exercise training in lowering blood pressure; a meta-analysis of randomised controlled trials of 4 weeks or longer. J. Hum. Hypertens. **11:** 641–649. Search date 1996; primary sources Medline, Embase, Science Citation Index.

229. EBRAHIM, S. & G. DAVEY SMITH. 1998. Lowering blood pressure: a systematic review of sustained non-pharmacological interventions. J. Public Health Med. **20:** 441–448. Search date 1995; primary source Medline.

230. ENGSTOM, G. *et al.* 1999. Hypertensive men who exercise regularly have lower rate of cardiovascular mortality. J. Hypertens. **17:** 737–742.

231. APPEL, L.J. *et al.* 1997. A clinical trial of the effects of dietary patterns on blood pressure. N. Engl. J. Med. **336:** 1117–1124.

232. BELIN, L.J. *et al.* 1996. Alcohol and hypertension: kill or cure? J. Hum. Hypertens. **10**(suppl 2): 1–5.

233. CAMPBELL, N.R.C. *et al.* 1999. Recommendations on alcohol consumption. Can. Med. Assoc. J. (Suppl. 9): 13–20. Search date 1996; primary source Medline.

234. GRAUDAL, N.A. *et al.* 1998. Effects of sodium restriction on blood pressure, renin, aldosterone, catecholamines, cholesterols, and triglyceride. JAMA **279:** 1381–1391.

235. WHELTON, P.K. *et al.* 1998. Sodium reduction and weight loss in the treatment of hypertension in older persons: a randomized controlled trial of non pharmacologic interventions in the elderly (TONE). JAMA **279:** 839–846.

236. MIDGLEY, J.P. *et al.* 1996. Effect of reduced dietary sodium on blood pressure. JAMA **275:** 1590–1597.

237. ALDERMAN, M.H. *et al.* 1995. Low urinary sodium associated with greater risk of myocardial infarction among treated hypertensive men. Hypertension **25:** 1144–1152.

238. BRAND, M.B. *et al.* 1998. Weight-reducing diets for control of hypertension in adults. *In* The Cochrane Library, Issue 4. Update Software. Oxford, UK.

239. WHELTON, P.K. *et al.* 1997. Effects of oral potassium on blood pressure: meta-analysis of randomized controlled clinical trials. JAMA **277:** 1624–1632.

240. MORRIS, M.C. *et al.* 1993. Does fish oil lower blood pressure? A meta-analysis of controlled clinical trials. Circulation **88:** 523–533.

241. GRIFFITH, L.E. *et al.* 1999. The influence of dietary and nondietary calcium supplementation on blood pressure. Am. J. Hypertens. **12:** 84–92.

242. GUEYFFIER, F. *et al.* 1996. New meta-analysis of treatment trials of hypertension: improving the estimate of therapeutic benefit. J. Hum. Hypertens. **10:** 1–8.

243. STAESSEN, J.A. *et al.* 2000. Risks of untreated and treated isolated systolic hypertension in the elderly: meta-analysis of outcome trials. Lancet **355:** 865–872.

244. STAESSEN, J.A. *et al.* 1997. Randomised double-blind comparison of placebo and active treatment for older patients with isolated systolic hypertension. Lancet **350:** 757–764.

245. THE HEART OUTCOMES PREVENTION EVALUATION STUDY INVESTIGATORS. 2000. Effects of an angiotensin-converting-enzyme inhibitor, ramipril, on cardiovascular events in high-risk patients. N. Engl. J. Med. **342:** 145–153.

246. HANSSON, L. *et al.* 1998. Effects of intensive blood pressure lowering and low-dose aspirin in patients with hypertension: principal results of the hypertension optimal treatment (HOT) trial. Lancet **351:** 1755–1762.

247. GROSSMAN, E. *et al.* 1999. Does diuretic therapy increase the risk of renal cell carcinoma? Am. J. Cardiol. **83:** 1090–1093. Search dates 1966 to 1998; primary sources Medline.

248. BETO, J.A. & V.K. BANSAL. 1992. Quality of life in treatment of hypertension: a meta-analysis of clinical trials. Am. J. Hypertens. **5:** 125–133. Search date 1990; primary sources Medline, ERIC.

249. CROOG, S.H. *et al.* 1986. The effects of antihypertensive therapy on quality of life. N. Engl. J. Med. **314:** 1657–1664.

250. PSATY, B.M. *et al.* 1997. Health outcomes associated with antihypertensive therapies used as first line agents: a systematic review and meta-analysis. JAMA **277:** 739–745. Search date 1995; primary source Medline.

251. MESSERLI, F.H. *et al.* 1998. Are beta blockers efficacious as first-line therapy for hypertension in the elderly? A systematic review. JAMA **279:** 1903–1907. Search date 1998; primary source Medline.
252. HANSSON, L. *et al.* 1999. Effect of angiotensin-converting-enzyme inhibition compared with conventional therapy on cardiovascular morbidity and mortality in hypertension: the captopril prevention project (CAPP) randomised trial. Lancet **353:** 611–616.
253. HANSSON, L. *et al.* 1999. Randomized trial of old and new antihypertensive drugs in elderly patients: cardiovascular mortality and morbidity the Swedish trial in old patients with hypertension-2 study. Lancet **354:** 1751–1756.
254. THE ALLHAT OFFICERS AND COORDINATORS FOR THE ALLHAT COLLABORATIVE RESEARCH GROUP. 2000. Major cardiovascular events in hypertensive patients randomized to doxazosin vs chlorthalidone: the antihypertensive and lipid-lowering treatment to prevent heart attack trial (ALLHAT). JAMA **283:** 1967–1975.
255. NEATON, J.D. *et al.* 1993. Treatment of mild hypertension study: final results. JAMA **270:** 713–724.
256. MATERSON, B.J. *et al.* 1993. Single drug therapy for hypertension in men. N. Engl. J. Med. **328:** 914–921.
257. PHILIPP, T. *et al.* 1997. Randomised, double blind, multicentre comparison of hydrochlorothiazide, atenolol, nitrendipine, and enalapril in antihypertensive treatment: results of the HANE study. BMJ **315:** 154–159.
258. WRIGHT, J.M. *et al.* 1999. Systematic review of antihypertensive therapies: does the evidence assist in choosing a first line drug? Can. Med. Assoc. J. **161:** 25-32.
259. CUTLER, J.A. 1998. Calcium channel blockers for hypertension—uncertainty continues. N. Engl. J. Med. **338:** 679-680.
260. ANTIPLATELET TRIALISTS' COLLABORATION. 1994. Collaborative overview of randomised trials of antiplatelet therapy – 1: prevention of death, myocardial infarction, and stroke by prolonged antiplatelet therapy in various categories of patients. BMJ **308:** 81–106.
261. HART, R.G. 2000. Aspirin for the primary prevention of stroke and other major vascular events. Meta-analysis and hypotheses. Arch. Neurol. **57:** 326–332.
262. MEDICAL RESEARCH COUNCIL'S GENERAL PRACTICE RESEARCH FRAMEWORK. 1998. Thrombosis prevention trial: randomised trial of low-intensity anticoagulation with warfarin and low dose aspirin in the primary prevention of ischaemic heart disease in men at increased risk. Lancet **351:** 233–241.
263. PETO, R. *et al.* 1988. Randomised trial of prophylactic daily aspirin in British male doctors. BMJ **296:** 313–316.
264. STEERING COMMITTEE OF THE PHYSICIANS' HEALTH STUDY RESEARCH GROUP. 1989. Final report on the aspirin component of the ongoing physicians' health study. N. Engl. J. Med. **321:** 129–135.
265. BURING, J.E. *et al.* for the WOMEN'S HEALTH STUDY GROUP. 1992. Women's health study: summary of the study design. J. Myocardial Ischemia **4:** 27–29.
266. KATEMDAHL, D.A. & W.R. LAWLER. 1999. Variability in meta-analytic results concerning the value of cholesterol reduction in coronary heart disease: a meta-meta-analysis. Am. J. Epidemiol. **149:** 429–441.
267. FROOM, J. *et al.* 1998. Measurement and management of hyperlipidemia for the primary prevention of coronary heart disease. J. Am. Board Fam. Pract. **11:** 12–22.
268. EBRAHIM, S. *et al.* 1999. What role for statins? A review and economic model. Health Technol. Assess. **3:** 1911–91.
269. LAROSA, J.C. *et al.* 1999. Effect of statins on risk of coronary disease: a meta-analysis of randomized controlled trials. JAMA **282:** 2340–2346.
270. DOWNS, J.R. *et al.* 1998. Primary prevention of acute coronary events with lovastatin in men and women with average cholesterol levels: results of the AFCAPS/TexCAPS. JAMA **279:** 1615–1622.
271. SCANDINAVIAN SIMVASTATIN SURVIVAL STUDY GROUP. 1995. Randomized trial of cholesterol lowering in 4444 patients with coronary heart disease: The Scandinavian Simvastatin Survival Study (4S). Lancet **344:** 1383–1389.

272. LONG-TERM INTERVENTION WITH PRAVASTATIN IN ISCHEMIC DISEASE (LIPID) STUDY PROGRAM. 1998. Prevention of cardiovascular events and death with pravastatin in patients with coronary heart disease and a broad range of initial cholesterol levels. N. Engl. J. Med. **339:** 1349–1357.

273. SACKS, F.M. *et al.*, for the CHOLESTEROL AND RECURRENT EVENTS TRIAL INVESTIGATORS. 1996. Effect of pravastatin on coronary events after myocardial infarction in patients with average cholesterol levels. N. Engl. J. Med. **335:** 1001–1009.

274. SHEPHERD, J. *et al.*, for the WEST OF SCOTLAND CORONARY PREVENTION STUDY GROUP. 1995. Prevention of coronary heart disease with pravastatin in men with hypercholesterolemia. N. Engl. J. Med. **333:** 1301–1307.

275. GOULD, A.L. *et al.* 1998. Cholesterol reduction yields clinical benefit: impact on statin trials. Circulation **97:** 94–52.

276. BUCHER, H.C. *et al.* 1999. Systematic review on the risk and benefit of different cholesterol-lowering interventions. Arterioscler. Thromb. Vas. Biol. **19:** 187–195.

277. CARLSSON, C.M. *et al.* 1999. Managing dyslipidaemia in older adults. J. Am. Geriatr. Society **47:** 1458–1465.

278. ANONYMOUS. 2000. Colesevelam (Welchol) for hypercholesterolemia. The Medical Letter **42:** 102–104.

279. KWAH, B. *et al.* 2000. Statins as a newly recognized type of immunomodulator. Nat. Med. **6:** 1399–1402.

280. PALINSKI, W. 2000. Immunomodulation: a new role for statins? Nat. Med. **6:** 1311–1312.

281. MARTINEZ, E. *et al.* 2001. Risk of lipodystrophy in HIV-1-infected patients treated with protease inhibitors: a prospective cohort study. Lancet **357:** 592–598.

282. ANONYMOUS. 2000. Drugs for HIV infection. Med. Lett. **42:** 1–6.

283. PISCITELLI, S.C. & K.D. GALLICANO. 2001. Interactions among drugs for HIV and opportunistic infections. N. Engl. J. Med. **344:** 984–996.

284. FISHER, S.D. & S.E. LIPSHULTZ. 2000. Cardiovascular abnormalities in HIV-infected individuals. *In* Heart Disease, 6th edit. E. Braunwald *et al.*, Eds. Chapter 68: 2211–2222. W.B. Saunders Co. Philadelphia, PA.

285. FISHER, S.D. & S.E. LIPSHULTZ. 2001. AIDS and the cardiovascular system. *In* Harrison's Internal Medicine Online. E. Braunwald, Ed. McGraw Hill. New York.

286. FISHER, S.D. & S.E. LIPSHULTZ. Cardiac disease. *In* AIDS Therapy, 2nd edit. R. Dolin, *et al.*, Eds. Churchill Livingston. New York. In press.

Catheter-Related Bloodstream Infections in HIV-Infected Patients

EMANUELE NICASTRI,[a] NICOLA PETROSILLO,[a]
PIERLUIGI VIALE,[b] AND GIUSEPPE IPPOLITO[a]

[a]Istituto Nazionale per le Malattie Infettive,
"Lazzaro Spallanzani"—IRCCS, 00149 Rome, Italy

[b]Clinica di Malattie Infettive e Tropicali, Università degli Studi di Brescia, Italy

ABSTRACT: Bloodstream infections (BSI) constitute a significant public health problem and represent an important cause of morbidity and mortality in hospitalized patients, with an approximate incidence of one episode per hundred hospital admissions. Studies on BSI in HIV+ patients have identified central venous catheters (CVC) as a risk factor, with an attributable mortality rate of 10–20%. The long-term CVC-related infection risk appeared to be 5 to 10-fold higher with respect to the infection rates among HIV- patients. CVC associated infection rate ranges from 1.3 to 12 infections per 1,000 catheter-days. *Staphylococcus aureus* is the most common etiologic agent causative of CVC-related BSI, likely the result of the high skin and nasal carriage of this organism among HIV+ patients, mostly intravenous drug users. Coagulase-negative staphylococci are also frequently identified as cause of CVC-related BSI, likely the result of breaches in infection control measures and in antiseptic technique during CVC management. Treating bacteremia without catheter removal would be optimal, but the reported efficacy of systemic antibiotic therapy alone is only 25–32%. Conversely, recent studies have shown that, using an antibiotic-lock procedure, up to 90% of HIV-infected and uninfected patients achieved complete eradication of catheter-related BSIs without catheter removal. Clinical trials using new materials such as covalently linked heparin on the CVC surface, electrically charged CVC, novel topical agents that interfere with bacterial colonization, antiadhesin molecules and agents that block the gene expression involved in the biofilm formation, are all needed to reduce the high catheter-related infection risk among HIV+ patients.

KEYWORDS: bloodstream infections; HIV/AIDS; central venous catheter; nosocomial infection

INTRODUCTION

Bloodstream infections (BSI) constitute a significant public health problem and represent an important cause of morbidity and mortality in hospitalized patients,[1] with an approximate incidence of one episode per hundred hospital admissions.[1] The

Address for correspondence: Emanuele Nicastri, M.D., Dipartimento di Epidemiologia, Istituto Nazionale per le Malattie Infettive, "Lazzaro Spallanzani"—IRCCS, Via Portuense, 292, 00149 Rome, Italy. Voice ++39-06-55170942; fax ++39-06-5582825.
craids@tiscalinet.it

excess hospital cost associated with BSI in surviving intensive care unit (ICU) patients was estimated to be 40,000 US$ per patient.[2]

The incidence of primary nosocomial BSI increased two- to threefold during the 1980s mostly related to central venous catheter (CVC) infections.[3] CVC are commonly used in critically ill patients and HIV[+] subjects in advanced phases of disease, often requiring a long-term CVC device to administer fluids, blood products, drugs and parenteral nutrition. Studies on BSI in HIV[+] patients have repeatedly identified intravenous catheters as a risk factor, thus emphasizing its clinical relevance in both the in- and out-patient setting, for HIV[+] patients[4–6] with an attributable mortality rate ranging from 10–20%, mostly due to septic shock.[2,7]

A prospective study estimated an incidence of 170 BSI per 10,000 person-years in HIV[+] subjects, with values ranging up to 3,200 per 10,000 person-years in AIDS patients.[8] Comparing CVC-related BSI (CR-BSI) rates among HIV[+] ICU patients with those among patients admitted to National Nosocomial Infections Surveillance (NNIS) system medical ICU, the rate was significantly higher in HIV[+] patients (12.1 vs. 6.8 per 1,000 catheter-days, $p < 0.05$).[9]

Relatively little information is available regarding how HAART has changed the epidemiology, the determinant factors, and the prognosis of CR-BSI in HIV[+] patients since 1996 when the extensive use of highly active antiretroviral therapy (HAART) began. The purpose of this review is to describe the pathogenesis, contributing factors, microbiology, infection rate, diagnosis, treatment and prevention of CR-BSI in HIV[+] patients.

DEFINITIONS

Catheter-related bloodstream infection is a systemic infection emanating from the venous catheter, with the same organism isolated from peripheral blood and specimens representative of the catheter (such as surface swabs, tip cultures, or quantitative blood culture taken through the catheter).[10] No other source of infection should be present. The Centers for Diseases Control and Prevention (CDC) of Atlanta, GA, USA, suggest that in the absence of laboratory confirmation, defervescence after removal of an implicated catheter from a patient with BSI may be considered indirect evidence of CR-BSI.[11]

Localized intravascular catheter infection should be used only to refer to clinical or microbiologically proved infection at the catheter exit site: periorificial cellulitis, purulence, tunnelitis, and pocket infection (for totally implantable devices).[10]

Catheter colonization means that the cultured catheter segment (hub, tip, subcutaneous segment) grows a significant number of bacteria according to the culture methods used: greater than 15 colony-forming units (CFU) for the semiquantitative roll-plate method, or greater than 1000 CFU for quantitative techniques in the absence of accompanying clinical symptoms of BSI.[10]

Catheter contamination is the process whereby micro-organisms reach the catheter, adhere to its surface, and proliferate below the significant number of bacteria by previously described methods.[10]

RISK FACTORS FOR CATHETER-RELATED BLOODSTREAM INFECTIONS

General Population

Several factors have been associated with an increased risk of catheter-related infections. The risk of BSI is higher with CVC (1–20%) than with peripheral cannulas, Swan-Ganz or arterial catheters.[12,13] Other well-known risk factors include the frequent manipulation of catheters,[14,15] prolonged catheterization time,[16] repeated catheterization, presence of an infectious focus elsewhere in the body, violation of aseptic techniques for insertion and maintenance of catheters by inexperienced personnel.[17,18]

Several studies suggest that triple-lumen CVC are associated with a higher risk of infection than single-lumen CVC,[19–21] but a prospective randomized trial failed to demonstrate any significant difference.[22,23] Actually, triple-lumen CVC are larger, stiffer, have grooves between the lumens, are manipulated more often and are likely to be inserted in sicker patients who are at a higher risk of developing CR-BSI.

Furthermore, the insertion site of the catheter could affect predisposition to infection: internal jugular CVC are more likely to become infected than subclavian catheters with a risk ratio as high as 2.7.[24,25]

HIV Immunocompromised Population

HIV infection is characterized by a progressive depletion of CD4 T lymphocytes, which play a key role in the host immune system. They are involved in the induction of cytotoxic T cell activity, natural killer function, activation of macrophages and induction of B cell maturation. Therefore, depletion of CD4 cells has a profound effect on the host immune response that increases the risk of life-threatening infections caused by bacteria, fungi, protozoa, and other viruses. Furthermore, the breakdown of the integrity of the skin barrier leads to increased susceptibility to infection by *Staphylococcus* spp. and *Candida* spp.

The long-term CVC infection risk appears to be at least 5- to 10-fold higher with respect to the infection rates among cancer patients matched for sex, age and Karnofsky performance status, as evidenced in a recent survey by Astagneau *et al.*[26] This suggests that the attributable risk ratio of HIV$^+$ persons with respect to HIV$^-$ ones, could be exactly identified in the immune system impairment.[26]

Conversely, in consideration of the possible protective role of antimicrobial prophylaxis towards such bacterial infections, a nested case control was conducted comparing prior exposure to antimicrobials in patients with *S. aureus* bacteremia.[27] Only rifabutin was associated with the diminished risk of BSI at univariate analysis but not at multivariate analysis.[27]

Among 209 French HIV$^+$ patients, the long-term CVC infection risk increased with the long-term CVC handling, from 3.04 per 1,000 catheter-days for 20–40% manipulation-days to 5.07 for 80–100% manipulation-days.[26] Similarly, all of the following factors were statistically associated to higher infection risk: changing the CVC extension set or the dressing more frequently than once per week, high APACHE III score, low CD4 cell count, administration of total parenteral nutrition and bacterial infections within the month prior to CVC implantation.[26,28]

In a multicentric Italian study 8 infections per 1,000 device-days were reported overall with an increased rate of CR-BSI associated with short-term CVC (less than 14 days, 17.6%) as compared to long-term CVC (greater than 14 days, 5%).[6] Surprisingly, several studies failed to report any significant correlation between the CR-BSI and the risk factors for acquiring HIV infection, particularly for i.v. drug use.[5,6,26,28]

ETIOLOGIC AGENTS

Since the mid-1980s, an increasing proportion of hospital acquired BSIs reported to U.S. NNIS have been due to Gram-positive, rather than Gram-negative, organisms. The increase reported to NNIS was largely due to 4 pathogens: *Staphylococcus aureus,* coagulase-negative staphylococci (CoNS), *Candida* species, and enterococci.[29]

S. aureus is the most common agent found in CR-BSI studies on HIV[+] patients,[4,30,31,32] even though in some non-randomized European studies, a higher incidence of CoNS has been reported.[26,28,33] Skin and nasal colonization rates with *S. aureus* appear to be higher in HIV[+] patients compared to uninfected controls, and this correlates with an increasing rate of *S. aureus* BSI.[34] Although *Pneumocystis carinii* prophylaxis with cotrimoxazole and the prophylactic administration of other antibiotics such as rifabutin, rifampicin and quinolones are associated with reduced colonization rates, no significant reduction of *S. aureus* BSI were reported in these patients compared to patients without any prophylaxis.[27]

Candida albicans, followed by *Candida parapsilosis*, accounts for most of the *Candida* species causing catheter-related infections.[29] From 1980 to 1990, NNIS hospitals reported a nearly fivefold increase in the rate of nosocomial fungal BSI (1 to 4.9 per 10,000 discharges).[35] This increasing isolation rate is particularly evident among patients receiving total parenteral nutrition (TPN).[36] This secular trend appears to be confirmed among HIV[+] patients also. The recognition that *Candida* species can be, in half of the cases, an exogenous infection, transmitted from the hands of healthcare workers, is of importance to infection control. Furthermore, the emergence of non-*albicans Candida* species and of imidazole- and amphotericin B-resistant fungi is of great concern.

Gram-negative bacilli acquired from the hospital environment, such as *Acinetobacter* species, *Pseudomonas* species, and *Stenotrophomonas maltophilia*, have also been reported to cause catheter-related sepsis.[37] Several studies have suggested an increased risk of nosocomial BSI due to enteric gram negative bacilli.

Moreover, a cohort of hemodialysis HIV[+] patients had a fivefold increased risk of gram-negative BSI in comparison to uninfected controls.[38] *Pseudomonas aeruginosa* was found to be the predominant gram-negative organism (26.4%) in a population of 680 HIV[+] children and was highly associated with a previous diagnosis of AIDS and/or severe immunosuppression,[39] to the disruption of specific barriers, and previous administration of large spectrum antibiotics.[40] Other enteric organisms, such as *Escherichia coli* and *Klebsiella pneumoniae,* rarely cause catheter-related infections.[29] It has been suggested that clusters of gram negative BSI should raise suspicion of a common source, such as contaminated pressure monitoring devices or i.v. solutions.

Furthermore, it was reported that as the number of infectious complications increased (such as a second or third infectious event in the same patient), there was a shift towards an increasing frequency of mixed gram-positive and gram-negative CR-BSI.[30]

Few authors have investigated the changing pattern of etiologic agents of BSIs among HIV$^+$ patients during HAART. A statistically significant reduction in the incidence of nosocomial bacteremia caused by CoNS and gram-negative bacteria, particularly evident for nontyphoid *Salmonella* ($p = 0.02$), compared to patients treated with one or two antiretroviral drugs has been reported.[31] The HAART-induced immune restoration, the shortened hospitalization stays, and the decreased incidence of AIDS-related infections and cancers are all clearly associated with the reduction of the prevalence of BSI.[31]

PATHOGENESIS

The pathogenesis of catheter-related infections is multifactorial and complex, but available scientific data show that short term (< 14 days) catheter-related infections usually result from migration of skin organisms at the insertion site into the cutaneous catheter tract with extraluminal colonization of the catheter tip.[41,42] Conversely, contamination of the catheter hub is an important contributor to intraluminal colonization of long-term catheters (greater than 14 days).[43–46]

Other important pathogenic determinants of catheter-related infections are the material of which the device is made and the intrinsic properties of the infecting organism. *In vitro* studies show that catheters made of Teflon, silicone elastomer, or polyurethane appear to be less susceptibile to the adherence of micro-organisms.[47]

The adherence properties of a given micro-organism are also important in the pathogenesis of catheter-related infection. For example, *S. aureus* can adhere to host proteins (e.g., fibronectin) commonly present on catheters,[48] and CoNS adhere to polymer surfaces more readily than do other common nosocomial pathogens such as *Escherichia coli* or *S. aureus*.[49] Additionally, certain strains of CoNS produce an extracellular polysaccharide often referred to as "slime." This extracellular matrix may be separated into primary attachment of bacteria to native or modified polymer surfaces followed by proliferation of attached bacterial cells leading to accumulation of multi-layered cell-clusters and glicocalyx formation.

In the presence of catheters, this slime potentiates the pathogenicity of CoNS by allowing them to withstand host defense mechanisms[50,51] (e.g., acting as a barrier to engulfment and killing by polymorphonuclear leukocytes) or by making them less susceptible to antimicrobial agents[52] (e.g., forming a matrix that binds antimicrobials before their contact with the organism cell wall). Similarly, certain *Candida* species, have surface receptors that allow adherence to the thrombin biofilm that forms on the catheter, and coagulase production by *Candida* spp. may further contribute to the formation of biofilm; second, hydrophobic interactions between *Candida* surface proteins and the plastic itself may also promote adherence.[53]

CATHETER-RELATED BLOODSTREAM
INFECTION RATE IN HIV⁺ PATIENTS

The incidence rate of CR-BSI among HIV infected patients ranges from 1.3 to 12 per 1,000 catheter-days[5,6,9,26,28,30,32,33,38] varying considerably with the type of device in use (see TABLE 1).

1. **Nontunneled central venous catheters (NTCVC).** Nontunneled, percutaneously inserted, CVC are the most commonly used central catheters and account for an estimated 90% of all CR-BSI.[11] Among 142 HIV⁺ patients with NTCVC, 26 catheters (18.3%) were infected: the total and serious

TABLE 1. Catheter-related bloodstream infection rate in HIV⁺ patients according to the type of device

Device	Infection Rate	Number of patients with catheter[a]	Reference
Nontunneled central venous catheters	2.8	87	Skiest, J. AIDS 1998
	3.2	100	Petrosillo, AIDS 2000
	12	212	Tacconelli, J. Hosp. Infect. 2000
Peripherally inserted central venous catheters	1.3	—	Prichard, South Med. J. 1988
	1.3	66	Skiest, Clin. Infect. Dis. 2000
Tunneled central venous catheters	4.7	44	Raviglione, Am. J. Med. 1989
	1.8	63	Mukau, J. Parenter. Enteral Nutr. 1992
	3.81	209	Asteagneau, Infect. Control Hosp. Epidemiol. 1999
	2.23	40	Mokrzycki, J. Am. Soc. Nephrol. 2000
Totally implantable intravascular devices	1.3	51	van der Pijl, AIDS 1992
	2.2	8	Dega, J. AIDS Human Retrov. 1996
	3.39	209	Asteagneau, Infect. Control Hosp. Epidemiol. 1999
CVC without device specification	2	72	Stanley, J. AIDS 1994
	1.25	102	Sweed, Am. J. Infect. Control 1995
	6.5–1.21[b]	1339	Stroud, Infect. Control Hosp. Epidemiol. 1997
	3.3	338	Thorne, AIDS 1998

[a] Per 1000 CVC-days.
[b] Patients in intensive care unit.

infectious rate were 2.8 and 1.4 per 1,000 device-days with a mean time to a serious infection of 407 days.[32] Conversely in two Italian survey, a CVC-related sepsis developed in 13% and 19% of devices with a total infectious rate of 8 and 12 per 1,000 device-days, respectively.[6,28] These apparently discordant data appear to be related to the more advanced phase of HIV infection in these patients.

2. **Peripherally inserted central venous catheters.** Peripherally inserted CVC (PICC) provide an alternative to subclavian or jugular vein catheterization. PICC are easy to maintain and are associated with fewer mechanical complications (e.g., thrombosis, hemothorax), lower rates of infection (range 0–1.5 per 1,000 catheter-days) and lower costs.[54,55] Similarly, in HIV+ patients a low infection rate compared to historical controls was reported: the total and serious infection rate was 1.3 and 0.8 per 1,000 device-days, respectively, with the mean time to a serious infection of 310 days.[5,56]

3. **Tunneled central venous catheters (TCVC).** Surgically implanted central catheters, including Hickman, Broviac, Groshong, and Quinton, commonly have a tunneled portion exiting the skin and a Dacron cuff just inside the exit site providing a natural anchor for the catheter. In general, the rates of infections reported with the use of tunneled catheters have been significantly lower than those reported with the use of nontunneled CVC. A large clinical trial with a prospective examination of 1431 devices in cancer patients demonstrated an infection rate of 2.77 per 1,000 device-days.[29] Consistent with these data, in a population survey of HIV+ patients from a hemodialysis service in the United States, a 2.23 BSI rate per 1,000 TCVC was found, very similar to the HIV− control population rate (2.5 per 1,000 device-days).[38]

4. **Totally implantable intravascular devices (TID).** TIDs are tunneled beneath the skin with a subcutaneous port accessed by needle puncture through intact skin. Similarly to TCVC, TID have the lowest reported rates of CR-BSI (about 0.21 infections per 1,000 device-days)[29] possibly because they are located beneath the skin with no orifice for ingress of micro-organisms.

A retrospective study in 84 consecutive HIV+ patients reported an infection rate of 2.2 per 1,000 device-days with a mean time to onset of infection of 82 days.[33] A recent survey of a population of 209 French HIV+ patients showed no differences between tunnelled-CVC and TID with a 3.81 versus 3.39 infection rate per 1,000 catheter-days ($p = 0.79$), although a crude infection rate was higher in TCVC than tunnelled catheters (36.1% versus 20.3%, $p < 0.02$).[26] On the other hand, a retrospective study on a North-American population of AIDS patients treated for cytomegalovirus retinitis, showed that TID had an increased risk of sepsis when compared to single-lumen TCVC.[30] This result, which differed from others,[7,26] is partially explained by the single lumen of TCVC and by the reduced manipulation of TID with respect to TCVC.

Probably, only a large longitudinal multicentric clinical trial could answer the question of what type of device shares the lowest infective complications rates in

HIV$^+$ patients. However, at this time, the selection of a given device for long-term intravenous access should depend on the intended use, the clinical condition of the patient, the expertise of the medical group, and patient-practitioner preference.

DIAGNOSIS OF CATHETER-RELATED BLOODSTREAM INFECTIONS

More than 90% of nosocomial BSI are associated with CVC and the diagnosis of these infections remains difficult.[1] Several definitions of CR-NBSI are used in clinical practice; for HIV$^+$ patients, the modified CDC definitions[11] are as follows[6]:

> Isolation of the same organism from blood culture and either from a catheter tip by the Maki roll plate technique (at least 15 CFU/ml) or the Cleri technique (at least 1000 CFU/ml) or in association with purulence, erythema, and growth of the same organism from the skin exit site; or primary bacteremia with positive blood culture (at least two positive blood cultures for CoNS) and presence of a CVC; or clinical sepsis that is refractory to antibiotics but resolves after CVC removal.

Which method is best for the diagnosis of CR-BSI is controversial. Seligman first proposed the use of quantitative culture of the catheter segment in 1974.[57] Several years later, Maki *et al.*, demonstrated that the roll-plate semiquantitative catheter segment culture was more accurate than the qualitative culture of the catheter,[58] and probably, it still remains the simplest and most commonly used method.

Recently, the result of a large meta-analysis[59] confirmed the superiority of quantitative techniques for catheter segment cultures. Quantitative catheter segment culture is the most accurate method, being the only one with pooled sensitivity and specificity above 90%.

Although it is plausible that the greater accuracy of the quantitative methods may derive from quantitation of the bacterial load, it may also be related to the variable pathogenesis of CR-BSI, which can arise from luminal or extraluminal infection. Quantitative catheter segment culture by using sonication, ultrasonication, and/or vortex techniques, permits detection of bacteria from both surface and lumen of the catheter, whereas the semiquantitative technique detects only organisms on the external surface of the catheter.

The paired quantitative method by culturing both simultaneous peripheral and central blood, seems to show a high performance in terms of accuracy with a 10:1 colonies forming units ratio between CVC and peripheral vein, indicative of CR-BSI. In consideration of the difficulty to perform quantitative blood cultures, the different bacteria growth kinetics between peripheral and central blood cultures (using a cut-off of 120 min as differential time to positivity) appears to be a valid alternative to the paired quantitative method for the diagnosis of CR-BSI in patients with long-term CVC.[60,61]

Recently, the gram stain and acridine-orange leukocyte cytospin (AOLC) test was investigated to obtain a rapid diagnosis of BSI; the test is a simple, inexpensive and rapid method, requiring only 100 microliter of catheter blood and the use of light and ultraviolet microscopy. Furthermore, it can permit early targeted antimicrobial therapy. The sensitivity of the gram stain and AOLC test is 96%, the specificity is 92%, with a positive predictive value of 91% and a negative predictive value of 97%, compared with the paired culture quantitative method.[62]

Treatment

Treatment of CR-BSI should take into account the organisms more frequently isolated, CoNS and *S. aureus,* among others. Since many of these organisms are hospital acquired, and the frequency of methicillin-resistance is likely to be high, an empirical initial treatment should consider the use of glycopeptides with or without the addition of a gram-negative coverage, depending on the local prevalence and resistance patterns.[63,64]

The reported efficacy of systemic antibiotic therapy alone is only 25–32% and the substitution of the catheter with or without replacing it at an alternative site is still considered standard practice.[11,63,65] Over time, with several catheter changes, vascular access sites may become limited.

Exchange procedures over a guidewire is frequently adopted to save the catheter and to reduce the patients' suffering. However, the CDC suggest that the exchange procedure should not be done in the setting of documented catheter-related infection.[11]

However, in a prospective study on HIV[+] patients, exchange of CVC by guidewire technique did not significantly correlate with an increased risk of CR-BSI and/or with major technical complications (e.g., pneumothorax, thrombosis, etc.) and allowing the culture of the catheter tip.[28] Indeed, the data in this study indicated that the incidence of established infections is much lower (19%) than that of suspected ones (33%), so it is unlikely to exchange in the course of a catheter-related infection.

Treating bacteremia without catheter removal would be optimal. Using systemic antimicrobial therapy in an attempt to salvage the CVC has become widespread practice, although this approach has never been subjected to a randomized controlled trial.[66] Some authors had encouraging results in the treatment of CR-BSI without CVC removal[67,68] but only one study evaluated the recurrence of infection: during a 12-months follow-up period, the bacteremia recurred in 20% of the patients whose catheters remained in place, compared with only 3% of those whose catheters were removed.[69] Furthermore, in the presence of CR-BSI caused by fungal agents or gram-negative organisms, the more conservative approach without CVC removing, showed a significantly lower cure rate;[70,71] particularly, the mortality rate in patients with CR-candidemia was significantly higher in patients in whom the CVC was retained.[71]

More recently attempts have been made to salvage the catheter by using high concentrations of antibiotic injected into the catheter and then "locked in" (antibiotic lock technique). Up to 90% of patients receiving home TPN achieved eradication of CR-BSI without catheter removal, using an antibiotic-lock procedure with or without systemic antibiotics.[72,73] In addition, in hemodialysis patients, a 4-hour continuous antibiotic infusion followed by an antibiotic-lock (vancomycin or ciprofloxacin 100 μg/ml in 5% sodium heparin) successfully eradicated all 13 cases of catheter-related sepsis without catheter removal.[74]

Similarly, in two longitudinal studies of 68 and 12 consecutive AIDS patients with TIDs, the antibiotic lock technique was associated in both cases with decreased device loss, when compared with systemic antibiotic therapy alone.[75,76] Furthermore, few studies confirmed the same antibacterial efficacy without major complications using a mixed lock solution of heparin (5000 UI/ml), in addition to antibiotics to improve the access to the infected catheter.[77,78] The spectrophotometrical analysis of the mixed antibiotic-heparin lock solution confirmed a good stability at 24-hour intervals.[79]

PREVENTIVE METHODS

Infusion-Therapy Team and Maximal Sterile Barriers

The infection rate of micotic and bacterial CR-BSI in TPN has been reduced 5- to 8-fold by the following measures: preparing solutions in laminar flow rooms with rigid aseptic techniques and routine bacteriological testing, dedication of catheters to TPN, and the use of a TPN team to perform all the necessary manipulations.[11,55] Moreover, the availability of an experienced infusion-therapy team has determined an exceptionally low rate of infection of nontunneled, noncuffed, silastic CVC used in a large population of immunosuppressed patients, that is 1.3 infections per 1000 catheter days.[55]

The level of barrier precautions needed to prevent infection during insertion of CVC still represents a source of debate. The usual procedure involves wearing gloves and using a small drape. A large drape and wearing sterile gloves, mask, gown, and cap represent a maximal sterile barrier. A randomized, longitudinal trial, comparing the CR-BSI rate for CVC inserted with maximal sterile barrier precautions versus the usual technique showed a 6-fold reduction. Most BSI (67%) in the control group occurred in the first week postinsertion, whereas all BSI in the sterile-barrier group occurred more than 2 months following insertion ($p < 0.01$).[80]

Antibiotics: Topical Ointment and Coated Catheters

Comparative studies of cutaneous antisepsis have largely examined its efficacy in eradicating bacterial flora from the hands of hospital personnel.[81,82] Povidone-iodine ointment applied to the insertion site has not been shown to significantly decrease the rate of catheter-related infections.[81]

Topical antibiotics (such as polymyxin-neomycin-bacitracin) do significantly decrease the total risk of acquiring catheter-related bacterial infections, but this occurs at the expense of an increased risk of fungal colonization and infection.[81]

A sustained-release chlorhexidine gluconate patch has been introduced as a dressing for catheter insertion sites. In one randomized trial of epidural catheters, the use of these patches significantly reduced the incidence of catheter colonization.[83] In a three-arm trial, the effectiveness of 70% alcohol, 10% povidone-iodine, and 2% chlorhexidine gluconate was compared.[82] The rate of CR-BSI was almost four-fold lower in the chlorhexidine arm than in the other two arms.

Coating catheters with antibiotics or antiseptics may be even more protective, particularly if both external and internal surfaces of the catheter are coated. The use of CVC coated with minocycline and rifampin was associated with a 30% reduction in catheter colonization and no CR-BSIs among patients with coated catheters.[84] Similarly, the use of CVC coated with chlorhexidine-silver sulfadiazine (CSS) was associated with a 44 and 79% reduction in catheter colonization and CR-BSI, respectively.[85]

A recent study reported that patients with catheters impregnated with minocycline and rifampin had a 3-fold lower infection rate compared to patients with CSS-coated catheters.[86] On the other hand, a randomized clinical trial reported no additional reduction in the CR-BSI rate by using CSS-coated catheters compared to non- antimicrobial–impregnated CVC in the presence of strict infection control measures.[87]

Silver Cuff

Several studies have shown that an attachable silver-impregnated cuff can reduce the CR-BSI among critically ill patients: catheters inserted with the cuff were threefold less likely to be colonized than were control catheters (28.9% versus 9.1%, $p = 0.002$) and were nearly fourfold less likely to produce bacteremia (3.7% versus 1.0%).[88,89]

Conversely, recent studies report that the silver cuff failed to prevent local CVC-related infections and CR-BSI in critically ill surgical, trauma and peritoneal dialysis patients.[90,91] Furthermore, silver-cuff material demonstrates a local cytotoxicity on hybrid cells and human fibroblasts *in vitro*. This finding may explain the observed

TABLE 2. Simple interventions to reduce the risk of catheter-related bloodstream infections

Continuing quality improvement programs aimed at improving compliance with catheter care guidelines are recommended.

Subcutaneous tunneling of short-term internal jugular or femoral vein CVCs is recommended if the catheters are not accessed for drawing blood.

Do not use antimicrobial drugs prophylactically before the insertion of and during the use of a CVC.

Prophylaxis with very-low-dose warfarin should be strongly considered for patients with long-term, indwelling intravascular catheters.

Use a single-lumen CVC, unless multiple ports.

Use subclavian, rather than jugular or femoral, sites for central venous catheter placement.

Use maximal barrier precautions for the insertion of CVC.

Chlorhexidine-containing antiseptics should be used, where approved, for skin preparation before catheter insertion.

Do not routinely apply antimicrobial ointment to central venous catheter insertion sites; but, povidone-iodine ointment to insertion sites of nontunneled, long term CVC in immunocompromised patients with heavy *S. aureus* carriage should be considered.

Wipe the catheter hub with an appropriate antiseptic before accessing the system.

In-line filters should be avoided.

Do not use guide wire–assisted catheter exchange whenever catheter-related infection is documented.

If CR-infection is suspected, but there is no evidence of local CR-infection, remove the existing catheter and insert a new catheter over a guide wire. Send the removed catheter for culture. Leave the newly inserted catheter in place if the catheter culture result is negative. If the catheter culture indicates colonization or infection, remove the newly inserted catheter, and insert a new catheter at a different site.

Consider use of a silver-impregnated collagen cuff or an antimicrobial- or antiseptic-impregnated CVCs if, despite full adherence to infection control measures, there is still an unacceptably high rate of infection.

Do not routinely replace nontunneled CVCs as a method to prevent CR-BSI.

NOTE: Modified by Pearlson[11] and Mermel.[94]

phenomena of decreased anchorage and inadvertent removal of catheters with silver-impregnated collagen cuffs.[92]

Flush and Antibiotic Flushes

Flush solutions with anticoagulants are designed to prevent thrombi and fibrin deposits on catheters, which may serve as a nidus for microbial colonization of the intravascular devices.[10] Using a mixed solution of heparin and vancomycin to flush tunneled CVC decreased the frequency of CR-BSI caused by gram-positive organisms colonizing the catheter lumen[93] during chemotherapy-induced neutropenia in patients with hematologic malignancy.[78] Nevertheless, either a potential superinfection with gram-negative bacilli and *Candida* spp. and/or the emergence of glycopeptide-resistant gram-positive cocci could be caused by heavy prophylactic use of vancomycin.[94]

In addition, there are reports of patient-to-patient transmission of organisms by using multidose vials.[95]

Major infection control measures for the management of CVC are shown in TABLE 2.

CONCLUSION

In order to carry out an effective program to reduce the catheter-related colonization, the CR-BSI and the emergence and dramatic spread of polymicrobic-drug resistance in the hospital setting, the following points should be made for the future:

- The procedure of catheter change over a guidewire is not recommended as an infection-control measure.[11] However, in consideration of the good results among HIV+ subjects,[28] the technique of catheter change over a guidewire should be further investigated.

- In consideration of the potential emergence of resistance to single antibiotic agents impregnated to catheters,[83] coated-catheters should not be used unless all other recommendations for preventing CR-BSIs are followed. If institutions still experience substantial CR-BSI rates despite adherence to all recommendations, then such catheters should be considered.

- Prophylaxis with glycopeptides during CVC insertion has not been demonstrated to reduce the incidence of CR-BSI and definitely should not be recommended.[94]

- In consideration of recent reports of limited studies,[72–79] lock antibiotic techniques should be further investigated in large prospective studies.

Finally, longitudinal randomized clinical trials experimenting with materials without incorporation of antimicrobial agents such as covalently linked heparin on the CVC surface, electrically charged CVC, novel topical agents (such as lytic enzymes, peptides, and antibodies) that interfere with bacterial colonization, anti-adhesin molecules that block the fibronectin-binding protein adhesin of *S. aureus* and agents that block the expression of open reading frames that mediate the *S. epidermidis* autoaggregation and biofilm formation, are all needed to reduce the high CR-infection risk among HIV⁺ patients.

ACKNOWLEDGMENT

This work was supported by III Italian AIDS Project-ISS 20C.10.

REFERENCES

1. WIDMER, A. 1993. IV-related infections. *In* Prevention and Control of Nosocomial Infections. R.P. Wenzel, Ed.: 556–579. Williams & Wilkins, Baltimore.
2. PITTET, D., D. TARARA & R.P. WENZEL. 1994. Nosocomial bloodstream infections in critically ill patients. Excess length of stay, extra cost, and attributable mortality. JAMA **271:** 1598–1601.
3. BANERJEE, S.N. *et al.* 1991. Secular trends in nosocomial bloodstream infections in the United States, 1980–1989. Am. J. Med. **91:** 87S–89S.
4. OMEÑACA, C. *et al.* 1999. Bacteremia in HIV-infected patients: short term predictors of mortality. J. AIDS **22:** 155–160.
5. SKIEST, D.J., M. ABBOTT & P. KEISER. 2000. Peripherally inserted central catheters in patients with AIDS are associated with a low infection rate. Clin. Infect. Dis. **30:** 949–952.
6. PETROSILLO, N. *et al.* 2000. Nosocomial infections in HIV infected patients. AIDS **13:** 559–605.
7. CORONA, M.L. *et al.* 1990. Infections related to central venous catheters. Mayo Clin. Proc. **65:** 979–986.
8. MEYER, C.N., P. SKINHOJ & J. PRAG. 1994. Bacteremia in HIV-positive and AIDS patients: incidence, species distribution, risk-factors, outcome, and influence of long-term prophylactic antibiotic treatment. Scand. J. Infect. Dis. **26:** 635–642.
9. STROUD, L. *et al.* 1997. Nosocomial infections in HIV-infected patients: preliminary results from a multicenter surveillance system (1989-1995). Infect. Control Hosp. Epidemiol. **18:** 479–485.
10. GOSBELL, I.B. 1994. Central venous catheter-relate sepsis: epidemiology, pathogenesis, diagnosis, treatment and prevention. Int. Care World **11:** 54–58.
11. PEARSON, M.L. 1996. Guideline for prevention of intravascular device-related infections. Hospital Infection Control Practices Advisory Committee. Infect. Control Hosp. Epidemiol. **17:** 438-73. Available at: http://www.cdc.gov/ncidod/hip/iv/iv.htm.
12. ARNOW, P.M., E.M. QUIMOSING & M. BEACH. 1993. Consequences of intravascular catheter sepsis. Clin. Infect. Dis. **16:** 778–783.
13. RELLO, J. *et al.* 1997. Specific problems of arterial Swan-Ganz and hemodialysis catheters. Nutrition **13:** 2S–8S.
14. SNYDMAN, D.R. *et al.* 1982. Total parenteral nutrition-related infections: prospective epidemiologic study using semiquantitative methods. Am. J. Med. **73:** 695–699.
15. HAMPTON, A.A. & R.J. SHERERTZ. 1988. Vascular-access infections in hospitalized patients. Surg. Clin. North. Am. **68:** 57–71.
16. MORO, M.L., E. FRANCO & A. COZZI. 1994. The central venous catheter-related infections study group: risk factors for central venous catheter-related infections in surgical and intensive care patients. Infect. Control. Hosp. Epidemiol. **14:** 153–159.
17. ARMSTRONG, C.W. *et al.* 1986. Prospective study of catheter replacement and other risk factors for infection of hyperalimentation catheters. J. Infect. Dis. **154:** 808–816.
18. SITZMANN, J.V. *et al.* 1985. Septic and technical complications of central venous catheterization: a prospective study of 200 consecutive patients. Ann. Surg. **202:** 766–770.

19. HILTON, E. *et al.* 1988. Central catheter infections: Single vs. triple-lumen catheters; influence of guidelines on infection rates when used for replacement of catheters. Am. J. Med. **84:** 667–672.

20. YEUNG, C. *et al.* 1988. Infection rate for single-lumen vs. triple-lumen subclavian catheters. Infect. Control Hosp. Epidemiol. **9:** 154–158.

21. MANTESE, V.A. *et al.* 1987. Colonization and sepsis from triple-lumen catheters in critically ill patients. Am. J. Surg. **154:** 597–601.

22. MACCARTHY, M.C. *et al.* 1987. Prospective evaluation of single and triple lumen catheters in total parenteral nutrition. J. Parenter. Enteral Nutr. **11:** 259–262.

23. FARKAS, J.C. *et al.* 1992. Single- versus triple-lumen central catheter-related sepsis: A prospective randomized study in a critically ill population. Am. J. Med. **93:** 277–282.

24. MERMEL, L.A. *et al.* 1991. The pathogenesis and epidemiology of catheter-related infection with pulmonary artery Swan-Ganz catheters: a prospective study utilizing molecular subtyping. Am. J. Med. **91**(Suppl. 3B): S197–S205.

25. GIL, R.T. *et al.* 1989. Triple- vs single-lumen central venous catheters. A prospective study in a critically ill population. Arch. Intern. Med. **149:** 1139–1143

26. ASTEAGNEAU, P. *et al.* 1999. Long-term venous catheter infection in HIV-infected and cancer patients: a multicenter cohort study. Infect. Control Hosp. Epidemiol. **20:** 494–498.

27. STYRT, B.A., R.E. CHAISSON & R.D. MOORE. 1997. Prior antimicrobials and staphylococcal bacteremia in HIV-infected patients. AIDS **11:** 1243–1248.

28. TACCONELLI, J. *et al.* 2000. Morbidity associated with central venous catheter use in a cohort of 212 hospitalized subjects with HIV infection J. Hosp. Infect. **44:** 186–192.

29. GROEGER, J.S. *et al.* 1993. Infectious morbidity associated with long-term use of venous access devices in patients with cancer. Ann. Intern. Med. **119:** 1168–1174.

30. THORNE, J.E. *et al.* 1998. Catheter complications in AIDS patients treated for cytomegalovirus retinitis. AIDS **12:** 2321–2327.

31. TUMBARELLO, M. *et al.* 2000. HIV-associated bacteremia: how it has changed in the highly active antiretroviral therapy (HAART) era. J. AIDS **23:** 145–151.

32. SKIEST, D.J., P. GRANT & P. KEISER. 1998. Nontunneled central venous catheters in patients with AIDS are associated with a low infection rate. J. AIDS **17:** 220–226.

33. DEGA, H. *et al.* 1996. Infections associated with totally implantable venous access devices (TIVAD) in human immunodeficiency virus-infected patients. J. AIDS Hum. Retrovirol. **13:** 146–154.

34. CRAVEN, D.E. *et al.* 1993. Risk factors for nasopharyngeal colonization in with *Staphylococcus aureus* in HIV-infected outpatients. Abstract S51 The 3rd annual meeting of Society of Hospital Epidemiology of America, Chicago.

35. BECK-SAGUÈ, C.M. & W.R. JARVIS. 1993. Secular trends in the epidemiology of nosocomial fungal infections in the United States, 1980–1990. J. Infect. Dis. **167:** 1247–1251.

36. BRANCHINI, M.L. *et al.* 1994. Genotypic variation in slime production among blood and catheter isolates of *Candida parapsilosis*. J. Clin. Microbiol. **32:** 452–456.

37. SEIFERT, H. *et al.* 1993. Vascular catheter-related bloodstream infection due to *Acinetobacter johnsonii* (formerly *Acinetobacter calcoaceticus* var. *lwoffi*): Report of 13 cases. Clin. Infect. Dis. **17:** 632–636.

38. MOKRZYCKI, M.H. *et al.* 2000. Tunneled-cuffed catheter associated infections in hemodialysis patients who are positive for the human immunodeficiency virus. J. Am. Soc. Nephrol. **11:** 2122–2127.

39. RONGKAVILIT, C. *et al.* 2000. Gram-negative bacillary bacteremia in human immunodeficiency type-1 infected children. Pediatr. Infect. Dis. J. **19:** 122–128.

40. DUSE, A.G. 1999. Nosocomial infections in HIV-infected/AIDS patients. J. Hosp. Infect. **43:** S191–S201.

41. SNYDMAN, D.R. *et al.* 1982. Predictive value of surveillance skin cultures in total parenteral nutrition-related infection. Prospective epidemiologic study using semiquantitative cultures. Lancet **2:** 1385–1388.

42. COOPER, G.L. & C.C. HOPKINS. 1985. Rapid diagnosis of intravascular catheter-associated infection by direct gram staining of catheter segments. N. Engl. J. Med. **312:** 1142–1147.

43. DECICCO, M. *et al.* 1989. Source and route of microbial colonization of parenteral nutrition catheters. Lancet **2**(8674): 1258–1261.

44. SALZMAN, M.B. *et al.* 1993. A prospective study of the catheter hub as the portal of entry for microorganisms causing catheter-related sepsis in neonates. J. Infect. Dis. **167:** 487–490.

45. SITGES-SERRA, A. *et al.* 1985. A randomized trial on the effect of tubing changes on hub contamination and catheter sepsis during parenteral nutrition. J. Parenter. Enteral Nutr. **9:** 322–325.

46. RAAD, I. *et al.* 1993. Ultrastructural analysis of indwelling vascular catheters: a quantitative relationship between luminal colonization and duration of placement. J. Infect. Dis. **168:** 400–407.

47. ASHKENAZI, S. *et al.* 1986. Bacterial adherence to intravenous catheters and needles and its influence by cannula type and bacterial surface hydrophobicity. J. Lab. Clin. Med. **107:** 136–140.

48. HERRMANN, M. *et al.* 1988. Fibronectin, fibrinogen, and laminin act as mediators of adherence of clinical staphylococcal isolates to foreign material. J. Infect. Dis. **158:** 693–701.

49. MACK, D. 1999. Molecular mechansms of *Staphylococcus epidermidis* biofilm formation. J. Hosp. Infect. **43:** S113–S125.

50. JOHNSON, G.M. *et al.* 1986. Interference with granulocyte function by *Staphylococcus epidermidis* slime. Infect. Immun. **54:** 13–20.

51. GRAY, E.D. *et al.* 1984. Effect of extracellular slime substance from *Staphylococcus epidermidis* on the human cellular immune response. Lancet **1**(8373): 365–367.

52. FARBER, B.F., M.H. KAPLAN & A.G. CLOGSTON. 1990. *Staphylococcus epidermidis* extracted slime inhibits the antimicrobial action of glycopeptide antibiotics. J. Infect. Dis. **161:** 37–40.

53. CALDERONE, R.A. & P.C. BRAUN. 1991. Adherence and receptor relationships of *Candida albicans*. Microbiol. Rev. **15:** 197–210.

54. RYDER, M.A. 1995. Peripheral access options. Surg. Oncol. Clin. N. Am. **4:** 395–427.

55. RAAD, I. *et al.* 1993. Low infection rate and long durability of nontunneled silastic catheters. Arch. Intern. Med. **153:** 1791–1796.

56. PRICHARD, J.C. *et al.* 1988. Infections caused by central venous catheters in patients with acquired immunodeficiency syndrome. South Med. J. **81:** 1496–1498.

57. SELIGMAN, S.J. 1974. Quantitative intra venous catheter cultures identify focus of bacteremia. Abstract M18 of the annual meeting of the American Society of Microbiology. American Society of Microbiology, Washington DC.

58. MAKI, D.G., C.E. WEISE & H.W. SARAFIN. 1977. A semiquantitative culture method for identifying intravenous-catheter-related infection. N. Engl. J. Med. **296:** 1305–1309.

59. SIEGMAN-SIGRA, Y. *et al.* 1997. Diagnosis of vascular catheter-related bloodstream infections: a meta-analysis. J. Clin. Microbiol. **35:** 928–936.

60. BLOT, F. *et al.* 1999. Diagnosis of catheter-related bacteraemia: a prospective comparison of the time to positivity of hub-blood versus peripheral-blood cultures. Lancet **354:** 1071–1077.

61. MALGRANGE, V.B., M.C. ESCANDE & S. THEOBALD. 2001. Validity of earlier positivity of central venous blood cultures in comparison with peripheral blood cultures for diagnosing catheter-related bacteremia in cancer patients. J. Clin. Microbiol. **39:** 274–278.

62. KITE, P. *et al.* 1999. Rapid diagnosis of central-venous-catheter-related bloodstream infection without catheter removal. Lancet **354:** 1504–1507.

63. MARR, K.A. *et al.* 1997. Catheter-related bacteremia and outcome of attempted catheter salvage in patients undergoing hemodialysis. Ann. Intern. Med. **127:** 275–280.

64. HURAIB, S. *et al.* 1994. Prevalence of infection from subclavian dialysis catheters with two different post-insertion catheter cares: a randomized comparative study. Angiology **45:** 1047–1051.

65. SWARTZ, R.D. *et al.* 1994. Successful use of cuffed central venous hemodialysis catheters inserted percutaneously. J. Am. Soc. Nephrol. **4:** 1719–1725.

66. OPPENHEIM, B.A. 2000. Optimal management of central venous catheter-related infections—what is the evidence? J. Hosp. Infect. **40:** 26–30.

67. FLYNN, P.M. *et al.* 1987. In situ management of confirmed central venous catheter-related bacteremia. Pediatr. Infect. Dis. J. **6:** 729–734.

68. SIMON, C. & M. SUTTORP. 1994. Results of antibiotic treatment of Hickman-catheter-related infections in oncological patients. Support Care Cancer **2:** 66–70.

69. RAAD, I. *et al.* 1992. Impact of central venous catheter removal on the recurrence of catheter related coagulase-negative staphylococcal bacteraemia. Infect. Control Hosp. Epidemiol. **13:** 215–221.

70. ELTING, L.S. & G.P. BODEY. 1990. Septicemia due to *Xanthomonas* species and non-*aeruginosa Pseudomonas* species: increasing incidence of catheter-related infections. Medicine (Baltimore) **69:** 296–306.

71. NGUYEN, M.H. *et al.* 1995. Therapeutic approaches in patients with candidemia. Evaluation in a multicenter, prospective, observational study. Arch. Intern. Med. **155:** 2429–2435.

72. BENOIT, J.L. *et al.* 1995. Intraluminal antibiotic treatment of central venous catheter infections in patients receiving parenteral nutrition at home. Clin. Infect. Dis. **21:** 1286–1288.

73. MESSING, B. *et al.* 1988. Antibiotic-lock technique: a new approach to optimal therapy for catheter-related sepsis in home parenteral nutrition patients. J. Enteral Parenteral Nutr. **12:** 185–189.

74. CAPDEVILA, J.A. *et al.* 1993. Successful treatment of haemodialysis catheter-related sepsis without catheter removal. Nephrol. Dial. Transplant. **8:** 231–234.

75. DOMINGO, P. *et al.* 1999. Morbidity associated with long-term use of totally implantable ports in patients with AIDS. Clin. Infect. Dis. **29:** 346–351.

76. VIALE, P.L. *et al.* 2000. Antibiotic-lock technique: an alternative therapeutic approach to central venous catheter related bacteremia. Abstract presented at the 4th decennial International Conference on Nosocomial and Healthcare-associated Infections. Infect. Control Hosp. Epidemiol. **21:** 98.

77. BOORGU, R. *et al.* 2000. Adjunctive antibiotic/anticoagulant lock therapy in the treatment of bacteremia associated with the use of a subcutaneously implanted hemodialysis access device. ASAIO J. **46:** 767–770.

78. CARRATALÀ, J. *et al. 1999.* Randomized, double-blind trial of an antibiotic-lock technique for prevention of gram-positive central venous catheter-related infection in neutropenic patients with cancer. Antimicrob. Agents Chemother. **43:** 2200–2204.

79. VERCAIGNE, L.M. *et al.* 2000. Antibiotic-heparin lock: in vitro antibiotic stability combined with heparin in a central venous catheter. Pharmacotherapy **20:** 394–399.

80. RAAD, I. *et al.* 1994. Prevention of central venous catheter-related infections by using maximal sterile barrier precautions during insertion. Infect. Control Hosp. Epidemiol. **15:** 231–238.

81. MAKI, D.G. & J.D. BAND. 1981. A comparative study of polyantibiotic and iodophor ointments in prevention of vascular catheter-related infection. Am. J. Med. **70:** 739–744.

82. MAKI, D.G., M. RINGER & C.J. ALVARADO. 1991. Prospective randomized trial of pov-idone-iodine, alcohol, and chlorhexidine for prevention of infection associated with central venous and arterial catheters. Lancet **338:** 339–343.

83. SHAPIRO, J.M., E.L. BOND & J.K. GARMAN. 1990. Use of a chlorhexidine dressing to reduce microbial colonization of epidural catheters. Anesthesiology **73:** 625–631.

84. RAAD, I. *et al.* 1997. Central venous catheters coated with minocycline and rifampin for the prevention of catheter-related colonization and blood stream infections. A randomized, double-blind trial. Ann. Intern. Med. **127:** 267–274.

85. MAKI, D.G. *et al.* 1997. Prevention of central venous catheter-related blood stream infections by use of an antiseptic-impregnated catheter. A randomized, controlled trial. Ann. Intern. Med. **127:** 257–266.

86. DAROUICHE, R.O. *et al.* 1999. A comparison of two antimicrobial-impregnated central venous catheters. N. Engl. J. Med. **340:** 1–8.

87. HEARD, S.O. *et al.* 1998. Influence of triple-lumen central venous catheters coated with chlorhexidine and silver sulfadiazine on the incidence of catheter-related bacteremia. Arch. Intern. Med. **158:** 81–87.
88. MAKI, D.G. *et al.* 1988. An attachable silver-impregnated cuff for the prevention of infection with central venous catheters: a prospective randomized multicenter trial. Am. J. Med. **85:** 307–314.
89. FLOWERS, R.H. III *et al.* 1989. Efficacy of an attachable subcutaneous cuff for the prevention of intravascular catheter-related infection. JAMA **261:** 878–883.
90. HASANIYA, N.W. *et al.* 1996. Efficacy of subcutaneous silver-impregnated cuffs in preventing central venous catheter infections. Chest **109:** 1030–1032.
91. POMMER, W. *et al.* 1998. Effect of a silver device in preventing catheter-related infections in peritoneal dialysis patients: silver ring prophylaxis at the catheter exit study. Am. J. Kidney Dis. **32:** 752–760.
92. HEMMERLEIN, J.B. *et al.* 1997. In vitro cytotoxicity of silver-impregnated collagen cuffs designed to decrease infection in tunneled catheters. Radiology **204:** 363–367.
93. SCHWARTZ, C. *et al.* 1990. Prevention of bacteremia attributed to luminal colonization of tunneled central venous catheters with vancomycin-susceptible organisms. J. Clin. Oncol. **8:** 591–597.
94. MERMEL, L.A. 2000. Prevention of intravascular catheter-related infections. Ann. Intern. Med. **132:** 391–402.
95. PETROSILLO, N. *et al.* 2000. Molecular epidemiology of an outbreak of fulminant hepatitis B. J. Clin. Microbiol. **38:** 2975–2981.

Risk of HIV and Other Blood-Borne Infections in the Cardiac Setting

Patient-to-Provider and Provider-to-Patient Transmission

VINCENZO PURO, GABRIELLA DE CARLI, PAOLA SCOGNAMIGLIO,
ROLANDO PORCASI, AND GIUSEPPE IPPOLITO,
ON BEHALF OF THE STUDIO ITALIANO RISCHIO OCCUPAZIONALE HIV[a]

*Dipartimento di Epidemiologia, Istituto Nazionale per le Malattie Infettive
"Lazzaro Spallanzani"—IRCCS, 00149 Rome, Italy*

ABSTRACT: Health care workers (HCWs) face a well-recognized risk of acquiring blood-borne pathogens in their workplace, in particular hepatitis B and C viruses (HBV/HBC) and human immunodeficiency virus (HIV). Additionally, infected HCWs performing invasive exposure-prone procedures, including in the cardiac setting, represent a potential risk for patients. An increasing number of infected persons could need specific cardiac diagnostic procedures and surgical treatment in the future, regardless of their sex or age. The risk of acquiring HIV, HCV, HBV infection after a single at-risk exposure averages 0.5%, and 1–2%, and 4–30%, respectively. The frequency of percutaneous exposure ranges from 1 to 15 per 100 surgical interventions, with cardiothoracic surgery reporting the highest rates of exposures; mucocutaneous contamination by blood-splash occurs in 50% of cardiothoracic operations. In the Italian Surveillance (SIROH), a total of 987 percutaneous and 255 mucocutaneous exposures were reported in the cardiac setting; most occurred in cardiology units (46%), and in cardiovascular surgery (44%). Overall, 257 source patients were anti-HCV[+], 54 HBsAg[+], and 14 HIV[+]. No seroconversions were observed. In the literature, 14 outbreaks were reported documenting transmission of HBV from 12 infected HCWs to 107 patients, and 2 cases of HCV to 6 patients, during cardiothoracic surgery, especially related to sternotomy and its suturing. The transmission rate was estimated to be 5% to 13% for HBV, and 0.36% to 2.25% for HCV. Strategies in risk reduction include adequate surveillance, education, effective sharps disposal, personal protective equipment, safety devices, and innovative technology-based intraoperative procedures.

KEYWORDS: blood-borne infections; health care workers; occupational exposures; provider-to-patient transmission

Address for correspondence: Dr. Vincenzo Puro, Dipartimento di Epidemiologia, Istituto Nazionale per le Malattie Infettive "Lazzaro Spallanzani"—IRCCS, Via Portuense, 292, 00149 Rome, Italy. Voice: +39 06 55170902; fax: + 39 06 55 82825.
puro@spallanzani.roma.it
[a]See APPENDIX for list of members.

INTRODUCTION

The risk of occupational blood-borne infections for health care workers (HCWs) has been reassessed in the last decades in relation to the spread of pathogens associated with significant morbidity and mortality, in particular hepatitis B virus (HBV), hepatitis C virus (HCV) and human immunodeficiency virus (HIV).[1] At-risk incidents have been identified as needlestick injuries or cuts with contaminated instruments, as well as blood contamination of open wound or of mucous membranes and possibly of a wide skin area with prolonged contact.[2,3] A series of recommendations for preventing and managing occupational exposures and infections have been issued and constantly updated, culminating in the Standard Precaution component of the Guideline for Isolation Precautions in Hospitals.[4]

The Studio Italiano Rischio Occupazionale da HIV (SIROH) is an Italian hospital network established in 1986, with ongoing enrollment, aiming to estimate the risk of transmission of HIV, HCV, and HBV to HCWs, following an occupational exposure to blood or other at-risk materials coming from infected sources. The SIROH protocol was expanded in 1994 to track all occupational exposures, regardless of the infectivity of the source, to identify high-risk devices, procedures, and jobs and therefore to study, monitor, and prevent the risk of occupational transmission of blood-borne pathogens in the health care setting.[3,5–7]

In the present study, we discuss the main findings from the literature and report results obtained by the SIROH, focusing on the risk of exposure in the settings of cardiology and cardiovascular surgery.

A specific paragraph is dedicated to recent public concerns regarding the risk of viral transmission from infected HCWs to the patients undergoing surgery or invasive exposure-prone procedures.[8,9]

THE OCCUPATIONAL RISK OF ACQUIRING HBV, HCV OR HIV INFECTION IN THE HEALTH CARE SETTING

The occupational risk of blood-borne infections in the health care setting mainly depends on three factors:
1. the prevalence of infected patients within the patient population,
2. the probability of acquiring a specific infection following a single occupational exposure, and
3. the frequency of at-risk exposures.[10]

Prevalence of HBV, HCV, and HIV Infection among Patients

The prevalence of HBV, HCV, and HIV infection among patients varies between, and within, different countries. This reflects the spread of these infections in the general population, and in sub-groups of populations who may serve as a reservoir for transmission in the health care setting.[1] Accordingly, prevalence amongst patients attending cardiology units or undergoing invasive cardiovascular procedures depends on how many people engage in behaviors at high risk for these infections, as well as for the development of cardiovascular diseases. For example, the majority of HIV[+] patients who need cardiac operations are intravenous drug abusers, mostly young-middle aged, because of the high incidence of endocarditis with a ruptured valve related to injection behaviors. This group is also characterized by a high prevalence of HBV and HCV infection.

In a designated AIDS treatment center in New York in 1992, the lowest prevalence of any blood-borne infection in patients having major surgery was found within those undergoing cardiothoracic surgery (2.7%: 0 for HIV, 1.1% for HBsAg and 1.5% for HCV), possibly due to the older age distribution of this population.[11]

However, over the past few years the pattern of HIV transmission has been changing, diffusion through the heterosexual route is increasing, and people seem to acquire the infection at an older age. Moreover, the incubation time for developing AIDS after the infection and the life-expectancy in people living with HIV infection and AIDS is growing owing to the beneficial effects of highly active antiretroviral therapy (HAART).[12–15]

In turn, because of the effects of prolonged HAART exposure on lipid metabolism,[16,17] treated HIV$^+$ patients may be at high risk of facing the cardiovascular complications associated with hyperlipidemia,[18] as reported elsewhere in this volume.

In industrialized countries, the prevalence of HCV$^+$ persons in the general population is usually higher than that of HIV$^+$ persons. In the USA, the highest prevalence of hepatitis C from 1988–1994 was found amongst people aged 30–49 years; similar findings have been observed in many parts of the world including most European countries.[19] Therefore, since HCV infection is a long-lasting chronic infection, the number of infected persons older than 50–60 years is thus expected to increase significantly in the next two decades.[20]

In conclusion, an increasing number of HCV$^+$ and/or HIV$^+$ persons could need specific cardiac diagnostic procedures and surgical treatment in the future. Therefore, this will determine an increase in the number of invasive procedures that expose cardiac personnel to the risk of acquiring blood-borne infections. Patients infected by one or more blood-borne pathogens can be observed in the cardiac services regardless of their sex or age, as found in all the other health care settings.[21] The need to follow the principles of Standard Precautions with all patients regardless of their known serostatus has been strongly recommended and is the object of several guidelines.[4]

Probability of Acquiring a Specific Infection following a Single Occupational Exposure

Several incidence studies have demonstrated that the risk of acquiring HIV and HCV infection after a single at-risk exposure averages less than 0.5%,[5] and about 1–2%, respectively.[3,22]

However, these reported rates represent an average, deriving from exposures at low as well as at high risk. Indeed, the multinational case-control study of HIV seroconversion in HCWs after percutaneous exposure to HIV-infected blood identified the following factors as being associated with HIV transmission: deep injury; injury by a device visibly contaminated with the source patient's blood; and injury by a device placed directly in a vein or artery.[23] These factors can be considered surrogate markers for the transmission of an increased volume of blood. In case of exposures involving two or more of these factors, then the risk could be much higher than 0.5%.

Although not formally studied, these factors are also likely to affect HCV transmission.

In the case-control study, terminal illness in the source patient, which can be considered a surrogate marker of an increased plasma HIV titer, has been found to be a further risk factor.[23] Indeed, viral load seems to be the major determinant influencing the source's efficiency in transmitting HIV and HCV, as observed in heterosexual and vertical cohort studies.[22,24–26]

Antiretroviral combination therapy strongly reduces the viral burden of HIV+ patients.[12,13] A similar effect is now occurring among HCV+ patients treated with currently available combination therapy.[22,27] By reducing the infectivity of source patients, these effects are likely to reduce the risk of transmission from treated patients to others, including occupationally exposed HCWs.

Apart from the particular and debatable case of viral variants, the risk of occupational HBV infection, which was previously estimated as ranging between 4–30% in incidence studies, should now be negligible because of the availability of effective post-exposure prophylaxis.[28]

In the above mentioned HIV case-control study, case-HCWs were significantly less likely to have taken post-exposure prophylaxis (PEP) with zidovudine than were control-HCWs, with a protective effect of this drug estimated to be approximately at 80%.[23] One must consider that if zidovudine alone has such a protective effect, currently recommended potent HIV PEP regimens including a combination of two or three antiretroviral agents, should further enhance the efficacy of PEP.[29]

Whether a similar effect could be reached by using available anti-HCV agents as post-exposure prophylaxis, needs further evaluation.[1,30] However, to date there have been no definitive and reliable data to support their use, apart from medical research.[21,22]

Frequency of At-Risk Exposures

The third determinant of the risk of acquiring an occupational infection—the frequency of exposures—has been the object of several surveillance studies in the surgical setting, which have observed rates of percutaneous exposure ranging from 1 to 15 per 100 interventions.[31–33] This rate varied within surgical specialties and occupation, with cardiothoracic surgery being included among those with the highest rates. The rate of mucocutaneous contamination by blood-splash during surgery has been estimated to be much higher, peaking at approximately 50% in cardiothoracic surgery.[34]

However, most of these studies relied on self-reported or recalled data from surgeons or other surgical staff, and are often based on observations of a small number of injuries from a single hospital, or derive from a short surveillance time. Under-reporting is well known as a potential bias in studies based on self-reported exposures, and physicians, particularly surgeons, are less reliable in reporting occupational exposures than other HCWs.[7,35] This could be at least in part due to the reluctance of surgeons to comply with the sort of continuous follow-up required because of the high frequency of exposure.

In 1990, Tokars and coworkers conducted a study in the US in which trained nurses or operating room technicians with no other duties in the operating room were present at 1,382 surgical procedures. Observers recorded data on percutaneous injuries occurring to operating room personnel in five surgical specialties.[36] Out of a total of 129 procedures which were performed in cardiac services, 12 procedures with at least one injury (9%) were documented.

Occupational exposures in cardiac care facilities are not limited to percutaneous or mucocutaneous exposures during invasive surgical procedures, and can also occur out of the operating room.[37,34]

In the following paragraph the frequency and characteristics of occupational exposures reported in the cardiac setting of hospitals enrolled in the SIROH will be presented. Some underreporting could have occurred in this study also, and selection bias could affect the data. However, the large number of participating hospitals recording a large number of injuries over a long surveillance time, make this study an important source of information regarding the circumstances of occupational exposures in the cardiac setting.

EXPOSURES IN THE CARDIAC SETTING: LESSONS FROM THE ITALIAN SIROH SURVEILLANCE

In 1986 the co-ordinating center of the SIROH began a multicenter, ongoing prospective study to estimate the transmission risk of HIV and other blood-borne pathogens to HCWs, following an occupational exposure to blood and other body materials.[3,5–7] Furthermore, this study aimed to identify high risk devices, procedures, and jobs in the health care setting. Since 1990, the coordinating center manages the Italian Registry of antiretroviral post-exposure prophylaxis in order to monitor its use and short-term toxicity.[7]

Hospitals are enrolled on a voluntary basis. At enrollment, hospitals are provided with two separate types of standardized forms (one for percutaneous and one for mucocutaneous exposures), as well as with a software for data entry and management. Participation is encouraged by inviting the members of the study group to an annual meeting where the main results of the program and new protocols are presented and discussed. At each participating hospital HCWs reporting an occupational exposure are interviewed, and data concerning the exposure are reported on the standardized forms. To participate in the study program, the HCWs' reporting of exposures should be actively encouraged in the hospital, and the presence of an employee health team, consisting of physicians, psychologists, and nurses, is required. The team is in charge of the management of the exposed HCW and of data collection, namely, interviewing the exposed HCW about circumstances of the exposure, counselling about the risk of occupational infections, offering prophylaxis, advising on the follow-up schedule, investigating each incident, and recording the exposure details. Follow up and post-exposure prophylaxis are provided according to current protocols.

Each hospital is also required to provide data on a yearly basis, in order to allow the calculation of specific rates of exposure by job category, work areas, the number of occupied beds, and health care activities (i.e., number of admissions in wards, day-hospital and emergency department; number of surgical interventions, deliveries, autopsies, dialysis treatments, etc.) and used supplies (i.e., needles, gloves, etc.).

As of December 1999, a total of 28,511 occupational exposures were recorded, 1,242 (4.3%) of which involved HCWs employed in the cardiac setting: 987/21,900 (4.5%) were percutaneous exposures, and 255/6,611 (3.8%) were mucocutaneous. Of all the 1,242 exposures in the cardiac setting, 570 (46%) exposures occurred in cardiology units, 63 (5%) in coronary care units (CCU), 547 (44%) in cardiovascular surgery, and 62 (5%) in pacemaker services.

The distribution of the reported exposures according to job category and service is shown in TABLE 1. Nurses reported 61% of the exposures, followed by resident physicians or surgeons (18%); of note, training personnel accounted for about 10% of the exposures reported in the cardiac setting.

Cardiology and Coronary Care Units

Most of the exposures that occurred in the cardiology units took place in the patient's room (49%) or immediately outside (i.e., hallway, nurses' station, etc., 15%). The remaining exposures occurred in the procedure room (i.e., during diagnostic examinations, 11%), and in the outpatient clinic (10%); about 5% of the incidents occurred in the operating room, related to minor surgical procedures (i.e., placement of a central venous catheter, etc.).

In cardiology, the procedures most frequently resulting in a percutaneous exposure were injections (23%), venous blood drawing (22%), and insertion/manipulation of a peripheral vascular catheter (21%). However, sampling collections (including venous or arterial blood drawing, fingerstick, and other body fluids collection) accounted cumulatively for 33% of exposures. The involved items were mainly disposable syringes (38%), winged steel needles (12%) and I.V. catheters (12%). Most exposures occurred during the use of these items (42%), while 21% involved items which had been used but not properly disposed of. About 13% occurred while recapping, and 17% were disposal-related accidents.

In CCUs 52% of percutaneous exposures occurred during sampling collection, 16% during insertion/manipulation of a peripheral vascular catheter, and 14% following an injection. Disposable syringes were involved in 36% of exposures, followed by I.V. catheters (12%) winged steel needles (10%) and vacuum tube phlebotomy sets (8%). Forty-six percent of exposures occurred during the use of the item and 16% after use and before disposal; recapping and disposal-related injuries accounted for 14% each.

Mucocutaneous exposures in cardiology resulted mainly from a direct exposure to the patient's blood or body fluids (56%), and from manipulating a leaking I.V. tubing (21%). On the contrary, in CCUs contamination occurred most frequently with a leaking I.V. tubing (54%), while in 31% of cases there was a direct exposure to the patient's blood.

More than 40% of the overall mucocutaneous exposures involved the conjunctiva; in 32% of cases there was broken skin contamination and in 26% an intact skin contamination. Almost 30% of the exposed HCWs had no protective garments at the time of the exposure; of the remaining, about 80% were wearing gloves, but less than 20% wore eye protection.

TABLE 1. Distribution of occupational exposures in the cardiac setting, by job category and working unit—SIROH, 1994–1999

Job Category	Cardiology Units		Coronary Care Unit		Cardiovascular Surgery		Pacemaker Services		Total		
	PC (%)	MC (%)	PC (%)	MC (%)	PC (%)	MC (%)	PC (%)	MC (%)	PC (%)	MC (%)	Total
Nurse	293 (65.4)	67 (54.9)	39 (78.0)	11 (84.6)	245 (56.1)	68 (61.3)	31 (58.5)	7 (77.8)	608 (61.6)	153 (60.0)	761 (61.3)
Student nurse	17 (3.8)	8 (6.6)	3 (6.0)	0	11 (2.5)	2 (1.8)	2 (3.8)	0	33 (3.3)	10 (3.9)	43 (3.5)
Resident	71 (15.8)	26 (21.3)	4 (8.0)	2 (15.4)	93 (21.3)	17 (15.3)	13 (24.5)	1 (11.1)	181 (18.3)	46 (18.0)	227 (18.3)
Intern	25 (5.6)	10 (8.2)	4 (8.0)	0	32 (7.3)	9 (8.1)	0	0	61 (6.2)	19 (7.4)	80 (6.4)
Housekeeper	35 (7.8)	3 (2.4)	0	0	43 (9.8)	8 (7.2)	5 (9.4)	1 (11.1)	83 (8.4)	12 (4.7)	95 (7.6)
Technician	4 (0.9)	5 (4.1)	0	0	5 (1.1)	4 (3.6)	1 (1.9)	0	10 (1.0)	9 (3.5)	19 (1.5)
Other	3 (0.6)	1 (0.8)	0	0	7 (1.6)	3 (2.7)	1 (1.9)	0	11 (1.1)	4 (1.6)	15 (1.2)
Total	448 (36.1)	122 (9.8)	50 (4.0)	13 (1.0)	436 (35.1)	111 (8.9)	53 (4.3)	9 (0.7)	987 (79.5)	255 (20.5)	1242 (100)

NOTE: PC: percutaneous; MC: mucocutaneous.

Cardiovascular Surgery and Pacemaker Services

Exposures in cardiovascular surgery occurred mainly in the operating room (58%); however, one third of exposures took place in the post-surgical ward (patient's room, 22%; hallways, 7%), and 10% in intensive care. Most exposures in cardiovascular surgery occurred while suturing (34%) and making an incision (13%); sampling collection accounted for 15% of injuries and the insertion/manipulation of a peripheral vascular catheter for 8%. Almost half of percutaneous exposures involved solid sharps: suture needles (32%), scalpels (15%), and other surgical instruments, more frequently suture or Kirschener's wire (5%). Hollow-bore needles, mainly disposable syringes, accounted for 30% of injuries. Sixty-three percent of injuries happened during the use of the device, one-fourth of which occurred while passing instruments, 15% after use and before disposal, and 8% were disposal-related; recapping accounted for 3%.

In pacemaker services, 21% of exposures occurred while performing subcutaneous or intramuscular injections and 15% while inserting/manipulating a peripheral vascular catheter; suturing and making an incision accounted for 13% each. Most injuries involved hollow-bore needles (62%), mainly disposable syringes (28%) and I.V. catheters (15%).

Solid sharps injuries accounted for 38% (scalpels, 19%; suture needles, 13%). Exposures occurred mostly during the use of the item (55%), half of which during a multi-step procedure, and with items used but not disposed of (23%); recapping and disposal-related injuries accounted for 6% each.

Mucocutaneous exposures resulted mainly from a direct exposure to the patient's blood or body fluids (55%) both in cardiovascular surgery and in the pacemaker service, involving mainly the conjunctiva (63%). Less than 20% of the exposed HCWs wore no protective garments; of the remaining, 78% wore gloves, but, again, only 21% wore eye protection.

Risk of Blood-Borne Infections in the Cardiac Setting

Overall, of all the exposures in the cardiac setting, 311 (25%) involved a blood-borne infected source: 243 (78%) patients were anti-HCV positive, 40 (13%) were HBsAg positive, 14 (5%) were positive for both markers; 14 source patients (5%) had HIV infection, 5 of whom were co-infected with HCV. However, in 134 cases (11%) the source was unknown, and in 252 (20%) the source was untested. Approximately 70% of the exposed personnel were already vaccinated against hepatitis B at the time of the exposure. No seroconversions either for HIV, HCV or HBV were observed after a mean follow-up of 6 months.

TRANSMISSION OF BLOOD-BORNE PATHOGENS FROM AN INFECTED HEALTH CARE WORKERS TO PATIENT

The report of transmission of viruses such as HIV, HBV and HCV from HCWs to patients have greatly alarmed public opinion, as well as public health managers.[8,9] On the basis of this evidence, beginning in the early nineties, industrialized countries have made recommendations for the prevention of blood-borne pathogen transmission from

HCWs to patients and for managing the case of an infected HCW.[8,9,37–40] In the worst case scenario, an HBV DNA- or HCV RNA-positive surgeon who performs exposure-prone procedures can be forbidden to continue operating if involved in a case of provider-to-patient transmission.

In the above-mentioned study by Tokars and coworkers, in 3% of the surgical procedures in the cardiac service the sharp instrument that had injured a worker re-contacted the patient's open wound, representing a potential risk of provider to patient transmission of infection.[36]

Up to December 2000, 10 reports have appeared in the English-language literature documenting transmission of HBV[41–49] or HCV[50,51] from infected health-care workers to patients during cardiothoracic surgery. None of the 3 cases of HCW to patient HIV transmission described in the literature occurred in the cardiac setting.[52–54]

The main characteristics of these reported cases of transmission of blood-borne pathogens from an infected health care worker to patient are discussed below and summarized in TABLE 2.

Hepatitis B Virus

Outbreaks of transmission of HBV from HCW to patient occurring in the cardiothoracic setting account for about 30% (14/47) of all such outbreaks reported in the literature from 1972 to December 2000. Moreover, cardiothoracic operations, especially those involving sternotomy and its suturing, are responsible for 17% of all patients acquiring HBV infection from an infected HCW reported in the literature (about 500).

The 14 outbreaks occurring in the cardiothoracic setting involved 12 HBV infected HCWs (9 cardiothoracic surgeons; 2 perfusion technicians, and 1 inhalation therapist) who transmitted the infection to approximately 107 patients (TABLE 2). As shown in TABLE 2, one perfusion pump technician,[42] and one cardiothoracic surgeon[47] were involved twice in 2 outbreaks in different periods. In seven of these cases the source HCW had chronic hepatitis and was HBeAg positive; 2 HCWs transmitted infection during the incubation period, 2 during acute hepatitis, and the remaining one a few months following acute hepatitis. The career outcome was reported for 7 of the 12 source HBV+ HCWs: 3 surgeons became HBsAg negative (one was successfully treated with α-interferon); 2 surgeons ceased to perform surgical procedures; and the 2 perfusion technicians were transferred to non-clinical work.

The 9 HBV+ cardiothoracic surgeons transmitted their infection to approximately 84 patients; for 64 of these patients information on the procedures involved was available: 26 coronary artery replacement/bypass; 9 other bypass surgery; 10 valve replacement; 8 unspecified open heart surgery; 4 orthotopic heart transplantation; 4 repair of congenital defects; 1 thymectomy; 1 open-lung biopsy; and 1 pneumonectomy (TABLE 2).

In many of these retrospective investigations the precise mode of transmission of the blood-borne virus from physician to patient remains unknown, but it was presumed to be caused by deficiencies in infection-control measures. However, in the HBV outbreak reported by Harpaz *et al.*[48] the investigation team excluded inadequate infection control. The authors reported that the cardiothoracic surgeon implicated in the outbreak often had pain over his index finger during prolonged suturing.

TABLE 2. Outbreaks of hepatitis B virus (HBV), or hepatitis C virus (HCV) infection transmitted by healthcare workers to patients, in cardiothoracic settings

Case No. ref.	Country	Occupation	Year	No. of Patients	Procedures	Clinical Stage of HCW and/or Serostatus
HBV						
1 [41]	Norway	cardiac surgeon	1978	5	open heart surgery	Incubation period
2 [42]	The Netherlands	cardiac surgeon	1979	3	open heart surgery	Acute hepatitis
3 [43, 44]	UK	cardiac surgeon	1980–83	5	not specified	Incubation period
4 [44, 45]	UK	cardiothoracic surgeon	1988	17	7 valve replacement; 9 coronary artery bypass; 1 other bypass surgery	Chronic hepatitis, HBeAg+
5 [44]	UK	cardiothoracic surgeon	1983–84	4	not specified	Chronic hepatitis, HBeAg+
6 [44, 46]	UK	gynecology, cardiothoracic and general surgery	1986	3	not specified	Chronic hepatitis, HBeAg+
7 [44]	UK	cardiothoracic surgeon	1990	5	not specified	Chronic hepatitis, HBeAg+
8 [47]	UK	cardiothoracic surgeon	1992	3	not specified	Chronic hepatitis, HBeAg+
8 [47]			1993	20	1 valve and coronary replacement; 17 coronary artery replacement (5 of whom as vein harvester); 1 aortic valve replacement; 1 pneumonectomy	

TABLE 2/continued.

Case No.ref.	Country	Occupation	Year	No. of Patients	Procedures	Clinical Stage of HCW and/or Serostatus
9 [48]	US	cardiothoracic surgeon	1991-92	19	8 bypass surgery; 4 heart transplantation; 4 repair of congenital defects; 1 valve replacement; 1 thymectomy; 1 open-lung biopsy	Acute hepatitis (5 months before the index case), followed by chronic infection HBeAg +
10 [49]	US	inhalation therapist	1974-75	6	arterial blood gas sample	
11 [42]	The Netherlands	perfusion pump technician	1979	6	use of the heart-lung pump	Chronic hepatitis, HBeAg+
11 [42]			1981	5	use of the heart-lung pump	
12 [43, 44]	UK	perfusion pump technician	1980-83	6	use of the heart-lung pump	Chronic hepatitis, HBeAg+
HCV						
13 [50]	Spain	cardiothoracic surgeon	1988-93	5	valve replacement	Chronic hepatitis, HCV-RNA positive
14 [51]	UK	cardiothoracic surgeon	1994	1	coronary artery replacement	Chronic hepatitis, HCV-RNA positive

Moreover, while participating in a 1-hour simulation of suture tying, the surgeon acquired paper-cut-like lesions on his fingers; HBsAg was detected in the saline used to rinse out the surgeon's gloves.

Hepatitis C Virus

Up to December 2000, 4 outbreaks of transmission of HCV from infected HCWs to patients have been reported in the literature,[50,51,55,56] and 2 others are still under investigation.[55,57]

Of the confirmed outbreaks, 2 (1 in Spain and 1 in the United Kingdom) occurred in the cardiothoracic setting.[50,51] Both surgeons were affected by chronic HCV, and had a high level of plasma HCV-RNA at the moment of investigation (22×10^6 and 10^6 genome equivalents per milliliter, respectively). The first surgeon left his practice and then resumed it after having been successfully treated with α-interferon plus ribavirin.[50] The second surgeon was required to cease performing exposure-prone procedures.[51]

The two cardiothoracic surgeons transmitted HCV infection to 6 out of 500 patients who underwent operations, were traced, and consented to be tested (out of a total of 996 patients operated on). Five patients acquired HCV infection during an operation of valve replacement, and one during coronary artery replacement (TABLE 2).

Estimated Rates of HCW to Patient Transmission

The observed cases of HCV, HBV, or HIV transmission cannot be used to estimate the average rate of transmission from an infected surgeon to an individual patient during an invasive procedure. This rate of transmission has been estimated both by the transmission rates observed during outbreaks, usually performed in the form of look-back investigations, and by mathematical models.

Look-back investigations have been performed starting from a patient or a surgeon case index. The aim is to trace as many patients as possible who underwent operations from the infected surgeon, and to test them for the infection markers. In outbreaks of HBV infection associated with cardiothoracic surgery, the transmission rate has been estimated to be between 5 and 13%.[44,45,47,48] The risk of transmission to patients exposed to an HCV$^+$ surgeon seems to be lower, ranging from 0.36% to 2.25%.[50,51]

However, look-back investigations involve intensive effort, are very expensive, and are often unreliable because of a high rate of patients lost to follow up. For this reason retrospective notification to patients exposed to an infected HCW is the object of debate. Notification should not be done routinely, but should be considered on a case-by-case basis, taking into account an assessment of risk, confidentiality issues, and available resources.[58,60]

Mathematical models consist of three parameters derived from the literature[61]: (A) the probability that an infected surgeon will sustain a percutaneous injury during an invasive procedure, (B) the probability that an instrument contaminated by the surgeon's blood will re-contact the patient, and (C) the probability of transmission of infection after a single exposure, which varies for each pathogen (30% for HBV, 0.3% for HIV, and 1% for HCV).[61]

Using the values reported in the above mentioned study by Tokars and coworkers[36] in the cardiac service (probability $A = 9$ injuries per one hundred procedures, and $B = 33$ re-contacts per one hundred injuries), the rate of transmission of a blood-borne pathogen from an infected cardiothoracic surgeon to a patient during exposure-prone procedures could be 0.009 per one hundred procedures for HBV, 0.0003 for HCV, and 0.00009 for HIV.

In a different mathematical model, the risk of transmission of HCV has been calculated based on the three probabilities described above, plus the probability that the surgeon is infected with HCV. The calculated risk for HCV transmission from a surgeon to a patient during a single procedure when the surgeon's state is unknown is $0.00018\% \pm 0.00002\%$ (mean $\pm$ SD); if the surgeon is HCV RNA positive the risk equals $0.014\% \pm 0.002\%$ (mean $\pm$ SD).[62]

DISCUSSION

Health care workers face a well-recognized risk of acquiring blood-borne pathogens in their workplace, among which HIV is considered one of the most serious. Additionally, HCWs infected with blood-borne pathogens may represent a risk for their patients, particularly in the case of invasive exposure-prone procedures.

About one hundred cases of documented occupational HIV infection in HCWs, have been reported in the literature world wide.[2] Surgeons are rarely or not represented among these cases, but are represented among the 170 cases of possible occupational infections—that is, cases in which the occupational HIV transmission could not be definitely established, mostly because the exposure was not reported at the time of the accident, or because the exposure was inapparent or unperceived and thus not reportable.

Cardiothoracic surgery is one of the settings at higher risk for occupational exposures.[31-36] Open heart operations using cardiopulmonary bypass represent the largest routine exposure to blood that occurs in clinical practice. The extensive use of sharp instruments, the large number of blood samples drawn, and the danger of splashing during cannulation and decannulation put cardiopulmonary surgical staff at high risk.

Good surgical outcomes both for patients and surgical teams are imperative in the blood-borne pathogen era. In the next decades, it can be anticipated that an increasing number of patients with blood-borne infections, mainly HCV and HIV, may require specific cardiac diagnostic procedures and surgical treatment. Cardiac personnel will therefore deal increasingly with this problem in the future. The efficacy of transmission of blood-borne agents through occupational exposures can nonetheless be expected to decrease for two main reasons: the lower infectivity of the sources, owing to more effective antiviral treatments; and, the availability of more effective prophylactic treatments against these agents.

However, efforts at prevention should focus not only on reducing the efficacy of transmission. Indeed, as the exposure is the basis of the potential patient-to-provider as well as provider-to-patient risk of transmission of blood-borne infections, efforts should be focused on eliminating, or at least minimizing, the causes of blood-borne exposures.

A combined set of strategies in risk reduction might be appropriate, including adequate surveillance, education,[63,64] more effective systems for sharps disposal,[64–66] availability and consistent use of personal protective equipment,[7] and innovative technology-based approaches to prevention, safer intraoperative technology and procedures.[67–70]

To make any surveillance system effective, efforts to minimize underreporting, including laws and hospital policies tailored to encourage HCWs to report all exposures, should continue. The positive safety climate created by such a program may increase the likelihood that the work environment will contain features that enable workers to comply with safer work practices.[71,72]

In order to minimize the risk of exposure, double gloving,[73] eye protection against blood splashes,[74] efficient gown wearing,[75] and general procedure recommendations[76] are suggested as standard precautions to be used and should become routine.

Effective surveillance systems for monitoring existing practices and methods, and gathering information about occupational risk, are essential in achieving a safer health care workplace.

This paper has shown that a standardized program, SIROH, can be implemented by a network of public hospitals, allowing significant data to be collected and monitored over a long period, thereby addressing many important questions concerning the safety of the HCW. From the analysis of the exposures recorded by the SIROH, the risk for HCWs differs greatly between cardiology and cardiothoracic surgery. Solid sharps injuries, which are more frequent in surgery, carry a lower risk of transmission than hollow-bore, blood-filled needlesticks, which are more prevalent in cardiology. On the contrary, the risk for the patients, due to infected HCWs performing invasive exposure prone procedures, appears to be higher in cardiothoracic surgery.

Several studies have shown that education and training programs have a positive impact on reducing exposures and enhancing exposure reporting.[63–65,77] Training courses directed to all hospital personnel could determine a global reduction of potentially preventable exposures, such as those occurring with improperly discarded needles or due to a lack of protective garments. However, it is necessary that education should be also focused on the characteristics which are unique to a specific setting, such as cardiology or cardiac surgery. Enhanced reporting rates can provide the opportunity for a consistent implementation of post-exposure prophylactic measures, as well as for counselling the exposed HCW on the hazardous patterns of his/her practice.

As most exposures occur during the use of the device, regardless of its design, engineering and management controls should be implemented in these settings. The widespread adoption of safer devices and changes towards safer surgical techniques, or even less invasive, alternative procedures should be implemented. On October 26, 2000, the US Congress approved the S 3067 Needlestick Safety and Prevention Act. This law mandates that the Occupational Safety and Health Administration (OSHA) Blood-borne pathogens Standard, be revised to require the use of "safety-engineered sharp devices."[78] The updated Standard clarifies the need for employers to select safer needle devices, as they become available, and to involve employees in identifying and choosing the devices. Although reports have been published on the effectiveness and performance of specific safety devices,[67,68,79,80] including for example blunt needles for suture,[79] the reports are few and their findings are in some cases inconsistent with each other. Whether these safety devices could have a further impact in reducing percutaneous exposure rates in all areas, and particularly in reducing exposures at higher risk of infection, needs to be further evaluated applying consistent and rigorous methods.

ACKNOWLEDGMENTS

Research presented here was supported by Italian Ministry of Health AIDS project and Ricerca Corrente IRCCS.

We wish to thank Zana Mariano for her assistance in reviewing the text, and Mariagrazie Martignoni for secretarial assistance.

REFERENCES

1. BELTRAMI, E.M., I.T. WILLIAMS, C.N. SHAPIRO, *et al.* 2000. Risk and management of blood-borne infections in health care workers. Clin. Microbiol. Rev. **13**: 385–407.
2. IPPOLITO, G., V. PURO, J. HEPTONSTALL, *et al.* 1999. Occupational human immunodeficiency virus infection in health care workers: worldwide cases through September 1997. Clin. Infect. Dis. **28**: 365–383.
3. PURO, V., N. PETROSILLO & G. IPPOLITO. 1995. Italian study group. Risk of hepatitis C seroconversion after occupational exposures in health care workers. Am. J. Infect. Control **23**: 273–277.
4. GARNER, J.S. & THE HOSPITAL INFECTION CONTROL PRACTICES ADVISORY COMMITTEE. 1996. Guideline for isolation precautions in hospitals. Infect. Control Hosp. Epidemiol. **17**: 53–80.
5. IPPOLITO, G., V. PURO, G. DE CARLI, *et al.* 1993. The risk of occupational HIV infection in health care workers: Italian Multicenter Study. Arch. Intern. Med. **153**: 1451–1458.
6. IPPOLITO, G., V. PURO, N. PETROSILLO, *et al.* 1999. Surveillance of occupational exposure to blood-borne pathogens in health care workers: the Italian national programme. Eurosurveillance **4**: 33–36.
7. IPPOLITO, G., V. PURO, N. PETROSILLO, *et al.* 1997. Prevention, management and chemoprophylaxis of occupational exposure to HIV. International Health Care Worker Safety Center Editor, Charlottesville, Virginia-USA.
8. CENTERS FOR DISEASE CONTROL. 1991. Recommendations for preventing transmission of human immunodeficiency virus and hepatitis B virus to patients during exposure-prone invasive procedures. Morbid. Mortal. Weekly Rep. **40**(RR-8): 1–9.
9. AIDS/TB COMMITTEE OF THE SOCIETY FOR HEALTHCARE EPIDEMIOLOGY OF AMERICA. 1997. Management of healthcare workers infected with hepatitis B virus, hepatitis C virus, human immunodeficiency virus, or other blood-borne pathogens. Infect. Control Hosp. Epidemiol. **18**: 349–363.
10. BEEKMANN, S.E., B.J. FAHEY, J.L. GERBERDING, *et al.* 1990. Risky business: using necessarily imprecise casualty counts to estimate occupational risk of HIV-1 infection. Infect. Control Hosp. Epidemiol. **11**: 371–379.
11. MONTECALVO, M.A., M. SUNG LEE, H. DEPALMA, *et al.* 1995. Seroprevalence of human immunodeficiency virus-1, hepatitis B virus, and hepatitis C virus in patients having major surgery. Infect. Control Hosp. Epidemiol. **16**: 627–632.
12. PALELLA, F.J. JR., K.M. DELANEY, A.C. MOORMANN, *et al.* 1998. Declining morbidity and mortality among patients with advanced human immunodeficiency virus infection. HIV Outpatients Study Investigators. N. Engl. J. Med. **338**: 853–860.
13. MOCROFT, A., S. VELLA, T.L. BENFIELD, *et al.* 1998. Changing patterns of mortality across Europe in patients infected with HIV-1. Lancet **352**: 1725–1730.

14. CASCADE COLLABORATION. 2000. Survival after introduction of HAART in people with known duration of HIV-1 infection. Lancet **355:** 1158–1159.
15. PEZZOTTI, P., P.A. NAPOLI, S. ACCIAI, *et al.* 1999. Increasing survival time after AIDS in Italy: the role of new combination of antiretroviral therapies. AIDS **13:** 249–255.
16. MAUSS, S. 2000. HIV-associated lipodystrophy syndrome. AIDS **14**(S3): 197–207.
17. PENZAC, S.R. & S.K. CHUCK. 2000. Hyperlipidemia associated with HIV protease inhibitor use: pathophysiology, prevalence, risk factors and treatment. Scand. J. Infect. Dis. **32:** 111–123.
18. FRIEDL, A.C., C.H. ATTENHOFER JOST, C. SCHALKER, *et al.* 2000. Acceleration of confirmed coronary artery disease among HIV-infected patients on potent antiretroviral therapy. AIDS **14:** 2790–2792.
19. ALTER, M.J., D. KRUSZON-MORAN, O.V. NAINAN, *et al.* 1999. The prevalence of hepatitis C virus infection in the United States, 1988 through 1994. N. Engl. J. Med. **341:** 556–562.
20. WONG, J.B., G.M. MCQUILLAN, J.G. MCHUTCHISON, *et al.* 2000. Estimating future hepatitis C morbidity, mortality, and costs in the United States. Am. J. Public Health. **90:** 1562–1569.
21. CHARACHE, P., J.L. CAMERON, A.W. MATERS, *et al.* 1991. Prevalence of infection with human immunodeficiency virus in elective surgery. Ann. Surg. **214:** 562–568.
22. CENTERS FOR DISEASE CONTROL AND PREVENTION. 1998. Recommendations for prevention and control of hepatitis C virus (HCV) infection and HCV-related chronic infection. Morbid. Mortal. Weekly Rep. **47**(RR 19): 1–39.
23. CARDO, D., D.H. CULVER, C. CIESELSKY, *et al.* 1997. A case-control of HIV seroconversion after percutaneous exposure. N. Engl. J. Med. **337:** 1485–1490.
24. OKAMOTO, M., I. NAGATA, J. MURAKAMI, *et al.* 2000. Prospective reevaluation of risk factors in mother-to-child transmission of hepatitis C virus: high viral load, vaginal delivery, and negative anti-NS4 antibody. J. Infect. Dis. **182:** 1511–1514.
25. MOFENSON, L.M., J.S. LAMBERT, E.R. STIEHM, *et al.* 1999. Risk factors for perinatal transmission of human immunodeficiency virus type 1 in women treated with zidovudine. N. Engl. J. Med. **341:** 385–393.
26. HISADA, M., R. T. O'BRIEN, P.S. ROSENBERG, *et al.* 2000. Viral load and risk of heterosexual of human immunodeficiency virus and hepatitis C virus by men with hemophilia. J. Infect. Dis. **181:** 1475–1478.
27. MCHUTCHISON J.G., S.C. GORDON, E.R. SCHIFF, *et al.* 1998. Interferon alpha-2b alone or in combination with ribavirin as initial treatment for chronic hepatitis C. N. Engl. J. Med. **339:** 1485–1492.
28. MAHONEY, F. J., K. STEWARD, H. HU, *et al.* 1997. Progress toward the elimination of hepatitis B virus transmission among health care workers in the United States. Arch. Intern. Med. **157:** 2601–2605.
29. CENTERS FOR DISEASE CONTROL AND PREVENTION. 1998. Public Health Service guidelines for the management of health care worker exposures to HIV and recommendations for post exposure prophylaxis. Morbid. Mortal. Weekly Rep. **47**(Suppl. RR-7).
30. PIAZZA, M., L. SAGLIOCCA, G. TOSONE, *et al.* 1997. Sexual transmission of hepatitis C virus and efficacy of prophylaxis with intramuscular immuneserum globulin. A randomized controlled trial. Arch. Intern. Med. **157:** 1537–1544.
31. SHORT, L.J. & D.M. BELL. 1993. Risk of occupational infection with blood-borne pathogens in operating and delivery room settings. Am. J. Infect. Control. **21:** 343–350.
32. POPEJOY, S.L. & D.E. FRY. 1991. Blood contact and exposure in the operating room. Surg. Gynecol. Obstet. **172:** 480–483.
33. KJAERGARD, H.K., J. THIIS & N. WIINBERG. 1992. Accidental injuries and blood exposure to cardiothoracic surgical teams. Eur. J. Cardiothorac. Surg. **6:** 215–217.
34. QUEBBEMAN, E.J., G.L. TELFORD, S. HUBBARD, *et al.* 1991. Risk of blood contamination and injury to operating room personnel. Ann. Surg. **214:** 614–620.
35. LYNCH, P. & M.C. WHITE. 1993. Perioperative blood contact and exposures: a comparison of incident reports and focused studies. Am. J. Infect. Control. **21:** 357–363.
36. TOKARS, J.I., D.M. BELL, D.H. CULVER, *et al.* 1992. Percutaneous injuries during surgical procedures. JAMA **267:** 2899–2904.

37. CANADA COMMUNICABLE DISEASE REPORT. 1998. Proceedings of the consensus conference on infected health care workers: risk for transmission of blood-borne pathogens. CCDR **24**(S4): 8–14.
38. UK HEALTH DEPARTMENTS. 1993. Protecting health care workers and patients from hepatitis B: recommendation of the Advisory Group on Hepatitis. London, The Stationery Office.
39. UK HEALTH DEPARTMENTS. 1998. AIDS/HIV infected health care workers: guidance on the management of infected health care workers and patient notification. London: UK Health Departments.
40. ISTITUTO SUPERIORE DI SANITÀ. 2000. Gestione intraospedaliera del personale HbsAg o anti-HCV positivo. Consensus conference. Rome, 28–29 October 1999. Rapporti ISTISAN Congressi **72**: 1–30.
41. HAEREM, J.W., J.C. SIEBKE, J. ULSTRUP, *et al.* 1981. HBsAg transmission from a cardiac surgeon incubating hepatitis B resulting in chronic antigenaemia in four patients. Acta Med. Scand. **210**: 389–392.
42. COUTINHO, R.A., P. ALBRECHT-VAN LENT, L. STOUTJESDIJK, *et al.* 1982. Hepatitis B from doctors. Lancet **i**: 345–346.
43. POLAKOFF, S. 1986. Acute hepatitis B in patients in Britain related to previous operations and dental treatment. Br. Med. J. **293**: 33–36.
44. HEPTONSTALL, J. 1991. Outbreaks of hepatitis B virus infection associated with infected surgical staff. Commun. Dis. Rep. CDR. Rev. **1**: R81–R85.
45. PRENTICE, M.B., A.J.E. FLOWER, G.M. MORGAN, *et al.* 1992. Infection with hepatitis B virus after open heart surgery. Br. Med. J. **304**: 761–764.
46. POLAKOFF, S. 1986. Acute viral hepatitis B: laboratory reports 1980–4. Br. Med. J. **293**: 37–38.
47. THE INCIDENT CONTROL TEAMS AND OTHERS. 1996. Lessons from two linked clusters of acute hepatitis B in cardiothoracic surgery patients. Commun. Dis. Rep. CDR. Rev. **6**: R119–R125.
48. HARPAZ, R., L. VAN SEIDLEIN, M. FRANCISCO, *et al.* 1996. Transmission of hepatitis B virus to multiple patients from a surgeon without evidence of inadequate control. N. Engl. J. Med. **334**: 549–554.
49. SNYDMAN, D.R., S.H. HINDMAN, M.D. WINELAND, *et al.* 1976. Nosocomial viral hepatitis B: a cluster among staff with subsequent transmission to patients. Ann. Intern. Med. **85**: 573–577.
50. ESTEBAN, J.I., J. GÓMEZ, M. MARTELL, *et al.* 1996. Transmission of hepatitis C virus by a cardiac surgeon. N. Engl. J. Med. **334**: 555–560.
51. DUCKWORTH, G.J., J. HEPTONSTALL, C. ALTKEN FOR THE INCIDENT CONTROL TEAM, *et al.* 1999. Transmission of hepatitis C virus from a surgeon to a patient. Commun. Dis. Public. Health. **2**: 188–192.
52. CIESIELSKI, C., D. MARIANOS, C.Y. OU, *et al.* 1992. Transmission of human immunodeficiency virus in a dental practice. Ann. Intern. Med. **116**: 798–805.
53. LOT, F., J-C. SÉGUIER, S. FÉGUEUX, *et al.* 1999. Probable transmission of HIV from an orthopedic surgeon to a patient in France. Ann. Intern. Med. **130**: 1–6.
54. GOUJON, C.P., V.M. SCHNEIDER, J. GROFTI, *et al.* 2000. Phylogenetic analyses indicate an atypical nurse-to-patient transmission of human immunodeficiency virus type 1. J. Virol. **74**: 2525–2532.
55. Two Hepatitis C look-back exercises—national and in London. 2000. Commun. Dis. Rep. CDR. Wkly. **10**: 125–128.
56. ROSS R.S., S. VIAZOV, T. GROSS, *et al.* 2000. Brief report: transmission of hepatitis C virus from a surgeon to an anesthesiology assistant to five patients. N. Engl. J. Med. **343**: 1851–1854.
57. Healthcare worker-to-patient transmission of HCV in the UK. 2000. Infect. Control Hospital Epid. **21**: 619.
58. OLIVER S.E., J. WOODHOUSE & V. HOLLYOAK. 1999. Lessons from patient notification exercises following the identification of hepatitis B e antigen positive surgeons in an English health region. Commun. Dis. Public. Health. **2**: 130–136.
59. DANILA, R.N., K.L. MACDONALD, F.S. RHAME, *et al.* 1991. A look-back investigation of patients of an HIV-infected physician. N. Engl. J. Med. **325**: 1406–1411.

60. DONNELLY, M., G. DUCKWORTH, S. NELSON, et al. 1999. Are HIV lookbacks worthwhile? Outcome of an exercise to notify patients treated by an HIV infected health care worker. Commun. Dis. Public Health. **2:** 126–129.
61. BELL, D.M., C.N. SHAPIRO, D.H. CULVER, et al. 1992. Risk of hepatitis B and human immunodeficiency virus transmission to a patient from an infected surgeon due to percutaneous injury during an invasive procedure: estimates based on a model. Infectious Agents and Disease. **1:** 263–269.
62. ROSS, R.S., S. VIAZOV & M. ROGGENDORF. 2000. Risk of hepatitis C transmission from infected medical staff to patients. Arch. Intern. Med. **160:** 2313–2316.
63. MCCORMICK, R.D., M.G. MEISCH, F.G. IRCINK, et al. 1991. Epidemiology of hospital sharps injuries: a 14-year prospective study in the pre-AIDS and AIDS eras. Am. J. Med. **91:** 301S–307S.
64. HAIDUVEN, D.J., T.M. DEMAIO, D.A. STEVENS. 1992. A five-years study of needlestick injuries: significant reduction associated with communication, education, and convenient placement of sharps containers. Infect. Control Hosp. Epidemiol. **13:** 265–271.
65. LINNEMANN, C.C., C. CANNON, M. DERONDE, et al. 1991. Effect of educational programs, rigid sharps containers, and universal precautions on reported needlestick injuries in health care workers. Infect. Control Hosp. Epidemiol. **12:** 214–219.
66. MAST, S.T, J.D WOOLWINE & J.L GERBERDING. 1993. Efficacy of gloves in reducing blood volumes transferred during simulated needlestick injury. J. Infect. Dis. **168:** 1589–1592.
67. ORENSTEIN, R., L. REYNOLDS, M. KARABAIC, et al. 1995. Do protective devices prevent needlestick injuries among health care workers? Am. J. Infect. Control. **23:** 344–351.
68. RUSSO, P.L., G. A HARRINGTON & D.W SPELMAN. 1999. Needleless intravenous systems: a review. Am. J. Infect. Control. **27:** 431–434.
69. DEJOY, D.M., C.A SEARCY, R.R. MURPHY, et al. 2000. Behavioral-diagnostic analysis of compliance with universal precaution among nurses. J. Occup. Health Psychol. **5:** 127–141.
70. DAVIS, M.S. 1996. Occupational hazard of operating: opportunities for improving. Infect. Control Hosp. Epidemiol. **17:** 691–693.
71. RAAHAVE, D. 1996. Operative precautions in HIV and other blood-borne virus diseases. Infect. Control Hosp. Epidemiol. **17:** 529–531.
72. PUGLIESE, G. 1993. Should blood exposure in the operating room be considered part of the job?. Infect. Control Hosp. Epidemiol. **21:** 337–342.
73. QUEBBEMAN, E.J., G.L. TELFORD, S. HUBBARD, et al. 1992. Double gloving. Protecting surgeons from blood contamination in the operating room. Arch. Surg. **127:** 213–217.
74. BREARLEY, S. & L.J. BUIST. 1989. Blood splashes: an underestimated hazard to surgeons. Br. Med. J. **299:** 1315.
75. SMITH, J.W. & R. LEE NICHOLS. 1991. Barrier efficiency of surgical gowns. Are we really protected from our patients' pathogens? Arch. Surg. **126:** 756–763.
76. JOINT WORKING PARTY OF THE HOSPITAL INFECTION SOCIETY AND SURGICAL INFECTION STUDY GROUP. 1992. Risks to surgeons and patients from HIV and hepatitis: guidelines on precautions and management of exposure to blood or body fluids. Br. Med. J. **305:** 1337–1343.
77. SELLICK, J.A., P.A HAZAMY & J.M. MYLOTTE. 1991. Influence of an educational program and mechanical opening needle disposal boxes on occupational needlestick injuries. Infect. Control Hosp. Epidemiol. **12:** 725–731.
78. Congress approves needlestick safety bill. 2000. Infect. Control Hosp. Epidemiol. **21:** 805-806.
79. CENTERS FOR DISEASE CONTROL AND PREVENTION. 1997. Evaluation of blunt suture needles in preventing percutaneous injuries among health care workers during gynecologic surgical procedures—New York City, March 1993–June 1994. Morbid. Mortal. Weekly Rep. **46:** 25–29.
80. CENTERS FOR DISEASE CONTROL AND PREVENTION. 1997. Evaluation of safety devices for preventing percutaneous injuries among health care workers during phlebotomy procedures—Minneapolis-St. Paul, New York City, and San Francisco, 1993–1995. Morbid. Mortal. Weekly Rep. **46:** 21–25.

APPENDIX

Members of the SIROH group are: G. Finzi, L. Gherardi, P. Cugini (*Policlinico S. Orsola-Malpighi, Bologna*); P. Bottura, G. Migliorino, R. Tambini, G. Marchetti (*Ospedale di Busto Arsizio*); I. Ferraresi, C. Sileo, R. Iuliucci (*Ospedali Riuniti di Bergamo*); A. Chiodera, P. Milini, L. Palvarini (*Spedali Civili di Brescia*); L. Pischedda, A. Lodi, G. Nurra, A. Rosati (*IRCCS L. Spallanzani, Roma*); M. Francesconi (*Ospedale San Sebastiano Martire, Frascati*); M. Daglio, D. Vlacos, M. Lanave (*Policlinico S. Matteo, Pavia*); M.L. Sodano, M.R. Cocco, D. Rosi, G. Nallira (*Azienda Ospedaliera S. Camillo-C. Forlanini, Roma*); M. Bombonato, B. Testini, I. Egger (*Ospedale Generale Regionale di Bolzano*); R. Bertucci, M. De Fazio, D. Zangrando, I. Berchialla (*Ospedale Amedeo di Savoia, Torino*); S. Maccarrone, C. Paradiso, T. Agosta (*Ospedale Vittorio Emanuele II, Catania*); G. Raineri, S. Pelissero, A. Vivalda, M. Ghio (*Azienda Ospedaliera S. Croce-Carle, Cuneo*); M. Desperati, M. Bergaglia (*Azienda Ospedaliera SS. Antonio e Biagio – C. Arrigo, Alessandria*); G. Micheloni (*Ospedale Niguarda, Milano*); P. Contegiacomo, E. Aspiro, B. Burrai (*Università Cattolica del S. Cuore – Policlinico A. Gemelli, Roma*); L. Battistella (*Ospedale di Cittadella*); C. Penna, M. Fulgheri, A. Argentiere, A. Ciucci (*Ospedale S. Martino, Genova*); G. Fasulo, M.C. Pirazzini, M. Tangenti, C. Libralato, C. Govoni, B. Bonfiglioli, A. Macchioni, G. Gualandi (*Ospedale Maggiore-C.A. Pizzardi, Bologna*); M.E. Bonaventura, V. Di Nardo (*Ospedale S. Camillo de Lellis, Rieti*); M. Massari, P. Rotelli, D. Bonvicini (*Arcispedale S. Maria Nuova, Reggio Emilia*); C. D'Anna, A. Materazzetti (*Ospedale S. Giuseppe, Marino*); P. Chiriacò, C. Poli (*Ospedale A. Di Summa, Brindisi*); A. Segata, G. Raponi, A.R. Boscolo, C. Tonelli (*Ospedale S. Maria Ausiliatrice, Rovereto*); P. Marchegiano, D. Tovoli, R. Bonini (*Azienda Ospedaliera Policlinico di Modena*); M. Lorenzani, R. Renusi (*Ospedale di Guastalla*); P. Masala, D. Sulas (*Ospedale G.B. Grassi, Ostia*); M. Perosino (*Ospedale S. Anna, Como*); W. Biagini, E. Teofilova, V. Belardinelli, L. Boanni (*Azienda Ospedaliera S. Maria, Terni*); G. Greco, F. Visani, V. Niccolai (*Presidio ospedaliero Misericordia, Grosseto*); L. Tavanti, I. Di Paola (*Presidio ospedaliero S. Donato, Arezzo*); M. Fiorio, M. Polidori (*Policlinico Monteluce, Perugia*); O. Lamanna, G. Piccini (*Presidio ospedaliero, Arco di Trento*); G. Simonini, G. Picelli, L. Cantarelli, R. Capellini (*Presidio Ospedaliero di La Spezia*); V. Mercurio, F. Soscia, R. Martiniello (*Ospedale S. Maria Goretti, Latina*); A. Zanon, E. Bellotto (*Ospedale di Vicenza*); F. Spazzapan (*Presidio ospedaliero di Monfalcone*); I. Pandiani, A. Aiello, B. Mattiacci (*Azienda ospedaliera SS. Annunziata, Taranto*).

Role of Guidelines in Clinical Practice for the Management of HIV-Related Diseases

FRANCESCO NICOLA LAURIA,[a] PAOLA VANACORE,[b]
AND MASSIMO CASCIELLO[c]

[a]Direzione Sanitaria, [b]Dipartimento di Epidemiologia delle Malattie Infettive,
Istituto Nazionale per le Malattie Infettive "Lazzaro Spallanzani"—IRCCS,
00149 Rome, Italy

[c]Ministero della Sanità-Servizio Vigilanza Enti, Rome, Italy

ABSTRACT: Several guidelines have been developed for the diagnosis, treatment and prevention of infectious diseases. Actually, evidence-based clinical practice guidelines provide physicians and other health care professionals with scientific information about the most appropriate strategy for the management of these patients, in order to avoid unnecessary or inappropriate interventions. As medical technology rapidly increases and becomes more complex, clinical guidelines can help health care providers to assess current practices and integrate new technological advances. Since AIDS was first recognized nearly 20 years ago, remarkable progress has been made in improving the quality and duration of life for HIV+ patients. In this area, clinical guidelines have been developed to manage patient care, focusing on: antiretroviral therapy, prevention of opportunistic infections, and treatment of tuberculosis. The quality of the guideline is notable when appropriate methodologies are applied. Different methods for developing guidelines are evaluated here: Agency for Health Care Policy and Research (AHPCR) methodology is designed to produce evidence-based guidelines that are valid, clinically applicable, and flexible. Finally, the problems associated with the implementation of guidelines for HIV-related diseases and other infectious diseases are examined.

KEYWORDS: guidelines; human immunodeficiency virus; HIV; management

INTRODUCTION

The term "recommendation", is a concept used to address members of a group, association, or an organization. Moreover, it is a concept which has been historically accepted as an identification criterion for features and purposes of the organization.

Peter A. Gross, from New Jersey Medical School, dates the first guidelines back to Moses and the Ten Commandments and believes that some examples of medical guidelines were already included in the Code of Hammurabi, King of Mesopotamia (1728–1686 B.C.). In fact, he noticed similarities between the Code of Hammurabi and the Health Assistance Organization in the USA: including programs of federal

Address for correspondence: Dr. Francesco N. Lauria, Direzione Sanitaria, Istituto Nazionale per le Malattie Infettive, "Lazzaro Spallanzani"—IRCCS, Via Portuense, 292, 00149 Rome, Italy. Voice: +39 06 551701; fax: +39 06 5594224.

lauria@spallanzani.roma.it

assistance (i.e., Medicare and Medicaid and Health Maintenance Organizations (HMOs).[1]

The concept of evidence-based medicine (EBM) is by now well accepted in the international scientific community, including Italy. The necessity to produce, spread and use guidelines in clinical practice has received such a high level of acceptance, that it has led to changes in the clinical setting.[2,3] Recently, the need to have adequate tools to support clinical decisions, has become an increasing priority, thus, guaranteeing a high standard of care, in spite of increasing costs due to the technological and organizational complexities found in health assistance.[1,4]

The health system in developed countries recently faced a serious financial and credibility crisis. This crisis has been an important factor in bringing about change, and does not include organizational criteria nor current public expenses in these countries.[4-6] Nevertheless, the need to combine the costs and quality of health assistance, should not be considered the only assumption to justify the adoption of a codified clinical practice. In fact, there are many valid reasons for the increasing interest in guidelines. It is often remarked that guidelines are used with contrasting intentions: social control tools versus professional tools; clinical tools for "decision making" versus guidelines to optimize business productivity; tools for restoring the standard of care found in medical organizations vs. guidelines to strengthen the "status quo" of the medical authority.[7,8]

A model can be represented by the management of patients with HIV infection. In recent years, increased knowledge has been reported in the area of infectious diseases with the development of biological markers of clinical progression, and an extended availability of drugs. As a result, it has been crucial to establish guidelines in the era of highly active antiretroviral therapy (HAART), especially when new antiretrovirals are constantly being introduced. Guidelines for the management of HIV infection have been produced in several European countries, as well as in Australia and United States. Their role is defined as follows:

- to promote a high standard of care for infectious diseases centers;

- to point out the strengths and weaknesses, and new, remarkable research acquisitions;

- to be a reference to evaluate funds allocated for the treatment of HIV+ patients;

- to be a reference for clinical evaluations for health care services; and

- to be a reference tool for clinicians who provide care to HIV+ patients.[9]

Occasionally, the incorrect use of the term "guideline" masks different objectives. These objectives are not always directed to offer decisional support to clinicians towards appropriate diagnostic and therapeutic choices. Incidentally, the management of HIV+ patients represents the opportunity to define a high quality standardized approach for the treatment of these patients.

The present paper is aimed to evaluate guidelines and protocols as valid tools for supporting clinical decision making, in order to define its characteristics, methodological standards, methods for implementation, as well as validation criteria.

GUIDELINES: GENERAL FEATURES

Guidelines should be consistent with medical literature, and the efficacy of recommendations should be explicit. Guideline drafting is supervised by organizations which have widespread medical credibility (i.e., scientific societies, research institution, etc.). In order to direct clinical practice and increase the knowledge and awareness of clinicians, selected experts review literature, interpret, and evaluate scientific evidence. Expert support is a necessary requirement, but is not essential to guarantee a good outcome. In fact, a specific work methodology is required to "force" experts to comply to scientific evidence. These methodological approaches can differ.[10]

Quality evaluation in guidelines is based on the following required features:

- scientific validity;

- validation, feasibility, clinical adaptability, and flexibility;

- comprehensible, multidisciplinary approach, and periodically revised.[1]

NECESSITY OF GUIDELINES FOR TREATMENT OF HIV INFECTION

Since the beginning of the HIV epidemic, the necessity for diagnostic and therapeutic recommendations in clinical practice has been evident. Initially, it was mainly necessary to spread information concerning the characteristics of the disease (i.e., epidemiology, pathogenesis and treatment), in order to transfer research results to clinical practice. Subsequently, remarkable results have been achieved in molecular biology, genetics and virology; new sophisticated diagnostic techniques have become available in clinical practice; and new potent drugs have been used for treatment.

Since AIDS was first identified, there has been remarkable progress in improving the quality and duration of life in HIV+ patients. During the first decade of the HIV epidemic, progress in research was mainly concerned with early diagnosis and treatment of opportunistic infections and tumors, as well as the primary and secondary chemoprophylaxis for opportunistic infections. The second decade has been marked by the introduction of HAART in 1996, which has drastically changed the natural history of HIV infection and significantly reduced morbidity and mortality for AIDS.

Furthermore, HAART has modified the occurrence of opportunistic infections (i.e., tuberculosis), the clinical presentation of diseases, and new clinical patterns related to immunological restoration have been made prevalent. The prolonged life of HIV+ patients has led to the recognition of several HIV-related diseases, such as cardiomyopathy and pulmonary hypertension and to an evaluation of concurrent HCV infections. Therefore, recommendations for the management of HIV+ patients have been updated to improve diagnostic and therapeutic practice. New recommendations for the diagnosis and treatment of diseases which were not previously considered or identified, have been pointed out.

Updated Recommendations

Antiretroviral Therapy

Since 1995, a panel of experts from 1) the International AIDS Society–USA and 2) National Institutes of Health–USA updated recommendations for antiretroviral therapy in HIV-infection. The review process has been performed to provide clinicians with a synthesis of progress in basic research, pharmacology and clinical research. The updated recommendations, have been achieved by integrating new scientific data on the pathogenesis of AIDS diseases, thus transferring the outcome to the therapeutic setting.

When considering updated recommendations, various factors have been examined:

- basic and clinical research, including controlled phase-3 studies;

- results of clinical, virological and immunological studies;

- *ad interim* analysis presented at national and international conferences; and

- research concerning HIV physiopathology.

New information has appeared since the publication of the first recommendations in 1996.[11] This includes HIV pathogenesis, viral load monitoring, and the impact of HAART. In 1997, these new data produced new recommendations strongly aimed at inducing earlier and more aggressive treatment.[12]

A careful individual selection of drugs for each patient clearly aims at achieving the best adherence and clinical results and is considered the basis for eradicating HIV infection. The concept of HIV eradication was based on the assumptions that the complete suppression of viral replication would be achievable and the medium half-life of chronically infected cells was between 10–14 days. This suggested the possibility of eradicating the infection within 2–3 years.[13] Scientific research has progressively identified the possibility of viral replication even when the viral load is undetectable (less than 50 copies/ml), and there is a longer CD4-infected half-life (6–44 months). Moreover, it was evident that a consistent immunological restoration could not be achieved using only HAART, which controls viral replication.

Clinical trials have shown several problems related to the complexity of HIV treatment, to the monitoring and adherence of therapy, and to the appearance of the long-term effects of therapy (i.e., lipodystrophy, etc.). Furthermore, a large number of patients present with a viral load below 50 copies/ml, which is undetectable.

With respect to this evidence and the availability of new treatments, new recommendations were published in January 2000. These recommendations were aimed at supporting clinicians in evaluating patients' adherence to therapy, taking into consideration the possibility of 1) long-term effects associated with therapy; 2) identifying therapeutic failures; 3) using new tools for monitoring patients; and 4) defining individual treatment.[14]

Similar recommendations have been published by the British HIV Association (BHIVA), whose expert panel has faced similar problems with a different methodology. A significant part of these recommendations is focused on data based on the biological credibility of surrogate markers. Experts believe that if only the best clinical evidence were considered, it would be impossible to create guidelines, since a large part of clinical practice has not yet been evaluated.

In fact, these recommendations are not only based on scientific evidence, but experts have also considered data published in abstracts, data on surrogate markers, study design, analysis of clinical trials, and notification of adverse reactions.[15]

Preventive Therapy for Opportunistic Infections

Recommendations regarding the preventive therapy of opportunistic infections in HIV+ patients were published in 1995 by the US Public Health Service and the Infectious Diseases Society of America (IDSA) and revised in 1997.[16]

The introduction of HAART has drastically reduced the incidence of opportunistic infections, and the increased longevity in HIV+ patients has indicated that more attention should be paid to the most essential preventive therapies. Nevertheless, problems concerning the adverse effects of treatment and the appearance of drug-resistant strains have made it difficult for the physician to select the most effective therapy. New data on preventive therapy of opportunistic infections have required a revision of the recommendations from March 1999.[17]

Experts have focused their attention on the possibility of discontinuing preventive therapy (primary and secondary) in patients with an increased number of CD4 cells after antiretroviral treatment. The following elements have been considered with regard to the discontinuation of preventive therapy:

- incidence of disease, morbidity and mortality rates;

- CD4 values associated with specific opportunistic infections;

- feasibility and cost/efficacy of preventive therapy;

- impact on the quality of life;

- toxicity and pharmacological interactions; and

- possible development of drug-resistance.

Furthermore, recommendations addressed HHV8 and HCV, two pathogens which had not been previously considered.

The revision of recommendations specifically pertained to:

(a) discontinuation of preventive therapy (for specific opportunistic infections) related to an increased CD4 count;

(b) new recommendations for HHV8 and HCV-infection;

(c) new recommendations for drug-users;

(d) new recommendations for a short course of antituberculosis preventive therapy in HIV+ patients having a positive Purified Protein Derivative (PPD) test;

(e) modification of a secondary preventive therapy (maintenance therapy for infection recurrence of MAC and CMV);

(f) special care for the administration of fluconazole during pregnancy; and

(g) administration of vaccines against chicken pox and rotavirus infections in HIV+ children.[17]

In 1994, guidelines for tuberculosis preventive therapy in HIV+ patients were published in Italy. In addition, a prospective observational study to evaluate the implementation of these guidelines was conducted in 1995 by GISTA (Gruppo Italiano per lo Studio della Tubercolosi e AIDS).[18]

Tuberculosis (TB) Treatment in AIDS Patients

The last Centers for Disease Control and Prevention (CDC) guidelines established that there must be a minimal duration of treatment of a six months. This should be extended to nine months, or stopped four months after the first negative culture, in patients showing a slow clinical and bacteriological response.[19] HAART has certainly improved the prognosis of HIV/TB co-infected patients, but has made their treatment more complex.

Recent scientific evidence allows for a better evaluation of: 1) susceptibility to TB-infection in HIV$^+$ patients, 2) possible modifications to the course of HIV infection induced by TB infection, and 3) clinical presentation of tuberculosis in HIV$^+$ patients.[20] We need updated recommendations concerning TB treatment in AIDS patients. This should take into account the last diagnostic methodologies, as well as the possible pharmacological interactions between antituberculosis and antiretroviral treatment, rifampin resistance, emerging multi-drug-resistant strains, and proper isolation measures for patients affected with bacillary TB.

Recommendations for the Treatment of HIV-related Diseases, Not Previously Considered

HIV/HCV Co-infection

Codified scientific evidence, regarding the progression of HIV infection in HIV$^+$ patients, has not been developed yet. Recent publications have looked at the case histories of patients treated for both HIV and HCV infections. HIV infection is considered an important factor for the progression of HCV disease, and research over the past few years has indicated that HCV could act as an opportunistic pathogen in HIV$^+$ patients.[21]

Introduction of HAART, which prolongs the survival rate of HIV$^+$ patients, has led to amendments in the treatment of HCV infection. The primary aim should be viral replication control and/or the elimination of HCV, since these patients are more susceptible to cirrhosis or liver carcinoma.[22] The secondary aim is to possibly delay liver damage and reduce the side-effects associated with HAART toxicity.

It is evident that HAART prolongs the survival rate of HIV$^+$ patients, but longevity increases mortality rates due to HCV-related diseases. Therefore, until longitudinal studies define the role of HAART in progressive and irreversible liver damage, it is necessary to standardize the treatment of these patients, and establish recommendations which support physicians in defining the priority of treatment:

- to identify co-infected patients and initiate an HCV-infection treatment before, or concurrently with HAART; and

- to identify the priority of treatment in case of simultaneous indications.

HIV-related Cardiovascular Diseases.

Recent literature identifies HIV-related cardiovascular diseases, characterized from a biological and clinical point of view:

- by means of experimental research in transgenic mice;

- the role of cytokines in developing HIV-associated cardiomyopathy and pulmonary hypertension; and

- association between dilatative cardiomyopathy and encephalopathy in HIV+ patients.

The role of antiretroviral therapy in the pathogenesis of HIV-related myocardial ischemia, and co-existing etiologic factors, involved in myocardial cell dysfunction, are frequently debated in medical literature. Specific recommendations have been recently discussed to guide physicians in the diagnosis and treatment of HIV-related cardiovascular disorders.

Methodologies for Drafting Guidelines

Different methods are used by Health Organizations and Clinical Centers to draft guidelines and spread recommendations. Methodologies are essentially concerned with ways to gain expert approval, by the criteria used to collect and classify evidence, and by how to define the strength of recommendations. Different methodologies are classified as follows:

- informal approval;

- formal approval;

- evidence-based guidelines; and

- development of explicit guidelines.[23]

Informal approval is the oldest and most common way of approaching methodologies, but such recommendations are usually of low quality with poor documentation.

Formal approval uses a systematic approach to evaluate expert opinions, in order to achieve consent about recommendations.

The development of evidence-based guidelines is strongly related to the quality of scientific evidence and its role has more emphasis than the opinions of experts. A classic example showing a strong correlation between guidelines and evidence-based quality was represented by a 1979 classification, introduced by the Canadian Task Force, to develop guidelines for preventive medicine services. A similar methodology has been used by the US Preventive Services Task Force.[24,25] The development of guidelines is intended to: 1) define potential benefits and damages, 2) evaluate the costs and feasibility of interventions, 3) assess results, and 4) take into account the patients' expectations.

The development of guidelines can be schematically represented as follows:

- initial decisions (i.e., selection of topics and expert groups, and a statement of aims);

- evaluation concerning an appropriate clinical approach (by reviewing scientific evidence and expert opinions);

- evaluation concerning health policies (i.e., resource restrictions and feasibility plans); and

- preparation of document and final evaluation.

METHODOLOGY OF THE
AGENCY FOR HEALTH CARE POLICY AND RESEARCH

A reference methodology is the one adopted by the Agency for Health Care Policy and Research (AHCPR) of the National Institutes of Health (NIH). Recommendations must meet criteria defined by the Institute of Medicine in Washington (see TABLE 1) and must have certain requirements.[26,27] Such criteria combine a list of requirements found in guidelines established by the American Medical Association (AMA) (see TABLE 2).[28]

AHCPR methodology refers to the following general features:

- recommendations must be based on scientific evidence, obtained from research, and a selection of medical literature;
- evidence quality must be confirmed by reporting literary sources; and
- the strength of the recommendations must be emphasized.

A general reference scheme for classifying evidence quality and strength, according to AHCPR methodology, is reported in TABLE 3.

Guidelines Requirements/Attributes for Accreditation by AHCPR

Specific requirements necessary for guideline accreditation by the National Guidelines Clearinghouse (NGC) and AHCPR are reported in a specific Summary Sheet. Guidelines must possess specific attributes/requirements to be classified into specific categories, thus defining the criteria and function of the recommendations (see TABLE 4).

Methods for Evidence Collection

Different methodologies for collecting and analyzing evidence have been identified. The referenced methodologies are based on the criteria identified by Sacks *et al.* and by L'Abbè.[29,30] Both authors identified criteria for evaluating available scientific evidence. In general, a systematic review of medical literature is preferred over a single clinical controlled and randomized trial (RCT); systematic review of

---

TABLE 1. Institute of Medicine, Washington: criteria required to accredit guidelines

Validity: a guideline has validity if correctly implemented and produces benefits (health or economic)

Reproducibility: different experts achieve the same conclusions deriving from the same scientific evidences and methodologies

Applicability: possibility to apply guidelines to distinct patient populations

Flexibility: possibility to manage outliers

Clarity: clear language to help its use

Multidisciplinary approach

Documentation: the scientific evidence considered and the methodologies used

Updating: circumstances requiring updating and its modalities

TABLE 2. Guideline attributes required by the American Medical Association (AMA)

1. Produced in co-operation with medical organizations
2. Using reliable methodologies to combine the most relevant evidence and the most significant clinical experiences
3. Accurate and exhaustive
4. Supported by current opinion
5. Widely diffused

an RCT with homogeneous results is preferred to studies with heterogeneous results; an RCT with a large sample size is favored in comparison to a smaller one; RCTs are preferred over cohort or case-control studies; prospective studies are preferred to retrospective ones; studies with a control group are preferred to studies without one; a high quality study is preferred to a single expert opinion.

Good quality recommendations generally apply these criteria, but it is not possible to be always compliant. In fact, an expert group, who organized the 1999 BHIVA antiretroviral therapy recommendations, believed that the best scientific evidence found in HIV infection, was not always immediately available and published. Often, there is a considerable lapse of time between the first data presentation (oral presentation, poster, abstract) and the final publication. Therefore, BHIVA experts based their recommendations on a different classification of evidence quality. They were based on the biological credibility of surrogate markers, expert opinion, abstract production over the previous three years, and aspects connected to the design study, taking into account the intention to treat and the time elapsed between the start of treatment and possible therapeutic failure.

TABLE 3. Recommendations

Strength of recommendations:

A. Good scientific evidence to support the recommendation for the utilization of procedures.

B. Fairly good scientific evidence to support the recommendation for the utilization of procedures.

C. Recommendations can be based on different considerations, if scientific evidence to support the recommendation for the utilization of procedures is insufficient.

D. Fairly good scientific evidence to support recommendations for the non-utilization of procedures.

E. Good scientific evidence to support recommendations for the non-utilization of procedures.

Quality of recommendations:

I. Documented evidence through well designed, controlled and randomized clinical trials, including meta-analysis.

II. Documented evidence through well designed observational studies, including controls (case- control and cohort studies).

III. Documented evidence by expert opinions, series of cases, case-reports, and studies including historical control groups.

Guidelines Implementation

Guideline implementation can be deduced through the observation of infectious diseases practice or different fields of internal medicine. Foremost, the receiver, as well as the guideline user, should be identified; second, there should be verification that every physician was able to provide appropriate care, based on a standardized reference. Recent studies indicate that general practitioners, without proper clinical experience, could provide inadequate care to HIV[+] patients.[31]

Some inexperienced physicians may not investigate patient sexual behavior, and probably do not offer counseling to low risk patients or identify signs of HIV-related infections through physical examination. On the contrary, a more experienced physician is more likely to prescribe an appropriate chemoprophylaxis or investigate, and treat a *P. carinii* pneumonia. Specific training in this medical field may not be necessary; however previous experience in treating HIV[+] patients is required to ensure a proper quality of care.[31]

Problems associated with the proper implementation of guidelines, have been studied and often reported in medical literature.[32] Some authors studied the association between the duration of antibiotic prophylaxis and the development of infection from a surgical wound. Experience over a long period, regarding antibiotic prophylaxis recommends its administration within 1–2 hours before a surgical operation. However, this procedure is not fully implemented, causing an economic impact and physical cost for patients.[33]

TABLE 4. **Guideline classification according to the Agency for Health Care Policy and Research (AHCPR) methodology**

Category	Example
A. Disease/Group of pathologies	HIV-related infections and neoplasms.
B. Guideline intervention area	Therapeutic recommendations and diagnostic procedures.
C. Guideline users	Specialists in infectious diseases and other specialists involved in the management of HIV infection.
D. Methods for revision of recommendations	Results of an external revision, comparison with other guidelines, pilot test, peer revision.
E. Methods for analyzing evidence	Meta-analysis: data analysis, observational studies, "Randomized Controlled Trials (RCT)", "Review" reporting scientific evidence. A protocol including: inclusion criteria of the studies, a list of analyzed trials, a list of trials not-included.
F. Methods used to evaluate quality and strength of evidence	Expert consensus, focus groups, subjective reviews.

A 1995 study documented that 20% of English cardiologists who performed invasive procedures had never been vaccinated against hepatitis B, there was no standard screening for HBV before an invasive procedure, and the information about occupational risk was inadequate in spite of specific national guidelines.[34] Another study documented that most health care workers (HCWs) agreed to an antituberculosis preventive therapy program, aimed to evaluate the level of positivity to tuberculosis infection.[35]

These studies suggest that the optimal implementation of guidelines could be achieved by HCWs who adapted guidelines to their setting. In 1995, a model for adapting and implementing guidelines was developed by the Michigan Medical Center and accepted by eight eminent organizations, such as: American Medical Association, American College of Physicians, Harvard Community Health Plan, and the most famous insurance society Blue Cross and Blue Shield Association.[36] This model consisted of:

- involving of physicians who followed recommendations;

- recurrence of previous recommendations as a basis for the discussion;

- review of historical medical literature to prevent incorrect definitions;

- focus on the adequacy of health care;

- simultaneous development of critical pathways;

- cost evaluation; and

- strong association with informative sources.

A main feature of this model is the elaboration of specific pathways associated with the implementation of recommendations. In fact, an optimal standard of health care also includes specific critical pathways. In other words, the first goal of a guideline is to promote an appropriate clinical practice, and the associated critical pathways are a means to improve its efficacy. Guidelines and critical pathways can be developed from two different work groups.[35]

The BHIVA guidelines for antiretroviral treatment is an example of the involvement between HCWs and patients. Implementation of guidelines includes[15]:

- a writing committee of physicians experienced in the treatment of HIV infection, with different specializations;

- a meeting with HIV⁺ patients and activist groups, which has been carried out— some representatives of these groups have become members of the writing committee;

- a draft set of guidelines which has been discussed at the annual conference, published on the internet with a comment request, and subsequently discussed at the annual conference;

- the final version of the guidelines will be submitted to reviewers, who will be allowed to publish their opinion about it; and

- after the publication of the final guidelines, a Web site will be available for open debate.

The above mentioned methodology has been applied by the National Institute for Infectious Diseases L. Spallanzani (INMI) in the area of severe infection,[37] nosocomial infection in Intensive Care Units,[38] and in the management of HCWs with HCV infection.[39] In the last two years, INMI developed a program for standardizing diagnostic procedures for opportunistic infections and neoplasms in HIV+ patients based on the following methodologies:

- specialist work groups have been created to draw up recommendations and diagnostic profiles;

- draft guidelines have been discussed at a special Consensus Conference;

- the implementation of the guidelines will be tested in a network of participating hospitals over a 12-month period; a follow-up form will be filled out for every patient treated in adherence with these recommendations and diagnostic profiles performed;

- the final draft will be defined in a second Consensus Conference, when the follow-up results will be evaluated;

- there will be a publication of recommendations on a Web site, to activate a debate over a 6-month period; and

- these recommendations will be validated and credited by an external committee who are in charge of peer revision.

CONCLUSIONS

The standardization process of diagnostic and therapeutic procedures, aimed at elaborating guidelines, has recently been promoted through the involvement of national and international agencies and research institutions. The main issue, which still needs further attention, is the usefulness of guidelines in improving the quality of care. Guidelines are often incorrectly delivered to the final users and inappropriately implemented. Updated knowledge about HIV and AIDS pathogenesis, availability of new treatments, emergence of resistant strains as well as the appearance of new clinical patterns of disease and previously unconsidered infections, make the management of HIV+ patients extremely complex. There is a pressing necessity to transfer scientific data into clinical practice by developing high quality and updated guidelines. Consequently, a marked improvement in the standards of care for HIV+ patients will be achieved through the implementation of guidelines in clinical practice.

ACKNOWLEDGMENT

Research reported here was supported in part by Ricerca Corrente degli IRCCS Ministero Sanità.

REFERENCES

1. GROSS, P.A. 1998. Practice Guidelines for infectious diseases: rationale for a work in progress. Clin. Infect. Dis. **26:** 1037–1041.
2. STEFANINI, A., M.P. FANTINI & M. ZANETTI. 1997. Linee Guida e razionamento dell'assistenza sanitaria. Oppurtunità e rischi. Epidemiol. Prev. **26:** 227–231.
3. BRADELY, F. & J. FLIED. 1995. Evidence-based medicine. Lancet **346:** 838–839.
4. KTIZHABER, J.A. 1993. Prioriting health services in a era of limits: the Oregon experience. *In* Rationing in Action. R. Smith, Ed. BMJ Publishing Group. London.
5. DIXON, J. 1997. Setting priorities New Zealand style. BMJ. **314:** 86–87.
6. DUNNIG, A.J. 1992. Choice in Health Care. Report by Affair Government Committee Health Care. The Netherlands Ministry of Health, Welfare, Culture.
7. LIBERATI, A. 1996. Linee-guida ed evidence-based medicine: l'importanza di distinguere i ruoli. Epidemiol. Prev. **20:** 277–278.
8. GRILLI, R. *et al.* 1996. Physicians' attitudes toward practice guidelines. Finding for a survey on Italian physicians. Soc. Sci. Med. **43:** 1283–1287.
9. SMITH, D. *et al.* 1997. Antiretroviral therapy for HIV infection: principle for use (standard of care guidelines). Clinical trials and treatments advisory committee booklet, October 1997.
10. AUDETT, A.M., S. GREENFLIED & M. FLIELD. 1990. Medical practice guidelines: current activities and future directions. Ann. Intern. Med. **13:** 709–714.
11. CARPENTER, C.J. *et al.* 1996. Antiretroviral therapy for HIV infection: recommendation of an international panel. JAMA **276:** 146–154.
12. CARPENTER, C.J. *et al.* 1997. Antiretroviral therapy for HIV infection. JAMA **277:** 1962–1969.
13. CARPENTER, C.J. *et al.* 1998. Antiretroviral therapy for HIV infection. JAMA **280:** 78–86.
14. CARPENTER, C.J. *et al.* 2000. Antiretroviral therapy in adults: update recommendations. JAMA **283:** 381–390.
15. POZNIAK, A. *et al.* 1999. Guidelines for the treatment of HIV-infected adults with the antiretroviral therapy. British HIV Association (BHIVA), December 1999.
16. USPHS/IDSA PREVENTION OF OPPORTUNISTIC INFECTIONS WORK IN GROUP. 1997. Guidelines for prevention of opportunistic infections in persons infected with human immunodeficiency virus. Ann. Intern. Med. **127:** 922–946.
17. USPHS/IDSA GUIDELINES FOR THE PREVENTION OF OPPORTUNISTIC INFECTIONS IN PERSONS INFECTED WITH HUMAN IMMUNODEFICIENCY VIRUS. MMWR **48:** No RR-10.
18. COMMISSIONE NAZIONALE PER LA LOTTA CONTRO L'AIDS. 1995. Linee-guida per chemioterapia preventiva della tubercolosi nei soggetti con infezione da HIV in Italia. Giornale Italiano dell'AIDS **6:** 27–29.
19. CDC. 1998. Prevention and treatment of tuberculosis among patients infected with human immunodeficiency virus: principles of therapy and revised recommendations. MMWR **47:** No. RR-20.
20. HAVLIR, D.V. & P.F. BARNES. 1999. Tuberculosis in patient with human immunodeficiency virus infection. N. Engl. J. Med. **340:** 367–373.
21. PIROTH, L. *et al.* 1998. Does HCV co-infection accelerate clinical and immunological evolution of infected patients? AIDS **12:** 381–388.
22. DIETRICH, D.T. 1999. HCV and HIV: clinical issues in co-infection. Am. J. Med. **338:** 853–860.
23. WOOLF, S.H. 1992. Practice guidelines, a new reality in medicine: methods on developing guidelines. Arch. Intern. Med. **152:** 946–952.
24. CANADIAN TASK FORCE ON THE PERIODIC HEALTH EXAMINATION. 1979. The periodic health examination. Can. Med. Assoc. J. **121:** 1193–1254.
25. WOOLF, S.H. & H.C. SOX. 1991.The expert Panel on Preventive Services continuing the work on the U.S. Preventive Services Task Force. Am. J. Prev. Med. **7:** 326–330.
26. WOOLF, S.H. 1991. Manual for Clinical Practice Guidelines development: A Protocol for Expert Panels Convened by the Office of the Forum for Quality and Effectiveness in Health Care. Agency for Health Care Policy and Research (AHPCR) Publication, pp. 91–107.

27. INSTITUTE OF MEDICINE, COMMITTEE TO ADVICE THE PUBLIC HEALTH SERVICE ON CLINI-CAL PRACTICE GUIDELINES. 1990. Clinical Practice Guidelines: Directions for a New Program. Washington DC. National Academy Press.
28. AMERICAN MEDICAL ASSOCIATION, OFFICE OF QUALITY ASSURANCE. 1990. Attributes to Guide the development of Practice parameters. American Medical Association. Chicago, IL.
29. SACKS, H.S. *et al.* 1987. Meta-analysis of randomized controlled trials. N. Engl. J. Med. **316:** 450–455.
30. L'ABBEÈ, K.A. *et al.* 1987. Meta-analysis in clinical research. Ann. Intern. Med. **107:** 224–233.
31. SHEFFIELD, J.V.L. & D.S. PAAUW. 1996. Primary HIV/AIDS care: how good it is? AIDS Reader **6:** 194–196.
32. EAGLE, K.A. *et al.* 1997. Guideline Implementation. IACC **29:** 1125–1148.
33. CLASSEN, D.C. *et al.* 1992. The timing of prophylactic administration of antibiotics and the risk of surgical wound infection. N. Engl. J. Med. **326:** 281–282.
34. PRENDERGAST, B.D. *et al.* 1995. Hepatitis B immunization among invasive cardiologist: poor compliance with United Kingdom guidelines. Br. Heart J. **74:** 685–688.
35. CAMINS, B.C. *et al.* 1996. Acceptance of isoniazid preventive therapy by health care workers after tuberculin skin test conversion. JAMA **275:** 1013–1015.
36. WISE, C.G. & J.E. BILLI. 1995. A model for practice guideline adaptation and implementation. J. Qual. Improv. **21:** 465–475.
37. GRUPPO ITALIANO DI STUDIO SULLE INFEZIONI GRAVI (G. IPPOLITO, Ed.). 1997. Le infezioni gravi- documento finale della Consensus Conference sulle infezioni gravi. (seconda edizione). Effetti Editore. Milano, pp. 1–111.
38. GRUPPO ITALIANO DI STUDIO SULLE INFEZIONI GRAVI (M. LANGER, Ed.). 1999. Infezioni in terapia intensiva. Effetti Editore. Milano, pp. 1–164.
39. ISTITUTO SUPERIORE DI SANITA, ISTITUTO NAZIONALE MALATTIE INFETTIVE LAZZARO SPALLANZANI, ASSOCIAZIONE ITALIANA STUDIO FEGATO. 2000. Gestione intraospedaliera del personale HBsAg o anti HCV positivo. ISTISAN rapporti **72:** 1–29.

Index of Contributors